SYMPOSIUM ON MYCOTOXINS
IN HUMAN HEALTH

SYMPOSIUM ON MYCOTOXINS IN HUMAN HEALTH

The Proceedings of a Symposium held in Pretoria from 2nd to 4th September 1970 under the auspices of the South African Medical Research Council with the collaboration of the South African Council for Scientific and Industrial Research.

Edited by

I. F. H. PURCHASE

Palgrave Macmillan

FIRST EDITION 1971

Published by
THE MACMILLAN PRESS LTD
London and Basingstoke
Associated companies in New York Toronto
Dublin Melbourne Johannesburg and Madras

SBN 333 13146 0

ISBN 978-1-349-01320-3   ISBN 978-1-349-01318-0 (eBook)
DOI 10.1007/978-1-349-01318-0

CONTENTS

v

INTRODUCTION

It was towards the end of the last century that scientists found that certain products of micro-organisms were responsible for various diseases in both man and animals. Further research during this century has increased the knowledge in the field of microbial toxins enormously and this is particularly so of bacterial toxins. We are in a position today of knowing not only the cause of these diseases, but also how to treat and prevent such diseases as botulism and salmonella, streptococcal and staphylococcal food-poisoning. The knowledge of mould-induced food-poisoning is much more scanty and research on causation and prevention of mould intoxication has far to go.

It is interesting to note that, although the general knowledge of mould toxicoses is limited, one of the oldest food-borne diseases recognised was a mould infection. Ergotism, known a thousand years ago as St Anthony's fire, was a disease which killed many thousands of people in Europe. This disease is caused by the fungus *Claviceps purpurea* which grows on rye. The rye grain becomes completely replaced by selerotia of the fungus and turns black. Ingestion of between 1 and 1·5 g of diseased rye grains daily can result in symptoms. Two types of the disease occurred, one in which the main syndrome was gangrene of the extremities caused by peripheral thrombosis of the arteries, and the other in which the syndrome was due to damage to the nervous system resulting in numbness, twitching, convulsions, blindness, deafness and paralysis. It was not for hundreds of years that the discoloured grain was recognised, as being the cause of the disease, by Kaspar Schwenckfeld in 1600. The disease continued to occur right into the 19th century in Europe and America and was last recorded on a large scale in Russia in the 1920s and 1930s.

More recently a disease known as alimentary toxic aleucia (A.L.A.) was recorded in the 1940s in Russia. In 1944 this was particularly severe in the Orenburg district where 10% of the population suffered from the disease. As the name suggests, the patients suffer from haemorrhagic diathesis, leucopenia, agranulocytosis and also necrotic skin lesions. There was widespread mortality at the time in all age groups but more particularly in malnourished people. The investigation of the disease showed that it was caused by mouldy grain. At first millet was thought to be the only source of infected material but later wheat and barley were shown to cause the disease. The conditions under which the disease occurs illustrate vividly that fungi can grow under the most unusual conditions. Three fungi were shown to be most important in causing the disease (*Fusarium pose*, *Fusarium sporotrichoides* and *Cladosporium epiphyleum*) and extensive laboratory investigation showed that these fungi produced their toxins only when the temperature dropped below freezing point. Under these conditions, although mycelial growth was limited, sporulation was profuse and the steroid-like toxin was produced. These facts fitted in well with the factors known to lead up to outbreaks of the disease. During the war years manpower was not always available to reap the harvest and as a result it was left standing in the fields during the winter. It was during this over-wintering that the fungus grew, became toxic and subsequently caused the epidemic in Russia.

Of course, animals are, in general, more likely to suffer from myco-toxicoses because of the way in which they are fed. This is reflected in the large number of diseases which are recognised in animals. Fungi are known to produce 'haemorrhagic syndrome' in poultry, nephrosis in pigs, stachybotrio-toxicoses in horses and many other diseases. Recently South African research workers were able to identify the fungus responsible for Lupinosis in sheep, a disease which has for many years been suspected of being a mycotoxicosis. All attempts to identify the fungus have been unsuccessful until recently and I am very pleased to see that a report on this most interesting syndrome is to be delivered at this symposium.

In spite of the fact that the major epidemics caused by mycotoxins occurred in Europe, it is no mistake that this symposium on mycotoxins in human health is being held in South Africa. Research in the last decade has been carried out by the CSIR and the newly formed MRC and I am not being unduly biased in saying that this South African research effort has contributed significantly to the basic knowledge which has been so carefully gathered. We are, however, very lucky to have such a large and distinguished overseas contingent at this symposium.

Japanese research workers have been involved in mycotoxin research for many years and their work on 'yellowsis' rice in the 1940s can probably be considered the forerunner of the work on carcinogenic mycotoxins. *Penicillium islandicum* later isolated from mouldy rice in Japan yielded toxins which have proved to be hepatocarcinogens in mice. This was truly an astounding discovery and it has been acclaimed as a fine piece of research work by all who know the field.

It is strange that the Japanese discovery had so little impact on research in the Western world. In spite of the fact that this work was published in the early '50s it was not until 1960 that work on other carcinogenic mycotoxins was undertaken. Most of this work occurred as a result of the so-called 'Turkey-X' disease which killed thousands of turkeys in Britain. The cause of the mortality was traced to a batch of Brazilian groundnut meal which contained a blue-fluorescent substance. This substance was later shown to be produced by the mould *Aspergillus flavus* and hence was given the name aflatoxin. It was found that several domestic animals including poultry, pigs and cattle, were susceptible to the toxin. Laboratory studies were soon initiated on the toxic effects of aflatoxin and it was found to be not only a hepatotoxin but also a potent hepatocarcinogen, producing liver tumours in rats, trout, ducks and pigs. This discovery, which resulted directly from the mortality in poultry, turned out to be the forerunner of a vast amount of research. It proved to be an important tool in studying the biochemical events leading up to cancer induction. The concept that a fungus could produce a metabolite which was a carcinogen stimulated numerous people for the first time to suggest that mycotoxins could be involved in the aetiology of liver cancer, in spite of the fact that a similar concept had been formulated in Japan nearly 10 years earlier. Impetus was given to this idea by subsequent findings which indicated that aflatoxin was not only a carcinogen, but that it was the most potent carcinogen known to man. A few hundred microgrammes are enough to produce tumours in a high percentage of test animals.

The suggestion that mycotoxins could be responsible for human liver cancer opened up a whole new field of investigation. The concept that mould-produced toxins could cause *chronic* disease in man was the major advance in thought, and it proved to be the trigger which has unleashed an avalanche of publications in this field until there are now nearly 1000 publications just on this subject.

In the particular context of human disease in South Africa, the idea that fungi might be responsible for chronic disease, and particularly liver cancer, received enthusiastic support. Liver cancer, like so many other cancers, has a variable distribution through the world and this variation suggested that it must be caused by an environmental agent. Many suggestions had been made which connected such diverse agents as virus infection, bilharzia and malnutrition with the high incidence of the disease. In each case, however, there was evidence which suggested that a direct causal relationship between these agents and the disease in man was unlikely. Mycotoxins appeared to be much more likely than any of the previously suggested agents to cause the disease. It was known that liver cancer occurred with high incidence in areas of high humidity and temperature and in relatively primitive populations. Fungi require high temperatures and humidity in which to grow and would grow in foods that were stored under primitive conditions. It seemed, therefore, that the ingestion of food contaminated with mycotoxins could provide a plausible explanation for the high incidence of liver cancer in certain areas in Africa.

There are a number of factors which make further study of this hypothesis uniquely difficult. In all the examples that I have mentioned of mycotoxins being responsible for a particular human or animal disease, the disease has been relatively acute with a short latent period between ingestion of the toxin and the development of lesions. It is, therefore, relatively easy to connect the development of the toxicity with the induction of the disease. In the case of liver cancer it is much more difficult. The latent period between ingestion of the toxin and development of the disease may be relatively long. Other toxin-induced cancers, such as bladder cancer resulting from industrial exposure to a carcinogen, have latent periods of 10-40 years. There is no reason to believe that liver cancer behaves differently, although in high-incidence areas children under the age of 10 do contract the disease. We are thus faced with the problem of identifying a toxin in the diet which is going to produce disease one or more decades hence.

A further complication is the rather variable way in which fungi produce their toxic metabolites. The acute diseases give us a good example of this variability. Ergotism occurred in isolated outbreaks, for example, that occurring in A.D. 943 in France which killed thousands of people. Similarly A.L.A. had a variable incidence in Russia and only occurred after temperatures had reached freezing point. The animal diseases, such as facial eczema in New Zealand, also had a very patchy and variable incidence. Aflatoxin itself is another good example. Studies by agriculturalists in groundnut-producing countries, including South Africa, have shown that the incidence of contaminated batches of groundnuts may vary from 0 to over 40% from one year to the next. In general the higher incidence occurs in drier years—a seeming paradox as the fungus requires high humidity in which to grow. The explanation is that in drier years insects damage the nuts with the result that a micro-climate is created in the damaged nuts which is conducive to mould growth. From these examples it can be seen that mycotoxins have a habit of behaving in a rather unexpected way which tends to result in marked variations in the amount present in a given food.

These two factors, namely a long latent period and a variable level of toxin in diets potentially infected with moulds, provide an extremely complicated background to the mycotoxin hypothesis. What at first appeared to be relatively simple now appears to be complicated and unfortunately vague. The hypothesis will, in fact, be extremely difficult to prove. One of the key questions to which there is as yet no answer is whether man himself is susceptible to the chronic or even acute effects of aflatoxin or other mycotoxins. In the absence of a direct answer to this question, circumstantial evidence will have to be accumulated to give us an idea of the susceptibility of man to these toxins. Careful studies are required which will measure the incidence of liver cancer and the intake of mycotoxins over relatively long periods. This will be required in a variety of environments so that populations with different levels of ingestion will be identified. In the final analysis, proof may be obtained only when it is shown that a reduction in the intake of the toxin is followed after a suitable latent period by a reduction in the incidence of the disease. Whether it will ever be possible to obtain all this information rests to a large extent with the scientists such as yourselves, who are involved in this complicated and challenging field of research.

I have outlined briefly the fascinating history of mycotoxin research. As in most research of this nature, the greatest development has occurred this century and the pace at which it is advancing continues to accelerate.

This symposium is the first of its type in the world where mycotoxins are being discussed purely from this point of human health. It comes at an opportune moment for it is the 10th anniversary of the first outbreaks of disease in turkeys, ducks, pigs and calves which resulted in the discovery of aflatoxin. Much research has been undertaken on the basic biochemistry and toxicology of aflatoxin and several field studies have been started. By coming together to discuss the results of these studies we hope that you will be able to learn a lot about the results and way of thinking of your colleagues from various parts of the world. We hope that you will learn also of the mistakes and misfortunes that they have encountered for this is where you will learn the most.

This symposium has the promise of being an occasion which will be remembered for many years for we have all the ingredients for success. We have the most dynamic research workers in this field from all over the world, we have a subject which is not only scientifically interesting but which is of great concern in many countries throughout the world, and to cap it all we now have the opportunity of exchanging ideas and learning. I wish you every success in your deliberations over the next three days.

—from the opening address by Dr the Honourable Carel de Wet, Minister of Health, Republic of South Africa.

PRETORIA, 1970

INTRODUCTIONS TO PAPERS

KEYNOTE ADDRESS: BIOCHEMISTRY SESSION
by
G. N. WOGAN
Massachusetts Institute of Technology, U.S.A.

In vivo studies have revealed that aflatoxin impairs RNA synthesis and that this could possibly be attributed to an inhibition of RNA polymerase. Furthermore, the results indicate that aflatoxin B_1 inhibits ribosomal RNA synthesis and also, to a significant degree, suppresses the synthesis of lower molecular weight RNA. The inhibition of RNA polymerase by aflatoxins possibly results from binding of the toxins to DNA in such a way as to impair its template activity. The inhibitory effects of aflatoxins B_1, G_1 and B_2 on RNA polymerase activity were compared and it was concluded that $B_1 > G_1 > B_2$.

In vitro results confirmed earlier findings that aflatoxin B_1 is inactive in inhibiting RNA polymerase when added to an *in vitro* system. In order to elucidate the action mechanism of aflatoxins on the enzyme, various *in vivo* studies were performed where chromatin was used as template. The combined results indicate that the inhibitory effects of aflatoxin B_1 on RNA polymerase *in vivo* results from interactions with some component or components of chromatin and not from a direct action on the enzyme. It seems, therefore, that the toxin must undergo metabolic transformation before interacting with chromatin.

THE METABOLISM AND SOME METABOLIC EFFECTS OF STERIGMATOCYSTIN
by
W. NEL
University College of Zululand
P. G. KEMPFF and M. J. PITOUT
South African Medical Research Council

Sterigmatocystin is a hepato-carcinogen in rats and there are indications that it may be carcinogenic to primates. This mycotoxin is a metabolite of a number of fungal species and was isolated, after culturing the fungus on a liquid growth medium or on maize meal, by extracting it with a chloroform-methanol mixture and purifying it on formamide impregnated columns.

^{14}C- and ^{3}H-labelled sterigmatocystin were administered to rats to study their uptake by the rat and their distribution in the intracellular liver fractions. No differences in the distribution of the radio-activity within the liver fractions could be detected between females and males. Non-fasted rats absorbed the radio-active moiety nearly twice as rapidly as fasted rats. It was found that the mitochondria, microsomes, nuclear sap and the acidic fractions of the nucleus of the non-fasted rats contained two to three times less radio-activity than in the corresponding fractions of the fasted rats.

The level of radio-activity in the livers of rats which received the carcinogen intraperitoneally was more than four times higher than in the rats which received the sterigmatocystin *per os*.

A study of the influence of sterigmatocystin on nuclear RNA indicated that the carcinogen had no effect on the total nuclear RNA content but it had an inhibitory effect on the synthesis of RNA.

THE EFFECT OF THE AFLATOXINS ON PANCREATIC DEOXYRIBONUCLEASE

by

J. C. SCHABORT

Rand Afrikaans University and

M. J. PITOUT

South African Medical Research Council

Aflatoxins B_1, B_2 and M_2 were found to be effective activators of pancreatic deoxyribonuclease activity in this order at concentrations lower than $80\mu M$. Difference spectroscopy and equilibrium dialysis indicated that these toxins bind to DNA with different affinities. Aflatoxin B_1 had the strongest and aflatoxin M_2 the weakest affinity for DNA. These toxins decreased the apparent Michaelis constant for DNA and thus increased the affinity of the enzyme for substrate (DNA as well as DNA-aflatoxin complex) in the order $B_1 > B_2 > M_2$.

Aflatoxins B_{2a}, G_{2a}, G_2 and M_1 were found to be non-competitive inhibitors of pancreatic deoxyribonuclease activity in this order. Difference spectroscopical studies showed that they bind to deoxyribonuclease. Their affinity for the enzyme was in the order $B_{2a} > G_{2a} > G_2 > M_1$. Aflatoxins B_{2a}, G_{2a}, G_2 and M_1 showed very weak binding to DNA. Inhibition constants were determined which also indicated different affinities of the different aflatoxins for deoxyribonuclease in the above order.

Aflatoxin G_1 did not show a definite activity or inhibiting effect on deoxyribonuclease activity.

The effect of the Δ^2-bond and the hydroxy groups in positions 2 and 4 of the terminal furane ring as well as the presence of another lactone ring (aflatoxins G_1 and G_2) in the molecular structure of the aflatoxins on the extent of their effect on deoxyribonuclease and their binding to DNA or deoxyribonuclease will be discussed. Results obtained during these studies will also be discussed in terms of the variation in their toxicity and carcinogenicity.

The interactions of aflatoxins B_{2a} and G_{2a} with pancreatic deoxyribonuclease was studied employing difference spectroscopy equilibrium dialysis and gel chromatography. Results obtained from these experiments and from studies on the differential interaction of these aflatoxins with amino acids indicated that 8 molecules of aflatoxin B_{2a} and G_{2a} bind per molecule of pancreatic deoxyribonuclease and most probably to the ε-amino group of lysine.

THE EFFECT OF AFLATOXIN B_1, AFLATOXIN B_2 AND STERIGMATOCYSTIN ON NUCLEAR DEOXYRIBONUCLEASES FROM RAT AND MOUSE LIVERS

by

M. J. PITOUT and H. McGEE
South African Medical Research Council and

J. C. SCHABORT
Rand Afrikaans University

Various results in the literature indicate an effect of certain carcinogens on the activity of pancreatic DNase I. In our laboratory it was shown that aflatoxin B_1 *in vitro* has an activating effect on the activity of pancreatic DNase I. In the light of these results, the effect of two mycocarcinogens, aflatoxin B_1 and sterigmatocystin on two nuclear DNases from rat liver was investigated.

In vitro studies were done with partially purified enzymes. DNase type II (pH opt. 4·7) was isolated from the nuclear sap and was purified using various procedures. It is fairly stable. On the other hand, DNase type I (pH opt. 8·0) which is associated with chromatin and is an acidic protein, could not be purified to the same extent as DNase II due to its instability. No significant interaction between aflatoxin B_1 and the two enzymes was observed. Sterigmatocystin is almost insoluble in aqueous solutions, and therefore, could not be used for *in vitro* studies.

In vivo experiments, however, clearly indicated a marked effect of aflatoxin B_1 on the total activity of DNase II. From these results it is suggested that aflatoxin B_1 could be a pre-carcinogen and that it may be converted, probably by microsomal enzymes, to the active carcinogenic compound. Alternatively, aflatoxin B_1 could react with the natural inhibitor, resulting in higher enzyme activity. In the normal cells activity of the enzyme must be under rigorous control in order to preserve the integrity of the genetic message. Abnormal circumstances causing release of activity might result in anomalies in the genetic expression mechanism. The negative result obtained with aflatoxin B_2 illustrates the fact that the double-bond of the terminal furane ring plays a vital role in determining the toxic and carcinogenic activity of aflatoxin B_1.

Sterigmatocystin produced no effect on either enzyme, suggesting that either the mechanisms of carcinogenic action of the two toxins are different; or the effect of sterigmatocystin may be slower; or that DNase activity is not implicated in carcinogenesis.

The fact that orally-dosed aflatoxin B_1 has no effect on the activity of DNase II from mouse liver nuclei supports the concept that the mouse is capable of converting the aflatoxin B_1 to non-carcinogenic metabolites.

AFLATOXIN METABOLISM
by
M. STEYN and I. F. H. PURCHASE
South African Medical Research Council

The reason for the greater resistance of female, as opposed to male, rats to the acute effects of aflatoxin B_1 has been investigated. Female rats absorbed slightly less aflatoxin from their stomachs and metabolised it to aflatoxin M_1 at a faster rate than did males. The metabolism to aflatoxin M_1 was hormone-dependent as it was shown that castration removed this sex difference. Treatment of castrated rats with male and female sex hormones had no effect on aflatoxin M_1 production. It was concluded that the female is capable of metabolising aflatoxin B_1 to M_1 at a faster rate than males because the female normally handles a greater quantity of steroid hormones than the male.

BIOCHEMICAL STUDIES ON OCHRATOXIN A

by

M. J. PITOUT

South African Medical Research Council

Ochratoxin A is one of three chemically related metabolites isolated from *Aspergillus ochraceus* and was found to be the major toxic metabolite. It has been structurally characterised as 7-carboxy-5-chloro-8-hydroxy-3,4-dihydro-3-R methylisocoumarin linked over its 7-carboxy group to L-β-phenylalanine.

The LD_{50} in rats dosed *per os* is 20 mg/kg and the toxin produces enteritis, renal necrosis and an increase in the quantity of glycogen in the liver. The route and time course of the metabolism of ochratoxin A was investigated by Nel and Purchase (*J.S.Afr. Chem. Soc.* XXI, 87, 1968) in view of the fact that the increase in glycogen only became evident 4 to 5 days after dosing. These authors concluded that ochratoxin A is metabolised to 7-carboxy-5-chloro-8-hydroxy-3,4-dihydro-3-R-methylisocoumarin (ochratoxin α). By means of thin-layer chromatography on silica gel and spectrophotometric methods such as difference and absorption spectra, it was found that ochratoxin A is hydrolysed by carboxypeptidase A and α-chymotrypsin. The results obtained indicate that ochratoxin A has a much greater affinity for carboxypeptidase A than for α-chymotrypsin. It is, therefore, possible that ochratoxin A is hydrolysed *in vivo* mainly by carboxypeptidase A to ochratoxin α and L-phenylalanine.

Ochratoxin A has an absorption peak at 380 mμ at pH 7·5 while ochratoxin α has an absorption peak at 330 mμ at the same pH. When ochratoxin A is hydrolysed by means of HCl or carboxypeptidase A the absorption peak at 380 mμ disappears while a peak at 330 mμ appears. Difference and absorption spectra indicate that the decrease of 380 mμ is much more sensitive than the increase of absorption at 330 mμ. This disappearance of absorption at 380 mμ was used as a spectrophotometric method to assay the activity of carboxypeptidase A from pancreas.

The inhibitory effect of certain dipeptides on carboxypeptidase A was investigated by Yanani and Mitz (*J. Amer. Chem. Soc.* **79**, 454, 1957) and they concluded that these dipeptides were effective competitive inhibitors, although their K_m values were substantially lower than that of carbobenzoxyglycyl-L-phenylalanine (0·03 M). Dipeptides are generally poor substrates of pancreatic carboxypeptidase. Since the structure of ochratoxin A resembles that of a dipeptide, it was found that the inhibitory action of the toxin resembles that of certain dipeptides.

A single dose of 10 mg of ochratoxin A/kg of body weight produced accumulation of glycogen in the liver of rats, an effect which is also seen after dosage with N-2 fluorenyldiacetamide. In man, hereditary glycogen storage disease results in the accumulation of glycogen in various organs. Electron microscopic studies showed that the changes induced by ochratoxin A in rat liver closely resemble those seen in certain types of glycogen storage disease. It was observed that ochratoxin A, *in vitro*, inhibited the phosphorylase enzyme system and it is probable that an increase in liver glycogen can result from an inhibition of certain enzymes in the enzyme complex.

PORPHYRIN METABOLISM IN PRIMARY HEPATOMA
by
J. M. SILVA and C. MANSO
University of Lourenço Marques

This study was done on 28 cases of primary hepatoma and 10 controls. The following parameters have been measured: proto- and coproporphyrins in the faeces, delta-aminolevulinic acid, porphobilinogen, uroporphyrins and coproporphyrins in the urine, coproporphyrins, protoporphyrins and haemoglobin in the blood. The following abnormalities have been found: an increased excretion of delta-aminolevulinic acid and of coproporphyrin in the urine; an increased concentration of protoporphyrin in the red cell together with a decrease in haemoglobin.

The data seem to point to an abnormality in the synthesis of delta-aminolevulinic acid, due either to increased production or decreased degradation. The possibility that toxic factors are responsible for the increase in red cell protoporphyrin with decreased haemoglobin formation is presented as an hypothesis.

SURVEYS FOR ALPHA-FETO-PROTEIN AMONG BANTU GOLD-MINERS
by

L. R. PURVES
South African Institute for Medical Research

The AFP test for primary liver cancer appears to be an absolute one at a level above 0·1 mg%. However, at much lower levels >0·002 mg% even some healthy Bantu goldminers appear to have discernible amounts of AFP in their blood. The significance of these results for the detection of the early stages of primary liver cancer is discussed.

KEYNOTE ADDRESS: MICROBIOLOGY SESSION
by

J. FORGACS
Good Samaritan Hospital, Suffern, New York, U.S.A.

Consumption of various portions of cycads has caused acute and chronic toxic symptoms in man and animals. Since some of the clinical and patho-logic manifestations have also been observed in some of the mycotoxicoses, various portions of 26 specimens of *Cycas circinalis* and 16 of *Zamia* species were examined for toxic fungi.

1. Macroscopically, practically all specimens of *C. circinalis* contained areas of discolouration typical of past or current fungal proliferation. Sliced, washed endosperms used for human consumption contained light brown to blue-black stria which penetrated into the subsurface layers, particularly along vacuolations within the megasporangium. All leaves and stems of the *Zamia* species contained numerous small, black spots embedded within necrotic lesions suggestive of phytopathogenic origin.

2. Microscopically, essentially all specimens of *C. circinalis* contained conidia, other fungal structures, and, particularly, proliferated mycelia which correlated closely with subsequent cultural findings. The leaves and stems of freshly-collected *Zamia* revealed a preponderance of pycnidia, pycniospores and some perithecia. On section, hyaline to sub-hyaline and amber mycelia were observed within various tissues, particularly within conducting vessels and adjacent tissues. Initially, the subsurface layers of the enlarged stem (root) showed no fungal bodies, but after 3 months storage at 24°C, numerous heavy-walled, dark brown to almost black mycelia, and black chlamydospores, and a few hyaline mycelia were detected.

3. Culturally, from 24 samples of *C. circinalis* (in one or more sites examined), the following fungi were isolated in decreasing order: *Aspergillus niger, Curvularia lunata, Phoma* spp., *Macrosporium* spp., *Aspergillus tamarii, Penicillium* spp., and a species of *Mucor*. When fresh seeds of this cycad were stored at 24°C for 4 months, there developed a sequential growth of fungal types. From the fresh leaves and stems of the *Zamia* plants, a fungus was isolated, tentatively identified as a species of *Mycosphaerella* which permeated into the interior tissues of the large stem within 4 months.

4. Homogenates prepared from both Czapek's solution and Mycophil agars on which had been cultured the *A. flavus, A. niger, A. tamarii, C. lunata, Macrosporium* spp., and *Phoma* spp. were toxic to mice, the *A. flavus* being the most toxic. The *Mycosphaerella* likewise was toxic when cultured on Czapek's solution agar.

FIELD SURVEY OF MYCOTOXIN-PRODUCING FUNGI CONTAMINATING HUMAN FOODSTUFFS IN JAPAN, WITH EPIDEMIOLOGICAL BACKGROUND
PART I: MYCOLOGICAL AND CHEMICAL ASPECTS OF THE DETECTION OF MYCOTOXIN PRODUCERS
by

H. Kurata, S. Udagawa, M. Ichinoe, S. Natori and S. Sakaki
National Institute of Hygienic Sciences, Tokyo, Japan

Studies on mycotoxin-producing fungi contaminating foodstuffs have been carried out with the aim of disclosing the possible causative agents of human disease, particularly of human cancer in Japan. Several areas showing relatively high incidence of liver and stomach cancer were selected for this project, including one rural city in central Japan (Honshu district) and three towns or villages in southern Japan (Kyushu district). Nutritional and epidemiological investigations were also performed in addition to the collection of the foodstuffs in these areas.

From samples of a wide variety of stored foods such as polished rice, wheat grains, wheat flour and the other flour-type products, cycad starch, legumes, miso (soybean paste), shoyu (soy sauce), moromi (mash), tsukemono (Japanese pickles), niboshi (dried small sardines), katsuobushi (dried bonito), edible seaweeds, noodle and the miscellaneous materials, a total of 2,940 strains of fungi have been isolated as food contaminants. The mycoflora of these foods mostly comprised two common mould genera, *Aspergillus* and *Penicillium*, which are generally called the storage fungi. From previous knowledge, the following 20 or more species of the isolates were at least suspected of having the potential of mycotoxin production: *Aspergillus clavatus, A. flavus, A. fumigatus, A. ochraceus, A. versicolor, Chaetomium globosum, Fusarium* spp., *Penicillium citreoviride, P. citrinum, P. purpurogenum, P. roqueforti, P. rugulosum, P. viridicatum,* and *Pithomyces chartarum*.

After the primary screening for fungal toxins on HeLa cells and mice, several strains belonging to *P. cyclopium, P. purpurogenum* and *C. globosum* were found to produce toxic metabolites. Thus, a large amount (3·5 g/1,000 ml) of rubratoxin B could be isolated chemically from the culture fluid of *P. purpurogenum*. This is the first record of rubratoxin production for this species. Further chemical survey on 33 strains of *A. ochraceus* showed that the toxic principle in these food contaminants was penicillic acid despite the first finding of ochratoxin production in the two of these Japanese strains.

ISOLATION OF *ASPERGILLUS OCHRACEUS* PRODUCING OCHRATOXINS FROM JAPANESE RICE

by

M. YAMAZAKI
University of Chiba, Japan

A survey of the toxigenic moulds growing of rice in Japan has been carried out. Fifty-eight out of 457 *Aspergillus ochraceus* strains were subjected to toxicity assay performed in mice and chick embryos and two strongly toxigenic and ochratoxin-producing strains were found. The nutritional factors affecting the toxin production by the two strains were investigated by a simple thin-layer chromatography-fluorodensitometric method. The production of a large amount of ochratoxin A in a nutrient solution containing 1% L-phenylalanine and 2% yeast extract was also proved.

PRODUCTION OF CITREOVIRIDIN, A NEUROTOXIC MYCO-TOXIN OF *PENICILLIUM CITREO-VIRIDE BIOURGE*

by

Y. Ueno

University of Tokyo, Japan

With the aim of disclosing the causal agent for Beriberi (Shoshin-kakke in Japanese) which was prevalent in Japan in the past, the isolation and purification of the neurotoxic mycotoxin of *Penicillium citreo-viride Biourge* moulded rice were carried out with the following results:

(1) *P. citreo-viride* produced on rice the neurotoxic agent which was chemically identical with citreoviridin.
(2) Ushinsky liquid medium proved to be a suitable culture medium for production of the toxin.
(3) The fungus was more toxic when cultured at rather lower temperatures.

STORAGE SURVEYS AND HOW THEY MAY BE USED BOTH TO DETECT AND ESTIMATE FUNGAL CONTAMINATION IN THE DIET

by

G. A. Gilman

Tropical Products Institute, London

Over the past two years a food storage and crop handling survey has been undertaken in E. Transvaal and Swaziland and where liver cancer incidence appears to vary. Selected villages were examined in detail to ensure a comparison between Bantu tribal groups, a full range of food crops and methods of handling and storage, as well as topographical and climatic differences. During this house-to-house survey, samples of grain and semi-prepared foodstuffs were collected for mycological and aflatoxin assessment using recognised sampling techniques. Storage practices which encourage microbiological deterioration will be discussed as well as methods for food preparation which may influence the removal of damaged grain prior to consumption.

KEYNOTE ADDRESS: TOXICOLOGY SESSION
by

W. H. BUTLER
Medical Research Council Laboratories, Carshalton, Surrey, England

Mycotoxins have been implicated in a wide range of clinical conditions in both man and animals and until recently most of these have been only poorly investigated. Many of these syndromes such as alimentary toxic aleukia are manifest in suppression of the bone marrow and diffuse haemorrhage. Other mycotoxins such as aflatoxin, sterigmatocystin, ochratoxin and rubratoxin induce pathological changes in many organs but, in particular, the liver. The toxicology of aflatoxin has been studied most extensively in a wide variety of both large farm and small laboratory animals. The sensitivity of the species to the acute lethal effects of the toxin varies considerably from the highly sensitive day-old duckling (LD_{50} 0·3 mg/kg) to the mature female rat (LD_{50} 17·9 mg/kg). The pattern of liver damage is also species-dependent and will be described.

The metabolism of aflatoxin has been studied in species of varying susceptibility but no consistent pattern is seen in the ability of the liver to produce a non-toxic metabolite and the susceptibility of the species. The acute effects of aflatoxin on the liver and its distribution have been studied in an endeavour to understand its mechanism of action. The ultrastructural changes which are induced leading to a large increase of smooth endoplasmic reticulum will be described.

The carcinogenicity of the aflatoxins for the liver is well established in the rat, duckling, trout and ferret. In the rat, either short-term damage or long-term feeding at very low doses induces hepatic carcinoma in the absence of cirrhosis. Aflatoxin B_1 is the most active of the aflatoxins while aflatoxin G_1 induces both hepatic and renal carcinoma. The carcinogenicity of aflatoxin B_2 and G_2 has not been conclusively established. Adenocarcinoma of the stomach has also been induced following feeding of mixed aflatoxins. The carcinogenicity of most of the other known mycotoxins is uncertain. However, the carcinogenicity of sterigmatocystin and the metabolites of *P. islandicum* is established and patulin on subcutaneous injection may induce sarcoma at the injection site.

HEPATIC AND RENAL PATHOLOGY INDUCED IN MICE BY FEEDING FUNGAL CULTURES

by

S. J. VAN RENSBURG, I. F. H. PURCHASE and J. J. VAN DER WATT
South African Medical Research Council

Twenty-two strains of fungi were grown on maize-meal which was then incorporated into the diet of groups of ten mice and fed for 36 days or less. Sections for histological examination were prepared from the liver and kidneys of the mice that died and also from all survivors at the end of the test period.

The histopathological changes found in each individual group are described. Every culture was found to be nephrotoxic to some extent and the majority also induced liver pathology. Hepatotoxic changes were found in several previously untested fungi and most frequently consisted of parenchymal degenerative changes and/or necrosis, proliferation of bile ductule cells and variations in the size of hepatocyte nuclei; these changes were particularly associated with chronic weight loss.

It may be concluded from the data that histopathological alteration in the organs of mice is a more sensitive and specific screening criterion for detecting potential hepatocarcinogens than the occurrence of mortality in mice or ducks, or the inducement of weight loss in test animals.

TOXICOLOGICAL AND BIOLOGICAL PROPERTIES OF FUSARENON-X, A CYTOTOXIC MYCOTOXIN OF *FUSARIUM NIVALE* Fn 2B

by

Y. UENO

University of Tokyo, Japan

Toxicological studies on fusarenon-X, a cytotoxic scirpene of *Fusarium nivale* revealed that the toxin was highly toxic to mice, rats, guinea-pigs, ducklings, fish, chicken embryo and a protozoan. No antibacterial, antifungal actions or prophage induction were observed. Biochemical studies proved that fusarenon-X as well as nivalenol, diacetoxyscirpenol and T-2 toxin inhibited protein synthesis in rat liver and reticulocyte ribosomal systems.

FIELD SURVEY OF MYCOTOXIN-PRODUCING FUNGI CONTAMINATING HUMAN FOODSTUFFS IN JAPAN, WITH EPIDEMIOLOGICAL BACKGROUND
PART II. BIOLOGICAL EFFECTS OF THE MYCOTOXINS PRODUCED BY THE FUNGI ISOLATED FROM FOODSTUFFS

by

M. SAITO, M. ENOMOTO, M. UMEDA, K. OHTSUBO

Institute of Medical Science, University of Tokyo and

T. ISHIKO

Kanto Communication Hospital and

S. YAMAMOTO and H. TOYOKAWA

Medical School, University of Tokyo

Approximately 250 fungi isolated from foodstuffs were used as the samples for the screening test for mycotoxins. From the results of the biological assay of the culture filtrates and extracts of the fungi both on animals (male mouse of DDD strain) and culture cells (HeLa), 31 kinds of fungi including 20 fungi producing known mycotoxins were characterised by their lethal or growth-inhibitory effects and their cytotoxic properties. The representative target effects of the mycotoxins shown in the present study will be presented together with the results of further investigation on their mode of action and chronic effects on animals.

The epidemiological and pathological aspects of the role of the semyco-toxins in human disease will be discussed.

EXPERIMENTAL EVIDENCE THAT LUPINOSIS OF SHEEP IS A MYCOTOXICOSIS CAUSED BY THE FUNGUS *PHOMOPSIS LEPTOSTROMIFORMIS* (KÜHN) BUBÀK

by

K. T. VAN WARMELO, W. F. O. MARASAS
Plant Protection Research Institute, Pretoria and

T. F. ADELAAR, T. S. KELLERMAN, I. B. J. VAN RENSBURG and J. A. MINNE
Veterinary Research Institute, Onderstepoort

During October, 1969 a severe outbreak of lupinosis occurred in the Cape Province amongst a flock of sheep which had grazed on a field of sweet white lupines (*Lupinus albus L.* cult. Pflugs Gela). Typical lupinosis was induced in Merino sheep fed either stems, seeds or pods of lupine plants from this field. The toxic lupine plants were found to be heavily infected with the pathogenic fungus *Phomopsis leptostromiformis* (Kühn) Bubàk. This fungus was readily isolated from infected discoloured pods and seeds. Typical lupinosis was induced in sheep fed pure cultures of *P. leptostromiformis* grown on autoclaved white lupine seeds. It is concluded that lupinosis of sheep is caused by a hepatotoxin produced by the fungus *P. leptostromiformis*.

AFLATOXIN CARCINOGENESIS IN RATS: DIETARY-EFFECTS

by

P. M. NEWBERNE and A. E. ROGERS
Massachusetts Institute of Technology, U.S.A.

Malnutrition, cirrhosis and liver carcinoma coexist in many geographic areas of the world. Recent evidence indicates that aflatoxin may be a significant contributing factor. It appears from animal experiments that there is an interaction between aflatoxin and dietary inadequacy which results in a response which neither exposure induces alone. Two strains of rats, purified aflatoxin B_1 and a marginal lipotrope diet have been used to illustrate the enhancing effect of diet on aflatoxin carcinogenicity. A severe lipotrope deficient diet diminished the carcinogenic effect of aflatoxin as did dietary penicillin. In contrast, a marginal lipotrope deficiency decreased acute toxicity but enhanced significantly the carcinogenicity of aflatoxin B_1. The marginal lipotrope diet alone decreased three drug-metabolising enzymes, two demethylases and one hydroxylase; AFB_1 in repeated doses increased the two demethylase enzymes and decreased the hydroxylase enzyme in control animals fed a normal diet. None of the enzymes was affected by repeated doses of AFB_1 to rats fed the marginal lipotrope diet. Total acid phosphatase was unaffected but the free fraction was elevated by AFB_1 in both dietary groups while glucose-6-phosphatase was depressed only in rats fed the low lipotrope and exposed to AFB_1. It is concluded that the metabolite responsible for toxicity differs from the carcinogen and that differences in enzyme concentrations as a result of dietary treatment may relate to the predominance of one or the other of these compounds. Furthermore, dietary treatment has a profound effect on nucleic acid metabolism, cell division, and the development of preneoplastic lesions, all of which correlate with the more rapid development and increased incidence of liver tumours in lipotrope-deficient animals. Since dietary inadequacies exist in all areas where liver cancer and aflatoxin coexist, it seems essential to consider dietary factors from infancy on if we are to make significant progress towards elucidation of endemic liver carcinoma about the world.

THE ACUTE AND CHRONIC TOXICITY OF STERIGMATO-CYSTIN

by

I. F. H. PURCHASE and J. J. VAN DER WATT

South African Medical Research Council

Sterigmatocystin, a metabolite of the moulds *Aspergillus nidulans, Aspergillus versicolor* and a *Bipolaris* species, has a chemical structure similar to that of aflatoxin, but biologically the effects of these two carcinogenic mycotoxins differ considerably. The acute LD_{50} of sterigmatocystin in

Wistar rats varies with the sex and route of administration, from as low as 60 mg/kg to as high as 166 mg/kg. In male vervet monkeys (*Cercopithecus aethiops*), the LD_{50} is 32 mg/kg after intraperitoneal injection. The main histological alterations observed in rats and monkeys after a single exposure occur in the livers where single cell necrosis precedes zonal necrosis or, at high dose levels, massive collapse and haemorrhage. The kidneys are similarly affected. The low dose groups show renal cortical haemorrhage, hyaline casts in collecting tubules, cortico-medullary degeneration and necrosis and, at higher doses, glomerular necrosis and hyalinisation of Bowman's capsule. Massive haemorrhage and necrosis of all renal components follow on doses greater than the LD_{50}. Less severe degenerative changes were seen in the other abdominal and thoracic organs. Daily exposure of rats over a period of 16 weeks resulted in hepatic changes which, histologically, closely resemble those alterations seen in human patients suffering from virus hepatitis. These tissue reactions are followed by diffuse nodular hyperplasia surrounded by degeneration and necrosis of hepatic parenchyma. Daily administration of sterigmatocystin to rats for 52 weeks results in liver neoplasia in all animals surviving this period.

Weekly administration to vervet monkeys for a similar period results in focal nodular hyperplasia. The interhyperplastic hepatic parenchyma consists of actively multiplying fibroblastic elements, marked increase in reticulin fibres and anaplastic hepatocytes. Proliferating mesenchymal cells (bile duct epithelial cells) are also observed.

In Wistar rats sterigmatocystin is not cirrhogenic but primarily hepatocarcinogenic. In contrast, in vervet monkeys the toxin induces an actively expanding type of portal fibrosis soon after initial exposure.

THE EFFECTS OF AFLATOXIN B_1 AND STERIGMATOCYSTIN ON TWO DIFFERENT TYPES OF CELL CULTURES
by
J. C. ENGELBRECHT
South African Medical Research Council

Confluent layers of primary monkey kidney cells were exposed to aflatoxin B_1 and sterigmatocystin for 24- and 48-hour periods. Both toxins proved to be extremely toxic to these cells and the effects produced by the toxins were similar, though not identical. Cells treated with medium containing 10 μg/ml aflatoxin B_1 or sterigmatocystin showed marked degenerative changes including karyorrhexis, pycnosis and increased cytoplasmic vacuolation. There were also more nuclei with folds indicating a loss of chromatin material. Other toxic effects were more specific; these included, formation of large cells, inhibition of mitosis and alterations in nucleolar morphology. Electron microscopic studies revealed that the nucleoli of treated cells were segregated into fibrillar, granular and amorphous areas.

In an additional series of experiments, confluent cell layers of a continuous mouse liver fibroblast cell line were exposed to aflatoxin B_1 and sterigmatocystin at a toxin concentration of 1·0 μg/ml medium for 24 hours. The cells exposed to the toxins showed no morphological changes after 24 hours treatment. On subculturing in fresh medium, numerous large cells and multinucleated giant cells appeared. The cells treated with sterigmatocystin were affected to a greater extent than those exposed to aflatoxin B_1. On continuous subculturing the large and giant cells disappeared. A second exposure to aflatoxin B_1 and sterigmatocystin caused the giant cells to reappear; sterigmatocystin treated cells were much more affected than those exposed to aflatoxin B_1. Cell cultures exposed to aflatoxin B_1 and sterigmatocystin for a second time after the tenth subculture displayed a pronounced disorientated growth pattern. Ultrastructural studies of the giant cells produced by sterigmatocystin treatment, showed no alterations in nucleolar morphology but many of these cells had numerous nuclei, areas of dilated endoplasmic reticulum, large dense inclusion bodies in the cytoplasm and numerous microvilli.

RECENTLY DISCOVERED METABOLITES WITH UNUSUAL TOXIC MANIFESTATIONS

by

B. J. WILSON

University of Nashville, Tennessee, U.S.A.

Recent research on mycotoxins and toxins from higher plants used as foods has revealed several metabolites with diverse and unusual toxicological manifestations. One of these is the tremorgenic-diuretic toxin produced on foods by *Penicillium cyclopium* and related species of common fungal contaminants of foodstuffs. In addition to a potent neurological effect evidenced by sustained trembling and convulsions, a diuresis is also noted in intoxicated animals resulting in loss of electrolytes and glucose.

Another unusual toxin, as yet unidentified, is the principle elaborated by *Fusarium moniliforme* growing on corn. This substance(s) characteristically produces a leukoencephalomalacia in equines, a disease entity which has been known for many decades in several parts of the world.

A different type of toxic metabolite is exemplified by the furanosesquiterpenes produced by the sweet potato (*Ipomoea batatas*) in response to fungus infection and other injurious phenomena. One of these substances is the well-known ipomearamone which is the enantiomer of ngaione, a normal metabolite of the Ngaio tree and other plants in Australia and New Zealand. A new toxin has been isolated from sweet potato tubers and named ipomeamaranol (hydroxyipomeamarone). This compound, like ipomeamarone and ngaione, is hepatotoxic. However, in most outbreaks of mouldy sweet potato poisoning in cattle the principal signs are rapid respirations and dyspnoea leading to death. These signs are referable to pulmonary adenomatosis and lung oedema evident at post-mortem. The disease has been reproduced in mice and the toxin responsible is a substance differing from ipomeamarone or ipomeamaranol. This compound has been isolated and characterisation studies are in progress. Methods for bioproduction of all three toxins using fungus inoculated sweet potatoes have been developed. Gas chromatography offers much promise for ultimate purification of all the abnormal metabolites of sweet potatoes.

KEYNOTE ADDRESS: EPIDEMIOLOGY SESSION

by

M. CRAWFORD

Biochemistry Department, Nuffield Institute of Comparative Medicine, London

In the people at risk to primary hepatoma in Uganda there is also a high incidence of bladder cancer which could have a dietary and chemical origin. The high incidence of bladder cancer in certain parts of Uganda is not explicable in terms of bladder schistosomiasis owing to absence of the parasite. We have demonstrated the possibility that chemical carcinogenesis may be important as a consequence of high titres of urinary orthoaminophenols, again a dietary phenomenon. The different tissue location of bladder and liver cancer could be attributed to the active renal transport of ortho-aminophenolic acids producing high urinary concentration and low systemic levels. Aflatoxin on the other hand is detectable only with difficulty in urine but is excreted in the bile. In the plasma it is largely protein bound and so may only be effective during the excretion process in the liver. But aflatoxin and possibly other similar toxins might also be free to act on the tissues of the oesophagus and gastro-intestinal tracts. These experiments could provide a rationale for tissue specificity. As the experimental model to test carcinogenesis only crudely reflects the human situation, it is possible that food carcinogens might be responsible for more diverse disorders in man than was originally thought.

In a specific examination of the occurrence of *Aspergillus flavus* in Uganda we studied 450 samples of groundnuts sold for human consumption; none were free from spores. Quantitative analysis of food does not provide an unequivocal answer to the question of whether people consume toxic or carcinogenic amounts of aflatoxin. Yet there is a real difference in the incidence of primary hepatoma in Europe and Africa.

Although a high incidence of primary liver cancer is found in parts of Africa and aflatoxin is known to induce cancer of the liver, the latest epidemiological information from East Africa suggests the correlation between primary hepatoma and consumption of mouldy groundnuts may not be as clear as was first thought. However, it is now known that toxin producing moulds can contaminate a wide variety of foods, particularly grains, and enquiries into the relationship of mycotoxins to primary hepatoma should no longer be confined to groundnuts.

Experiments with guinea-pigs show that low protein/low fat/high carbohydrate diets render them more susceptible to aflatoxin toxicity. Hence one must ask in what way is the nutritional plane in Africa relevant to the epidemiology. It is probable that in the human situation a variety of factors is likely to be integrated. It is also likely that the response of an individual tissue to different chronic insults is limited.

In the past much weight has been placed on the narrow definition. Efforts to isolate a single factor responsible for certain pathological processes have led to much confusion. It is probable that an understanding of human epidemiology will benefit from a far more integrated approach to the chemical environment of populations rather than attempts to delineate an isolated cause in an individual.

DIETARY AFLATOXIN LOADS AND THE INCIDENCE OF HUMAN HEPATOCELLULAR CARCINOMA IN THAILAND

by

R. C. SHANK

Massachusetts Institute of Technology, U.S.A.

A 22-month survey of market flood samples in Thailand indicated that fungal invasion and aflatoxin contamination of common foods and food-stuffs were frequent. *Aspergillus flavus* was the most common mould found to invade Thai foods, and groundnuts and maize were the most common source of the aflatoxins.

A 1-year pilot study was carried out to measure both the amount of aflatoxins consumed and the incidence of hepatocellular carcinoma in three selected Thai populations. The study population consuming the most aflatoxin also had the highest incidence of primary cancer of the liver. Liver cancer incidence was lowest in the population consuming the least amount of toxin. For the third study area, the aflatoxin consumption and liver cancer incidence levels were intermediate between the 'high-high' and 'low-low' areas. Aflatoxin consumption followed a seasonal variation, being highest in the rainy season. There was an approximate 35-fold difference in intake values between the high and low areas and a 5- to 10-fold difference in liver cancer incidence in the same areas. The data so far obtained offer some support to the hypothesis that aflatoxins may play a role in the aetiology of human hepatocellular carcinoma in Thailand.

PRELIMINARY RESULTS FROM FOOD ANALYSES IN THE INHAMBANE AREA

by

I. F. H. PURCHASE

South African Medical Research Council and

T. GONÇALVES

Lourenço Marques

An ideal area in which to study the aetiology of liver cancer can be defined as one which has a high incidence of liver cancer, which is relatively accessible and in which the population is stable. Moçambique has the highest reported incidence of liver cancer in the world and it seemed likely that it would be a good area in which to study the disease. An examination of the case records of the hospital at Chicuque in the Inhambane district revealed that 101 cases of liver cancer were seen in 1968. This gives a crude incidence rate of 16·1/100,000/annum. This area is accessible by a scheduled airline service but a proportion of the male population migrates to Lourenço Marques and the South African mines. Nevertheless it appears to be an excellent area for this study. Food samples were collected from the homes of liver cancer patients and from the homes of patients of the same age and sex who were not suffering from liver cancer. The samples were assayed for aflatoxin and sterigmatocystin content and tested for toxicity on day-old ducklings. Of the 171 samples received, 9 (5·25%) contained aflatoxin, none contained sterigmatocystin and 2, which contained aflatoxin, were toxic. No definite conclusions can be drawn from these results at this stage.

AFLATOXIN INGESTION AND EXCRETION BY HUMANS
by

T. C. CAMPBELL and L. SALAMAT
Virginia Polytechnic Institute, College of Agriculture, U.S.A.

Surveys of Philippine foods, during 1967-1969, indicate that the principal foods contaminated with aflotaxin are peanuts and corn. Of the various peanut preparations, peanut butter had the highest levels early in the survey (500 μg/kg mean), although recent measures instituted by government and industry indicate considerable improvement.

Examinations of human excreta taken from subjects known to have consumed aflatoxin demonstrate the presence of aflatoxin M_1 in urine when 24-hour collections are made following ingestion of at least 15 μg aflatoxin. No M_1 was found in faeces or human milk and no aflatoxin B_1 could be seen in urine, faeces or milk. Because of the absence of B_1 in all excreta and the presence of small amounts of M_1 in the urine, it is suggested that the human may be capable of metabolising aflatoxin fairly rapidly which should result in lower hepatotoxicity relative to other species. Because of the limited sensitivity for the detection of aflatoxin in human urine, the use of this type of examination in general survey for aflatoxin ingestion would be somewhat limited.

THE INCIDENCE OF FUNGI IN FOODSTUFFS AND THEIR SIGNIFICANCE, BASED ON A SURVEY IN THE EASTERN TRANSVAAL AND SWAZILAND

by

P. M. D. MARTIN, G. GILMAN and P. KEEN
South African Institute for Medical Research

Seventy-seven lots of foodstuffs, collected between 1966 and 1970 and comprising a total of 470 samples, were analysed in terms of fungal population. Strains of the commoner species of fungi were grown on maize meal and fed to day-old ducklings. It was found that there was a proportion of toxic strains for every fungal species tested, though some species could be reckoned as a general rule more toxic than others. Although there was a fairly large number of species found in common from different foodstuffs and various preparations of the same food-stuffs, there were nevertheless characteristic species or proportions of common species noted for each foodstuff. The significance of these findings is discussed.

BIOLOGICAL SCREENING AS A LABORATORY AID IN DETERMINING CANCER AETIOLOGY

by

I. F. H. PURCHASE and H. J. B. JOUBERT
South African Medical Research Council

The Bantu of the Transkei suffer from the highest recorded incidence of oesophageal cancer in the world. It has been shown by Burrell and co-workers that the high incidence of the disease occurs in families which consume foods grown in gardens with certain mineral deficiencies (Mo). It is not known, however, whether or how this mineral deficiency produces oesophageal cancer. On theoretical grounds, it appears that identification of the aetiological agent would be easier if a relatively non-specific bio-logical screening method was used than if a highly specific chemical method was used to detect it in the food.

Food was therefore collected from the mineral deficient gardens and fed to a susceptible strain of rats in order to ascertain whether the diet of the Bantu with a high incidence of oesophageal cancer contained any carcinogen. The rats fed a diet of maize and beans plus imifino (wild

B

vegetables) developed hepatocullelar carcinomas at 125 weeks. Those receiving the same diet, without imifino, did not develop tumours. It is not known whether this is a direct or indirect effect of imifino.

These results indicate that the relatively non-specific biological screening method used here can help to identify food-borne carcinogens.

EFFECTS OF AFLATOXINS ON *IN VIVO* NUCLEIC ACID METABOLISM IN RATS

by

Gerald N. Wogan

Massachusetts Institute of Technology, Department of Nutrition and Food Science, Cambridge, Massachusetts 02139

INTRODUCTION

The scientific background, control and implications of the aflatoxin problem are the subjects of a recent monograph (Goldblatt, 1969[11]) in which these various topics are comprehensively discussed. Studies on the biochemistry of aflatoxin-poisoned systems have received a great deal of investigation, with the general objective of elucidating their mechanisms of action (Wogan, 1969[19]). Among the various biochemical parameters that have been studied, alterations in RNA metabolism are among the earliest demonstrable effects that occur as a result of exposure of animals or cell cultures to aflatoxins. The mechanisms involved in this type of response have received a great deal of study. We have investigated a number of aspects of this response in rat liver, and our earlier findings are summarised elsewhere (Wogan, 1969[19]). This discussion will deal with more recent findings and their relationships to those of other workers. However, by way of background, it will be useful for the remaining discussion to summarise briefly the main lines of evidence that led up to more recent experiments.

Most of the available evidence deals with effects of aflatoxin B_1, which when administered *in vivo* to rats or placed into contact *in vitro* with liver slices causes rapid and dramatic inhibition of precursor incorporation into RNA, especially in the nucleus. These effects have been observed in regenerating rat liver (Lafarge *et al.*, 1966[12]), and in liver of intact rats (Clifford and Rees, 1966[3]; Sporn *et al.*, 1966[17]; Wogan, 1969[19]). LD_{50} doses of the toxin cause suppression of precursor incorporation amounting to 90% or more; the effect is evident within 15 minutes of dosing and persists for several days in animals that survive.

Similar inhibition has been noted in rat liver slices exposed to aflatoxins *in vitro* (Clifford *et al.*, 1967[6]). In this system, aflatoxins G_1 and B_2 also inhibit RNA synthesis, but with less potency than B_1.

That impaired RNA synthesis is due to inhibition of RNA polymerase activity has been shown by a number of investigators (Gelboin *et al.*, 1966[10]; Clifford and Rees, 1967[2]; Moule and Frayssinet, 1968[2]). Over the past several years, the characteristics of the RNA polymerase response to aflatoxins have been studied in some detail, and the remainder of the present discussion will deal with some of our recent findings along these lines.

GENERAL CHARACTERISTICS OF THE *IN VIVO* RESPONSE IN RATS

We have used the assay method of Widnell and Tata (1966[18]) for determining effects of aflatoxin on DNA dependent RNA polymerase activity in nuclei isolated from rat liver. This assay utilises two methods of activation, by Mg^{2+} or by Mn^{2+}–ammonium sulphate. Widnell and Tata have inferred that the former enzyme is responsible for ribosomal RNA synthesis, whereas the latter synthesises lower molecular weight DNA-like RNA. In our experience, a single sublethal dose (1 mg/kg) of aflatoxin B_1 inhibited both kinds of enzyme activity, with similar time-course characteristics (Pong and Wogan, 1970[15]). Enzyme activities were maximally (65%) suppressed for 15 minutes to 12 hours after dosing, and returned to pre-treatment levels by 36 hours.

Suppressed enzyme activity was accompanied by loss of RNA from the nucleus, as illustrated by nuclear RNA/DNA ratios in the same preparations as those used for enzyme determinations. Saline control values generally ranged from 0·20 to 0·25 in fed animals, and the aflatoxin vehicle (DMSO) was without effect on it. However, in aflatoxin-treated animals, the ratio was significantly reduced (25%) within 15 minutes and maximally lowered (30%) by 12 hours after dosing. Like the effect on enzyme activity, this response to aflatoxin reversed itself by 36 hours. Data from other experiments (Wogan, 1969[19]) indicated that a more prolonged loss of liver cytoplasmic RNA took place over several days following aflatoxin dosing.

Inhibition of RNA polymerase in rat liver was dose-dependent over a range of sublethal doses. The data showed that inhibition of activity of the Mn^{2+}–ammonium sulphate-activated polymerase was a linear function of the logarithm of the aflatoxin dose in rats killed 15 minutes after dosing. The correlation between the two parameters, and a no-effect dose was calculated to be 0·065 mg/kg. Similar dose-dependency was found for the Mg^{2+}–activated enzyme.

Electron microscopic studies of liver cell nuclei in these experiments yielded findings that correlated well with both time-course and dose-response characteristics of inhibition of RNA polymerase. Within 15 minutes of dosing, there was microsegregation of fibrillar and granular elements in the nucleolus. By 1 hour 'nuclear capping' (macrosegregation) had occurred. These changes reversed themselves on the same time scale as enzyme inhibition and changes in RNA/DNA ratio.

It seemed important to determine whether the observed suppression of RNA polymerase activity was selective with respect to the types of nuclear RNA synthesis affected, or whether the inhibition was equally effective for all types of nuclear RNA. We therefore carried out a series of experiments to determine the pattern of precursor incorporation into various nuclear RNA fractions during periods when RNA polymerase activity was maximally suppressed by aflatoxin B_1 (Friedman and Wogan, 1970[9]).

Sedimentation analysis and precursor incorporation into various fractions of nuclear RNA were carried out as follows: RNA was extracted from isolated nuclei with phenol, and was subsequently purified, layered on a 10-40% linear sucrose gradient and centrifuged for 16 hours at $105\,000 \times g$. RNA distribution was analysed by scanning at 260 nm. Animals were injected with ^{14}C-orotate 1 hour before they were killed, and incorporation into RNA fractions was determined. In the control animals that received DMSO, precursor incorporation was principally into the 28 S fraction, with less into the other two major peaks (18 S and 6 S).

The effects of aflatoxin B_1 became apparent in animals killed 45 minutes after aflatoxin B_1 dosing (at 0·5 mg/kg). Incorporation into the 28 S fraction was strongly inhibited with little apparent effect on the lower molecular weight fractions. These effects were even more clearly evident 12 hours after dosing. At this time, incorporation of precursor into the 28 S and 18 S peaks was almost entirely blocked and only small amounts of incorporation into the 6 S peak were observed.

Floyd *et al.* (1968[8]) studied the characteristics of RNA synthesised in the nucleoli of regenerating liver from aflatoxin-treated rats. They concluded that aflatoxin B_1 at a dose of 0·2 mg/kg or larger completely suppressed the synthesis of 45 S RNA. Taken together with the data summarised above, these findings indicate that aflatoxin B_1 inhibits ribosomal RNA synthesis and also, to a significant degree, suppresses the synthesis of lower molecular weight RNA.

STRUCTURE-ACTIVITY RELATIONSHIPS

Because of large differences in potency with respect to toxicity and carcinogenicity exhibited by the various aflatoxins, we became interested in studying the extent to which those differences could be correlated with *in vivo* effects on RNA metabolism.

It has been postulated by several investigators, and is generally assumed, that inhibition of DNA and RNA polymerases by aflatoxins results from binding of the toxins to DNA in such a way as to impair its template activity. Thus, binding to DNA is envisioned as the initial reaction in a sequence that results in impaired synthesis of nucleic acids and proteins. These assumptions were based originally upon similarities in the actions of actinomycin D and aflatoxins. Although direct experimental evidence for many aspects of this parallelism is not extensive, binding of aflatoxins to DNA has been shown by several groups using different techniques and it would be worth while to review their findings briefly.

Using as evidence the spectral changes induced in the aflatoxin spectrum in the presence of DNA, i.e. the shift in absorption maximum and hypochromism at 363 nm, and also an equilibrium dialysis technique, Sporn et al. (1966[17]) reported binding of aflatoxin B_1 to calf thymus DNA. Rees and co-workers (Clifford and Rees, 1967[4]; 1969[5]) also using spectral evidence, reported binding of aflatoxin B_1 to calf-thymus DNA and further indicated that aflatoxins G_1 and G_2 showed quantitatively smaller binding capability. More recently, Neely et al. (1970[14]) investigated aflatoxin-DNA interactions using fluorescent quenching and polarisation, and found the extent of binding to be linearly related to DNA concentration in mixtures of the two substances.

Details of the aflatoxin-DNA interaction have also been investigated but to a lesser extent. Schabort (1969[16]), using difference spectroscopy, studied binding of aflatoxins B_1, G_1, and G_2 to DNA from different sources and with different base compositions. He concluded that interaction of aflatoxins with DNA was more likely to depend on base sequence than on base composition. Clifford and Rees (1969[5]) reported results of further studies on aflatoxin-calf thymus DNA binding from which they concluded that the aflatoxins are associated with DNA in such a manner that binding is easily disrupted. Schabort (1969[16]) also commented upon the weakness of the association, particularly of aflatoxins G_1 and G_2.

Owing to the apparent ease with which reversal occurs in the binding of aflatoxins and DNA *in vitro*, and almost total lack of direct evidence of binding in intact systems, the extent to which binding *per se* can be associated with effects observed in intact systems is uncertain. We have recently completed a series of experiments that bears on this point. The studies were done in collaboration with Dr M. B. Sporn of the National Cancer Institute, N.I.H., and the principal findings will be summarised here. Details can be found in the full publications (Edwards et al., 1971[7]; Wogan et al., *Cancer Res.*, in press, 1971[7]).

Several aflatoxins and related compounds were studied. Their structures are shown in Figure 1. Various experiments were conducted using aflatoxins B_1, B_2, G_1, and also tetrahydrodeoxy B_1 (the reduction product), and three substituted coumarins related to B_1, without the furanofuran portion of the molecule. These latter compounds were synthesised by

Büchi's group (Asao *et al.*, 1965[1]) in the course of the aflatoxin structure-elucidation. We have studied 'compound 11' most extensively, as it most closely approximates the aflatoxin B_1 molecule.

Using equilibrium dialysis, Sporn compared the binding properties of aflatoxin B_1, B_2, tetrahydrodeoxy B_1, and compound 11 to calf thymus DNA. Each compound was studied over a 5-fold range of concentrations. After 4 days at 2°C, the concentration (c) of free compound and the number of moles of compound bound per mole of DNA phosphorus (r) were calculated. Reciprocal plots of $1/r$ vs $1/c$ were than made, which showed that the binding of any of these substances to DNA was increased with increasing concentration, and that $1/r$ was a linear function of $1/c$.

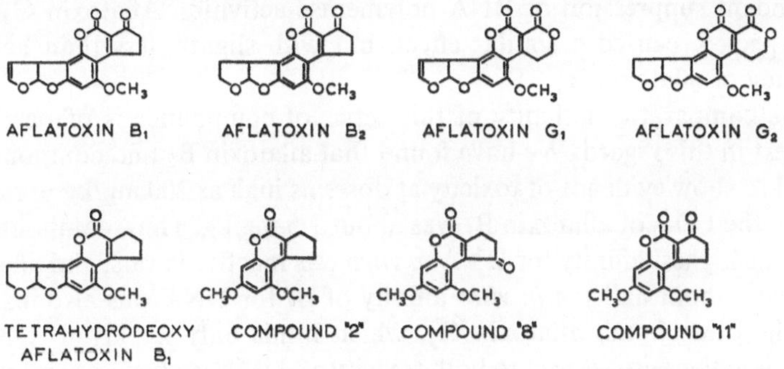

AFLATOXIN B₁   AFLATOXIN B₂   AFLATOXIN G₁   AFLATOXIN G₂

TETRAHYDRODEOXY   COMPOUND '2'   COMPOUND '8'   COMPOUND '11'
AFLATOXIN B₁

FIG. 1

It also became apparent that the limiting value (y-intercept) $1/r_{max}$ for all four compounds was approximately the same. Thus, although values of $1/c$ that would saturate DNA were not experimentally attainable, it can be calculated that the saturation binding value of these four compounds is about 1 mole of ligand per 25 mole of nucleotide.

Using the equation: $\text{slope} = \dfrac{1}{(r_{max})(K)}$, the association constant (K) of each compound with DNA was calculated. Compound 11 has the highest association constant $(5\cdot4 \times 10^4)$ followed, in decreasing order, by aflatoxin B_1 $(2\cdot1 \times 10^4)$, aflatoxin B_2 $(1\cdot2 \times 10^4)$ and tetrahydrodeoxy aflatoxin B_1 $(6\cdot9 \times 10^3)$. It is of interest to note that the K value for each member of the series differs from the one below it by a factor of about 2.

In view of the large differences in association constants, it was of interest to compare the biological activities of these compounds, especially their effects in rats, and we have done a series of such experiments. With respect to their abilities to inhibit RNA polymerase *in vivo*, we have compared aflatoxins B_1, B_2, and G_1.

Rats were dosed with aflatoxin B_1 (0·2 mg/kg), aflatoxin B_2 (200 mg/kg), or with steroid-suspending medium (SSM), the vehicle used to administer the aflatoxins. The animals were killed either 30 minutes or 3 hours after dosing; liver nuclei were isolated and assayed for RNA polymerase activity as described earlier. Aflatoxin B_1 had its expected inhibiting effect, causing about 40% reduction in activity by 30 minutes, and the inhibition was still greater after 3 hours. By contrast, B_2 had no demonstrable effect at either time, providing further evidence of its lack of acute activity in rats.

The comparative potency of aflatoxins B_1 and G_1 on RNA polymerase was also studied. Rats were injected with aflatoxin B_1 at doses of 0·2 or 0·5 mg/kg, or with aflatoxin G_1 at 0·55 mg/kg, or with SSM. They were killed 30 minutes after dosing and RNA polymerase activities assayed as before. Aflatoxin B_1 caused the predicted effects, resulting in a dose-dependent suppression of RNA polymerase activities. Aflatoxin G_1, also as expected, caused a similar effect, but with slightly less than half the potency of aflatoxin B_1.

The comparative lethality of this series of compounds is of particular interest in this regard. We have found that aflatoxin B_2 and compound 11 failed to show evidence of toxicity at doses as high as 200 mg/kg in rats for which the LD_{50} of aflatoxin B_1 was about 1·5 mg/kg. Thus, compound 11, with the highest affinity for DNA *in vitro* was inactive in rats, and aflatoxin B_2, with about half the *in vitro* affinity of B_1 for DNA was also inactive. On the other hand, aflatoxin G_1, which binds only weakly to DNA *in vitro*, is active with respect to both toxicity and RNA polymerase inhibition in rats, and has much higher potency than its binding properties would predict.

It would therefore appear, at least within this series of compounds, that *in vitro* binding characteristics are inadequate in their predictive value for *in vivo* toxicity to rats. Several mechanisms might account for this discrepancy, but little direct evidence is available to evaluate the alternatives. We have explored one obvious possibility that might explain the difference in potency between aflatoxins B_1 and B_2. The large difference might have been attributable to grossly different distribution and excretion of the two compounds. We therefore compared the tissue distribution and excretion pattern of aflatoxins B_1 and B_2 labelled with ^{14}C in the ring carbons.

Rats were injected with the compounds and killed 3 hours later. Tissues and excreta were analysed for ^{14}C, and the tissue distribution calculated as per cent of recovered [14]C (essentially equivalent to per cent of dose). In agreement with earlier findings on B_1 (Wogan *et al.*, 1967[20]) the liver contained a larger amount of ^{14}C than other tissues (22%). Animals dosed with B_2 had only about half as much ^{14}C in liver (11%), and this was the only significant difference between the two compounds. The lower amount of radio-activity from B_2 in the liver was accounted for by elevated urinary excretion.

Although this difference suggested that the smaller amount of B_2 in liver might partially account for its lower toxicity, the magnitude of the difference does not seem great enough to explain the factor of 2 in biological activity simply on the basis of concentration. The data do suggest, however, that differences in metabolic pathways might exist that would be more important in this regard. Unfortunately, the metabolites of B_2 have not yet been identified.

AFLATOXIN EFFECTS ON TEMPLATE ACTIVITY OF CHROMATIN

Despite the considerable amount of evidence that aflatoxins inhibit RNA polymerase when administered to rats, an interesting and important discrepancy exists between *in vivo* and *in vitro* responses. Several investigators have attempted to demonstrate that the template activity of DNA reacted *in vitro* with aflatoxin is diminished. For the most part, the results have been negative; i.e. DNA–aflatoxin complexes are transcribed as effectively as DNA alone.

The following systems have been studied: (1) calf-thymus DNA reacted *in vitro* with aflatoxin B_1 and transcribed by bacterial RNA polymerase, or rat testicular polymerase; (2) rat liver chromatin preparations reacted *in vitro* with aflatoxin (or isolated from aflatoxin-treated rats) and transcribed by bacterial enzyme. Similarly, direct addition *in vitro* of aflatoxin B_1 to isolated rat liver nuclei fails to inhibit RNA polymerase activity. Actinomycin D causes inhibition in all these systems.

These experimental models fail to duplicate *in vivo* conditions in several respects. Most important, they do not provide conditions for metabolic activation to occur, should this be a required step in the observed suppression of enzyme activity. Recent development of techniques to solubilise rat liver RNA polymerase in useful quantities made possible direct experiments dealing with this problem, and several such experiments utilising this technique have recently been completed in our laboratory (Edwards and Wogan, 1970[7]). Our approach was to separate rat liver chromatin and RNA polymerase in such a way that recombination produced enzyme activity, i.e. the enzyme was transcribing its own template. Cross-over experiments using materials isolated separately from treated and untreated rats then allowed evaluation of the effects of aflatoxin B_1 on enzyme and template independently.

We first repeated the *in vitro* incubation systems to verify earlier findings. Rat liver nuclei were isolated from untreated rats, and were placed in the usual RNA polymerase assay medium either with or without the presence of aflatoxin B_1. Aflatoxin had no effect on either type of enzyme activity under three different conditions. In one case, it was added at the same time as the assay was begun. In another case, the toxin was pre-incubated with the nuclei, in the absence of precursors, for either 1 hour at 0°C or 6 minutes at 37°C in an attempt to facilitate interaction. Under all of these conditions, no evidence of aflatoxin inhibition was seen. By contrast, actinomycin D, which was used as a positive control, showed its usual inhibitory properties.

These results confirmed many earlier findings that aflatoxin B_1 is inactive in inhibiting RNA polymerase when added to an *in vitro* system. We then proceeded to a series of *in vivo* experiments, in which one group of rats was dosed with aflatoxin B_1 at 0·5 mg/kg and were killed 30 minutes later. Other groups received aflatoxin B_2 at 200 mg/kg or actinomycin D. Chromatin preparations were made from nuclei isolated from the livers of these animals. The isolation technique was as gentle as possible to minimise the possibility of removal of aflatoxins that might be bound to chromatin. For control purposes, chromatin was also isolated from DMSO-treated rats.

In the first of two types of transcription experiments, the enzyme preparation used was rat liver polymerase isolated from untreated animals. Thus, untreated enzyme was transcribing either untreated or treated chromatin. In three separate experiments, aflatoxin B_1 caused about a 30-50% inhibition of polymerase activity, comparable in degree to that caused by actinomycin D. In contrast, aflatoxin B_2 at a dose of 200 mg/kg showed no evidence of inhibition. It was of particular interest that bacterial polymerase failed under the same conditions to detect the inhibition exhibited by the rat liver enzyme.

In the second type of cross-over experiment, RNA polymerase solubilised from livers of either aflatoxin-treated or control rats was allowed to transcribe untreated template. This was done in order to determine whether the aflatoxin had a direct action on the enzyme itself. Rats were dosed with 0·5 mg/kg aflatoxin B_1 or DMSO and were killed 30 minutes later. RNA polymerase solubilised from their liver nuclei was then allowed to transcribe either calf-thymus DNA or liver chromatin from untreated rats. No significant inhibition was evident under either condition when treated and control activities were compared.

These results permit several conclusions with respect to the mechanism through which aflatoxin inhibits RNA polymerase. The combined results of the cross-over experiment indicate that the inhibitory effects of aflatoxin B_1 on RNA polymerase *in vivo* results from interactions with some component or components of chromatin and not from a direct action on the enzyme. These findings, together with a lack of effect of the toxin when added to the *in vitro* system, strongly suggest that the toxin is effective only under *in vivo* conditions, where metabolic transformation is possible. The same conclusion has been reached by other investigators from different lines of evidence, and the subject of metabolism of aflatoxins will be discussed by other participants in the symposium.

I shall close this presentation by stating the obvious. Despite progress that has been made along some lines of investigation, we are a long way from understanding the mechanisms by which aflatoxins poison cells. We are still a longer way from understanding what, if anything, these short-term events have to do with the carcinogenic processes that take place in some species following chronic exposure. At least some further understanding of these phenomena will be required before a complete assessment of their significance to human health will be possible.

REFERENCES

1. ASAO, T., BÜCHI, G., ABDEL-KADER, M. M., CHANG, S. B., WICK, E. L. and WOGAN, G. N. (1965). The structures of aflatoxins B_1 and G_1. *J. Am. Chem. Soc.*, **87**, 882-886.
2. CLIFFORD, J. I. and REES, K. R. (1967). The action of aflatoxin B_1 on the rat liver. *Biochem. J.*, **102**, 65-75.
3. CLIFFORD, J. I. and REES, K. R. (1966). Aflatoxin: a site of action in the rat liver cell. *Nature*, **209**, 312-313.
4. CLIFFORD, J. I. and REES, K. R. (1967). The interaction of aflatoxins with purines and purine nucleosides. *Biochem. J.*, **103**, 467-471.
5. CLIFFORD, J. I. and REES, K. R. (1969). Investigations of the nature of the binding of aflatoxin B_1 with DNA. *Biochem. Pharmacol.*, **18**, 2783-2785.
6. CLIFFORD, J. I., REES, K. R. and STEVENS, M. E. M. (1967). The effect of the aflatoxin B_1, G_1, and G_2 on protein and nucleic acid synthesis in rat liver. *Biochem. J.*, **103**, 258-261.
7. EDWARDS, G. S. and WOGAN, G. N. (1970) Aflatoxin inhibition of template activity of rat liver chromatin. *Biochem. Biophys. Acta.*, **224**, 597-607.
8. FLOYD, L. R., UNUMA, T. and BUSCH, H. (1968). Effects of aflatoxin B_1 and other carcinogens upon nucleolar RNA of various tissues in the rat. *Exptl. Cell Res.*, **51**, 423-438.
9. FRIEDMAN, M. A. and WOGAN, G. N. (1970). Liver nuclear RNA metabolism in rats treated with aflatoxin B_1. *Life Sciences*, **9**, 741-747.
10. GELBOIN, H. V., WORTHAM, J. S., WILSON, R. G., FRIEDMAN, M. A. and WOGAN, G. N. (1966). Rapid and marked inhibition of rat-liver RNA polymerase by aflatoxin B_1. *Science*, **154**, 1205-1206.
11. GOLDBLATT, L. A. (1969). Aflatoxin—Scientific Background, Control and Implications. New York: Academic Press.

12. LaFarge, C., Frayssinet, C. and Simard, R. (1966). Inhibition preferentielle des syntheses de RNA nucleolaire provoquee par l'aflatoxine dans les cellules hepatiques du rat. *Comptes Rendus Academie Sciences Paris*, **263**, 1011-1014.

13. Moule, Y. and Frayssinet, C. (1968). Effect of aflatoxin on transcription in liver cell. *Nature*, **218**, 93-95.

14. Neely, W. C., Lansden, J. A. and McDuffie, J. R. (1970). Spectral studies on the deoxyribonucleic acid aflatoxin B_1 system. Binding interaction. *Biochemistry*, **9**, 1862-1866.

15. Pong, R. S. and Wogan, G. N. (1970). Time course and dose-response characteristics of aflatoxin B_1 effects on rat liver RNA polymerase and ultrastructure. *Cancer Res.*, **30**, 294-304.

16. Schabort, J. C. (1969). The differential interaction of aflatoxins B_1, G_1, and G_2 with deoxyribonucleic acids from different sources. *J. South African Chemical Institute*, **22**, 80-87.

17. Sporn, M. B., Dingman, C. W. and Phelps, H. L. (1966). Aflatoxin B_1: binding to DNA *in vitro* and alteration of RNA metabolism *in vivo*. *Science*, **151**, 1539-1541.

18. Widnell, C. C. and Tata, J. R. (1966). Studies on the stimulation by ammonium-sulfate of the DNA-dependent RNA polymerase of isolated rat-liver nuclei. *Biochim. Biophys. Acta.*, **123**, 478-492.

19. Wogan, G. N. (1969). Metabolism and biochemical effects of aflatoxins. In: *Aflatoxin—Scientific Background, Control, and Implications* (Ed. Goldblatt, L. A.), pp. 152-184. New York: Academic Press.

20. Wogan, G. N., Edwards, G. S. and Shank, R. C. (1967). Excretion and tissue distribution of radioactivity from aflatoxin B_1-^{14}C in rats. *Cancer Res.*, **27**, 1729-1736.

THE METABOLISM AND SOME METABOLIC
EFFECTS OF STERIGMATOCYSTIN

by

W. Nel
University College of Zululand

and

P. G. Kempff and M. J. Pitout
*Division of Toxicology, National Institute for Nutritional Diseases
South African Medical Research Council*

The influence of the metabolites of carcinogens and toxins on macro-molecules is becoming of increasing interest in the study of the biochemistry of tumours. Sterigmatocystin, with a chemical structure closely related to aflatoxin, is carcinogenic to rats[1] and there are indications that it may also be carcinogenic to Vervet monkeys.[2] The type of tumour produced experimentally with sterigmatocystin is morphologically similar to tumours seen in the Bantu races of Southern Africa.

The first stage of this study, which is still in progress, was to examine the distribution of radio-activity after labelled sterigmatocystin (dosed either intraperitoneally or *per os*) was administered to rats in a fasting or a non-fasting state. The influence of sterigmatocystin on the synthesis of RNA was the second aspect studied.

METHODS

1. The preparation, isolation and purification of sterigmatocystin

Unlabelled sterigmatocystin was prepared, isolated and purified by using the method of Holzapfel *et al.*[3]

2. Uptake experiments using ^{14}C-sterigmatocystin

[14]C-labelled sterigmatocystin was prepared by Mr N. P. Ferreira of the Microbiological Research Unit of the CSIR. The fungus *Aspergillus nidulans* (CSIR 106) produced sterigmatocystin in the following liquid growth medium: 30·0 g sucrose, 2·0 g sodium nitrate, 1·0 g potassium bisulphate, 0·5 g magnesium sulphate, 0·5 g potassium chloride, 0·05 g ferri sulphate, 0·05 g zinc sulphate, all dissolved in 1 litre distilled water. On the 8th and 10th day of incubation 100 μCi acetate-1-^{14}C were added. The sterigmatocystin containing medium was harvested on the 18th day of incubation. The isolation and purification was then performed using Holzapfel's method.

In the studies conducted on the distribution of ^{14}C-sterigmatocystin, 4 male Wistar-derived rats were each injected intraperitoneally with 6·4 mg sterigmatocystin dissolved in 0·25 ml dimethylsulphoxide (DMSO). This amount of toxin equalled 178,963 disintegrations per minute (d.p.m.). The rats were not fasted before dosing and were maintained in metabolism cages through which air was circulated after passing over calcium chloride. Twenty-four hours later the rats were killed by decapitation. The following organs were removed at post-mortem: brain, heart, lungs, liver, kidneys, spleen, testes and the gastro-intestinal tract with its contents. The faeces and urine were collected separately. The excretions and organs were homogenised individually in water with a blender and an aliquot was digested for 2 hours in 1 N NaOH and Hyamine 2389 (Rohm and Haas Company). This digested sample was added to Bray's cocktail[4] and then counted in a Beckman Scintillation System. The quenching factors for the various samples were determined by adding an internal standard of ^{14}C-N-hexadecane (obtained from the Radiochemical Centre, Amersham) to the samples. The entire experiment was repeated with 2 more rats over a period of 12 hours.

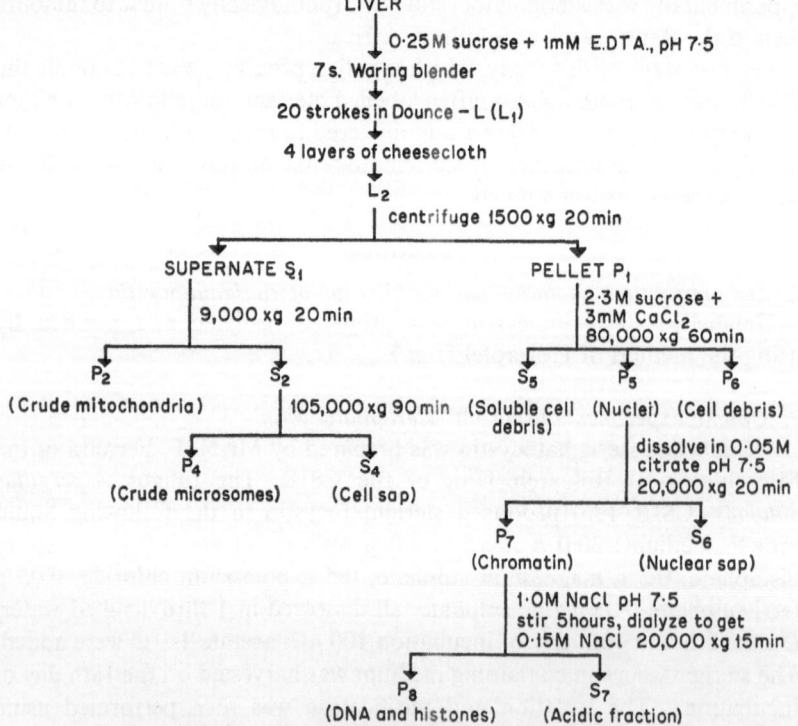

FIG. 1.   Flow diagram for intracellular liver fractions (Mahler and Cordes[5].)

3. Uptake and subcellular distribution experiments using ³H-sterigmatocystin

³H-sterigmatocystin with a much higher relative activity than ^{14}C-sterigmatocystin was prepared by the Radiochemical Centre by tritiating 99% pure sterigmatocystin resulting in 14.5×10^6 d.p.m./mg ³H-sterigmatocystin.

Three groups, each consisting of 2 rats weighing 200 ± 10 g each, were used in this study on the uptake and distribution of the tritiated sterigmatocystin. The radio-active carcinogen, dissolved in 0·5 ml DMSO, was administered *per os* at a dose of 1·41 mg/rat which equalled 20.5×10^6 d.p.m./rat. The rats were kept in metabolism cages for 16 hours with air flowing through the cages. In the first experiment the animals were not fasted but in two subsequent experiments the animals were fasted for a period of 6 hours before dosing them. During the experimental period the animals received no food but water *ad libitum*. The expired air was collected over anhydrous calcium chloride. After the 16-hour period the rats were killed by decapitation and the organs and excretions treated as mentioned before for determination of radio-activity in the liquid scintillation counter.

The excised livers were fractionated into subcellular components according to the method described by Mahler and Cordes.[5] The flow diagram was followed with the few modifications made for our own purposes (see Fig. 1). In preliminary runs it was found that the radio-activity in the lysosomal fraction could not be detected and therefore pellet P_2 was not fractionated any further.

4. The effect of sterigmatocystin on nuclear RNA synthesis[6]

Three groups, each consisting of 21 Wistar-derived rats, were used for these experiments. The first group was injected intraperitoneally with 50 mg/kg body weight, with sterigmatocystin in the form of a suspension in sodium carboxymethyl cellulose (Cellofos B) and water. The second group was injected intraperitoneally with a corresponding volume of Cellofos B in water and the third group was an untreated control group. Three animals from each group were killed $\frac{1}{2}$, 1, 2, 3, 4, 16 and 48 hours after treatment. Fifteen minutes before decapitating the animals, each rat was intraperitoneally injected with 5 μCi of 6-^{14}C-orotic acid (obtained from the Radiochemical Centre, Amersham). The livers were excised, chilled and the nuclei isolated by the method of Muramatso *et al.*[7] The nuclei were resuspended and lysed with 0·2% sodium lauryl sulphate in a Dounce homogeniser. Aliquots of the lysate were precipitated with 0·4 N perchloric acid and after standing for 15 minutes the precipitates were centrifuged. The concentration of RNA in the pellet was determined by the mild alkaline hydrolyses method of Fleck and Munro.[8] For the determination of the incorporation of the ^{14}C-orotic acid into the nuclear RNA, the hydrolysates were acidified, aliquots taken and added to Bray's cocktail for counting in the liquid scintillation system. The quenching of the samples was determined by adding ^{14}C-N-hexadecane as an internal standard.

RESULTS

1. The uptake and distribution of ^{14}C-sterigmatocystin

A pronounced decrease in radio-activity of the urine, faeces, gastro-intestinal tract and in the liver between 12 and 24 hours can be seen in

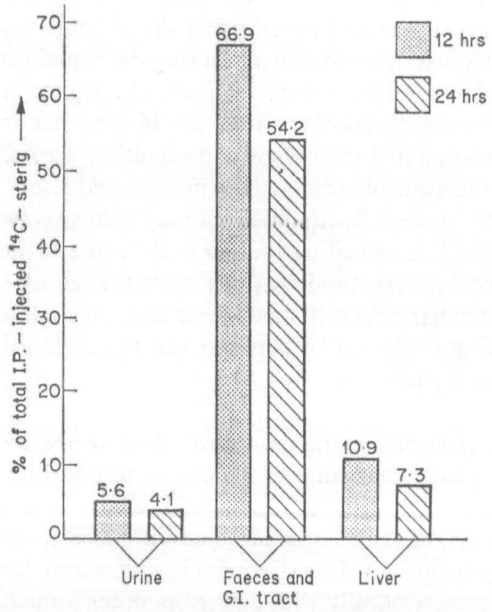

FIG. 2. Histogram of the percentage activity in the organs and excretions of non-fasted rats.

Figure 2. The radio-activity in the rest of the organs and carcass comprised a mere 1% of the total sterigmatocystin injected.

2. The uptake and subcellular distribution of ^{3}H-sterigmatocystin

In studies conducted on the distribution of ^{3}H-sterigmatocystin in female and male Wistar rats no difference could be detected. This was also found when using Wistar rats and comparing the radio-active distribution with BD IX Max Planck Institute (Freiburg) derived inbred black rats. Tritiated sterigmatocystin, dissolved in DMSO, administered intraperitoneally resulted in a much higher activity in the liver homogenate as was obtained after *per os* administration.   A mean of 2·3% of the total radio-activity injected was detected in the liver of *per os* administered rats

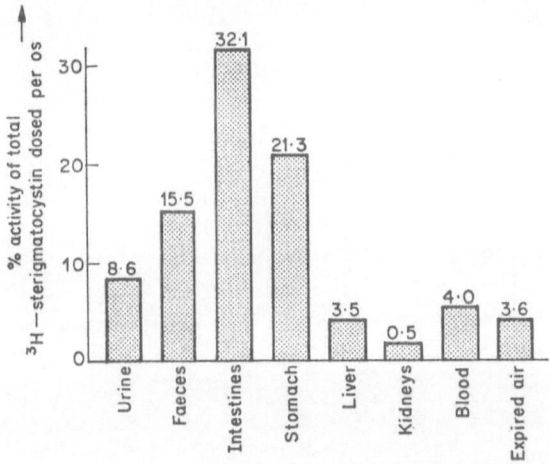

Total recovered activity 89·1%

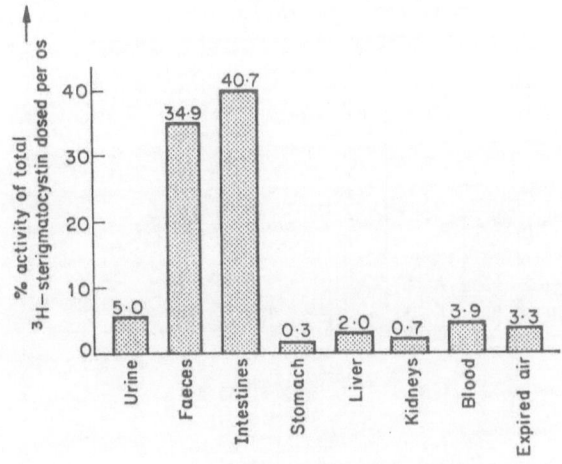

Total recovered activity 90·8%

FIG. 3. Histograms of the distribution of radio-activities in the organs and excretions of non-fasted (below) and fasted (above) rats.

in contrast to 14·3% after intraperitoneal administration. The differences between the distribution of radio-activity in the organs and excretions of fasted and non-fasted rats are shown in Figure 3.

By fractionating the livers into the different subcellular components a higher radio-activity in the mitochondria, microsomes, nuclear sap and

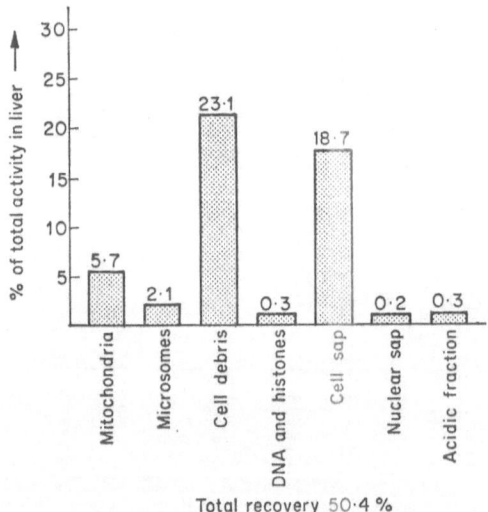

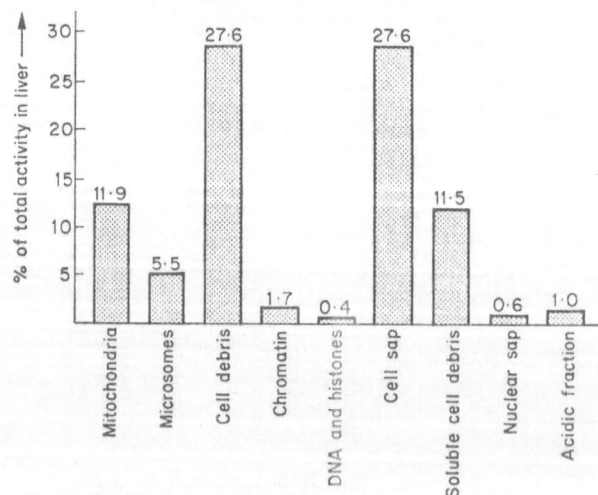

FIG. 4. Histograms of the distribution of radio-activities in the intracellular fractions of livers in fasted (above) and non-fasted (below) rats.

acidic fraction of the nucleus of the fasted rats in comparison to the non-fasted rats was found. This difference is illustrated in Figure 4.

3. The influence of sterigmatocystin on nuclear RNA synthesis

The intraperitoneal injection of sterigmatocystin had no effect on the total RNA content of the nuclei up to 48 hours after treatment and there

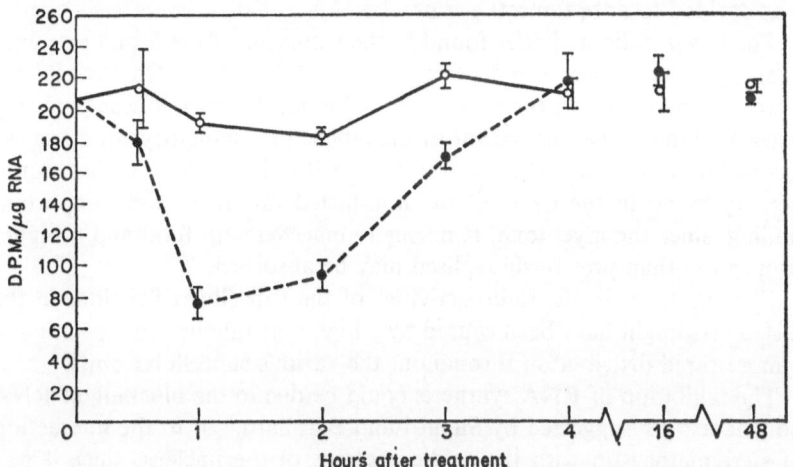

FIG. 5. Incorporation of ¹⁴C-orotic acid into nuclear RNA of normal liver from rats treated with Cellofos B (O —— O) and liver from rats treated with sterigmatocystin suspended in Cellofos B (● ---- ●). The mean value obtained from untreated controls (group 3 in this text) was 205 d.p.m.

was no difference detected between the incorporation of ¹⁴C-orotic acid into nuclear RNA of the untreated controls and in the Cellofos B treated rats. The intraperitoneal injection of sterigmatocystin had an inhibitory effect on the incorporation of ¹⁴C-orotic acid into nuclear RNA (Figure 5).

DISCUSSION

The decrease in the amount of radio-activity of the urine, faeces, gastro-intestinal tract and in the liver between 12 and 24 hours might have been caused by the catabolism of sterigmatocystin into metabolites such as ¹⁴CO₂ in the expired air. Another reason for the decrease may possibly be the evaporation of volatile ¹⁴C-compounds in the urine and faeces.

Sterigmatocystin, in contrast to aflatoxin, is insoluble in water and for administration to animals it has to be dissolved in an organic solvent of low toxicity to the rats. Dimethylsulphoxide (DMSO) was found to be the most suitable solvent for this application.

The low specific radio-activity (0.11×10^6 d.p.m./mg) of the ¹⁴C-sterigmatocystin did not yield satisfactory results. Therefore it was decided to use ³H-sterigmatocystin (14.5×10^6 d.p.m./mg).

With the intraperitoneal administration of DMSO-dissolved ^{3}H-sterig-matocystin a much higher radio-active count was detected in the liver (see results 2). This higher radio-activity was caused by the precipitation of the labelled carcinogen on the surface of the liver. To obviate this artifact it was decided to dose the rats *per os*.

The lower radio-activities found in the stomachs of the fasted rats were possibly due to more rapid passage into the intestines. Conversely, the lower radio-activity in the intestines of the non-fasted rats was probably caused by the slower movement of the labelled sterigmatocystin along the gastro-intestinal tract when it was filled with chyme. The higher radio-activity found in the livers of the non-fasted rats may be an important finding, since the mycotoxin is normally ingested with food and a higher proportion than previously realised may be absorbed.

The difference in the radio-activities of the subcellular fractions in the fasted rats might have been caused by a higher metabolic rate, resulting in a more rapid distribution throughout the various subcellular units.

The inhibition of RNA synthesis could be due to the blocking of RNA polymerase as suggested by Simard and Bernhard,[9] or to the interaction of sterigmatocystin with the acidic proteins of the nucleus, since it was shown by Paul and Gilmour[10, 11] that the acidic proteins of the nucleus have an effect on the synthesis of RNA.

REFERENCES

1. PURCHASE, I. F. H. and VAN DER WATT, J. J. (1968). *Fd. Cosmet. Toxicol.*, **6**, 555.
2. PURCHASE, I. F. H., VAN DER WATT, J. J. and VAN RENSBURG, S. J. (1970). Personal communication.
3. HOLZAPFEL, C. W., PURCHASE, I. F. H., STEYN, P. S. and GOUWS, L. (1966). *S.A. med. J.*, **40**, 1100.
4. BRAY, G. A. (1960) *Analyt. Bioch.*, **1**, 279.
5. MAHLER, H. R. and CORDES, E. H. (1967). In: *Biological Chemistry*, p. 394, Harper and Zow.
6. NEL, W. and PRETORIUS, H. E. (1970). *Bioch. Pharm.*, **19**, 957.
7. MURAMATSO, M., SMETENA, K. and BUSCH, H. (1963). *Cancer Res.*, **23**, 510.
8. FLECK, A. and MUNRO, H. N. (1962). *Biochem. Biophys. Acta*, **55**, 571.
9. SIMARD, R. and BERNHARD, W. (1966). *Int. J. Cancer*, **1**, 463.
10. PAUL, J. and GILMOUR, R. S. (1968). *J. Molec. Biol.*, **34**, 305.
11. PAUL, J. and GILMOUR, R. S. (1969). *J. Molec. Biol.*, **40**, 137.

THE EFFECT OF AFLATOXINS ON PANCREATIC DEOXYRIBONUCLEASE

by

J. C. Schabort
Rand Afrikaans University, Johannesburg

and

M. J. Pitout
Division of Toxicology, National Institute for Nutritional Diseases
South African Medical Research Council

Notwithstanding a close similarity in their chemical structures, the aflatoxins were found to have a wide variation in toxicity as well as a variation in their carcinogenicity.[1-5] Clifford, Rees and Stevens[6] found a correlation between the magnitude of spectral changes obtained in the DNA-aflatoxin interactions and inhibition of RNA synthesis in liver slices by aflatoxins B_1, G_1 and G_2 and postulated that the degree of interaction with DNA might determine their degree of toxicity. The inhibition of DNA dependent RNA-polymerase after aflatoxin B_1, poisoning supports the proposals that the inhibition of nuclear RNA synthesis by aflatoxin B_1 was the result of the toxin interacting with the DNA and thereby preventing a transcription of the DNA.

The effect of certain strong carcinogens on pancreatic deoxyribonuclease has recently been reported.[7] Melzer[7] reported that certain strong carcinogens had an activating effect on deoxyribonuclease whereas certain much weaker carcinogens had no effect and other weak carcinogens had an inhibitory effect on the activity of the enzyme *in vitro*. These effects are most probably due to their interaction with the enzyme molecule.

In this investigation a study was made of the relationship between the effect of aflatoxins B_1, B_2, G_1, G_2, M_1, M_2, B_{2a} and G_{2a} on pancreatic deoxyribonuclease and their interactions with DNA and deoxyribonuclease.

Activation of pancreatic deoxyribonuclease by aflatoxins B_1, B_2 and M_2

The assay method for deoxyribonuclease activity was based on the increase in absorption at 260 nm after removal of the unhydrolysed DNA and enzyme by precipitation with cold 1·4 M perchloric acid and centrifugation.[8] The activity was expressed as $\Delta A260$ nm/h.

The activation of deoxyribonuclease by aflatoxins B_1, B_2 and M_2 at two different concentrations, *viz.* 80 and 160 μM, are given in Table 1. The activating effect of aflatoxin B_2 was much more concentration dependent than the other two toxins and was the strongest activator at concentrations

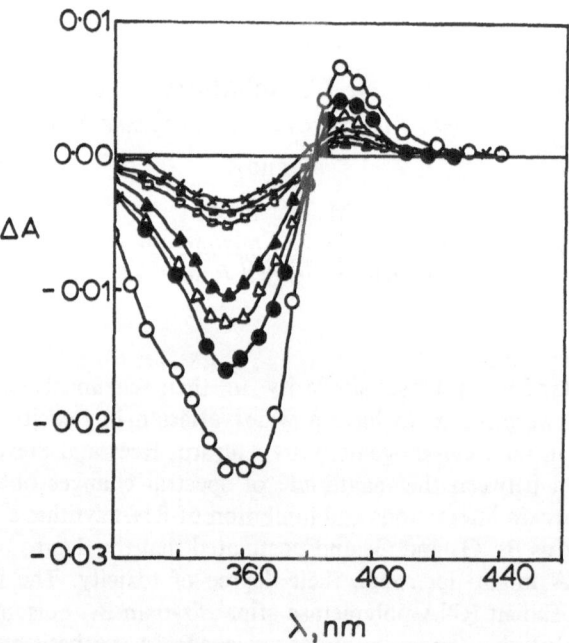

FIG. 1. Difference spectra of aflatoxins with calf thymus DNA. The concentration of each toxin was 10 μM and that of DNA 532 μM DNA-P. Aflatoxins B_1, B_2, M_2, G_1, G_2, M_1 and B_{2a} and G_{2a} are represented by $\bigcirc$, $\bullet$, $\triangle$, $\blacktriangle$, $\square$, $\blacksquare$ and x, respectively.

Table 1

Effect of Aflatoxins B_1, B_2 and M_2 on deoxyribonuclease Activity

Toxin	Toxin concn. μM	Final corr. $\Delta A260$ nm/h	Activation (%)
Aflatoxin B_1	160	0·745	24·2
Aflatoxin B_1	80	0·695	15·8
Aflatoxin B_2	160	0·870	45·0
Aflatoxin B_2	80	0·692	15·3
Aflatoxin M_2	160	0·785	30·8
Aflatoxin M_2	80	0·660	10·0
Control	—	0·600	—

higher than 80 μM. At lower concentrations, B_1 was the strongest activator and M_2 was the weakest.

Aflatoxins B_{2a}, G_{2a}, G_2 and M_1 were found to be inhibitors of deoxyribonuclease activity at all concentrations studied, whereas aflatoxin G_1 had no definite effect.

Interaction with DNA and the effect of the activating aflatoxins on the apparent Michaelis constants for DNA

It has been shown recently that aflatoxins B_1, G_1 and G_2 can bind to DNA most probably in this order of magnitude.[6, 9] According to difference spectroscopy and equilibrium dialysis, aflatoxin B_2 also binds to DNA nearly as strongly as aflatoxin B_1 (see Fig. 1). Aflatoxin M_2 binds weakly

Table 2

Effect of Aflatoxins B_1, B_2 and M_2 on the Apparent Michaelis Constant
for Deoxyribonuclease

Toxin	Toxin concn. mM	Apparent Km mM
Aflatoxin B_1	0·16	0·16
Aflatoxin B_1	0·12	0·18
Aflatoxin B_1	0·08	0·21
Aflatoxin B_1	0·04	0·24
Aflatoxin B_2	0·16	0·18
Aflatoxin B_2	0·08	0·24
Aflatoxin B_2	0·04	0·35
Aflatoxin M_2	0·07	0·30
Aflatoxin M_2	0·035	0·38
No toxin	—	0·40

to DNA. The inhibitors, aflatoxins B_{2a}, G_{2a}, G_2 and M_1, showed weak binding to DNA as indicated by Fig. 1.

The effect of different concentrations of aflatoxins B_1, B_2 and M_2 on the apparent Michaelis constant for DNA was determined by employing the double reciprocal plot of Lineweaver-Burk. The different apparent Michaelis constants obtained are given in Table 2.

The fact that all the plots had the same intercepts on the $1/v$ axis indicates that at high concentrations of DNA, the toxins had no effect on the deoxyribonuclease activity. At low concentrations, aflatoxin B_2 was much less effective in lowering the apparent Km than aflatoxin B_1. The order in which the aflatoxins should decrease the apparent Km and thus increase the affinity of the enzyme for the substrate (DNA) was $B_1 > B_2 > M_2$ at all concentrations of toxins studied. This corresponds with the order of their activating activity as well as the order in which they interact with DNA. Aflatoxins B_1, B_2 and M_2 showed no binding to the enzyme according to difference spectroscopy.

The apparent Km values are presumably complicated functions of constants like K_0 (dissociation constant of the substrate (DNA):aflatoxin complex), K_{AS} (dissociation constant of the enzyme:substrate:aflatoxin complex) and K_S (dissociation constant of the enzyme:substrate complex)[10]. Because in this case the enzyme most probably binds to the substrate (DNA) and substrate:activator complex with different affinities and the K_0 values for aflatoxins B_1 and B_2 are known, the K_{AS} values for these aflatoxins can be calculated from a mathematical relationship.[10]

The average K_{AS} values obtained for aflatoxins B_1 and B_2, determined at a DNA-P concentration of 80 μM and an aflatoxin concentration of 160 μM were 0.68×10^{-4}M and 1.26×10^{-4}M, respectively. The K_{AS} values are related to the normal affinity of the enzyme for the substrate-aflatoxin complex and according to the observed K_{AS} values, the affinity of the enzyme for the DNA-aflatoxin B_1 complex was approximately 1.85 times higher than that for the DNA-aflatoxin B_2 complex. It is clear that the affinity of the enzyme for these two DNA-aflatoxin complexes is much higher than for the DNA alone because these K_{AS} values are much lower than the K_S value (dissociation constant of the enzyme:substrate complex which was determined in the absence of aflatoxin) as well as the apparent Km values determined in the presence of 160 μM aflatoxin.

Table 3

Inhibition of Deoxyribonuclease Activity by Aflatoxins B_{2a}, G_{2a}, G_2 and M_1

Assay method as described under METHODS

Toxin	Toxin concn. μM	Final corr. ΔA260 nm/h	Inhibition (%)
No toxin	—	0.600	—
Aflatoxin B_{2a}	160	0.084	86.0
Aflatoxin B_{2a}	80	0.396	34.0
Aflatoxin G_{2a}	160	0.432	27.9
Aflatoxin G_{2a}	80	0.504	16.0
Aflatoxin G_2	160	0.500	16.7
Aflatoxin G_2	80	0.520	13.3
Aflatoxin M_1	160	0.484	19.3
Aflatoxin M_1	80	0.564	6.0

Inhibition of pancreatic deoxyribonuclease activity by aflatoxins B_{2a}, G_{2a}, G_2 and M_1

Aflatoxins B_{2a}, G_{2a}, G_2 and M_1 were found to be inhibitors of deoxyribonuclease activity in the order of magnitude of Table 3. Inhibition of deoxyribonuclease by aflatoxin B_{2a} showed the largest concentration dependence.

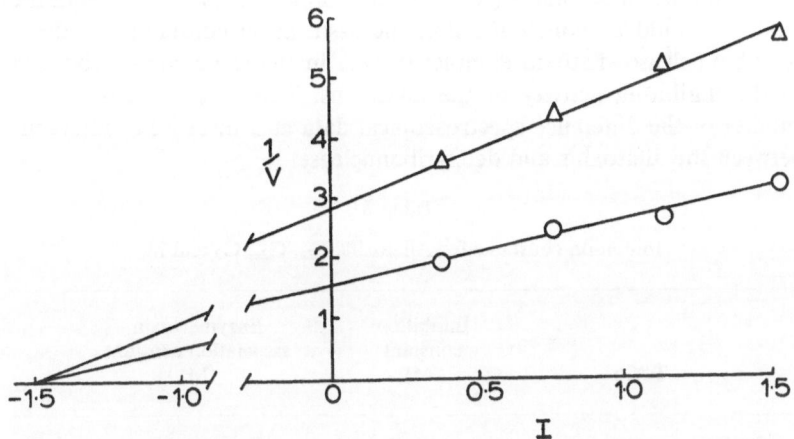

FIG. 2.   The inhibition of DNase by aflatoxin B_{2a} at DNA-P concentrations of 0·08 mM ($\triangle$) and 0·16 mM ($\bigcirc$), respectively.   v = reaction velocity in $\Delta A260$ nm/h and I = inhibitor (aflatoxin B_{2a}) concentration in 10^{-4}M.

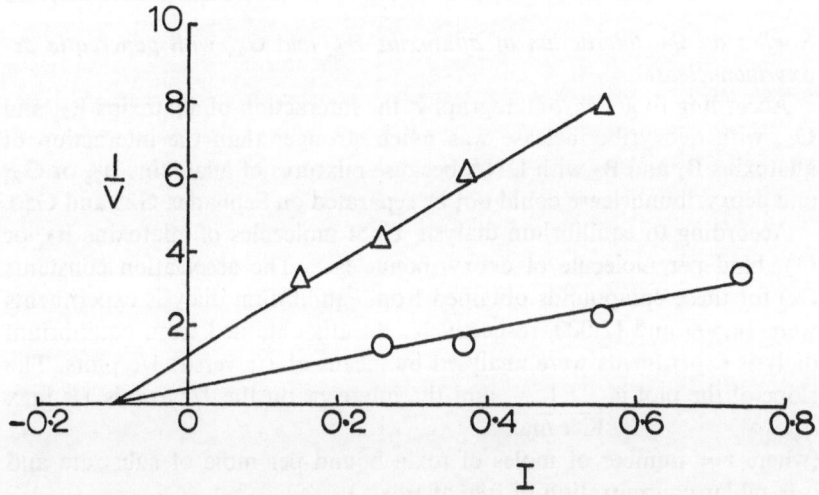

FIG. 3.   The inhibition of DNase by aflatoxin G_{2a} at DNA-P concentrations of 0·08 mM ($\triangle$) and 0·16 mM ($\bigcirc$), respectively.   Symbols v and I are similar to those described in the legend to Figure 2.

Dixon plots, given in Figures 2 to 5, illustrate that the mechanism of inhibition by all four aflatoxins was non-competitive.

According to difference spectroscopical studies (Fig. 6) these four aflatoxins bind to deoxyribonuclease most probably in the same order of magnitude as their inhibitory effect on the enzyme. These four toxins showed weak binding to DNA.

The inhibition constants (Ki) were determined (Table 4) and from these values it could be concluded that the association constants for the deoxyribonuclease-aflatoxin complexes were in the same consecutive order as the inhibiting activity of the aflatoxins. This also demonstrates the validity of the difference spectroscopical data as a measure of interaction between the aflatoxins and deoxyribonuclease.

Table 4

Inhibition constants for Aflatoxins B_{2a}, G_{2a}, G_2 and M_1

Toxin	Inhibition constant (M)	Enzyme:toxin association constant (M^{-1})
Aflatoxin B_{2a}	$1 \cdot 0 \times 10^{-5}$	100,000
Aflatoxin G_{2a}	$2 \cdot 9 \times 10^{-5}$	34,480
Aflatoxin G_2	$15 \cdot 0 \times 10^{-5}$	6,670
Aflatoxin M_1	$60 \cdot 0 \times 10^{-5}$	1,170

Studies on the interaction of aflatoxins B_{2a} and G_{2a} with pancreatic deoxyribonuclease

According to gel chromatography, the interaction of aflatoxins B_{2a} and G_{2a} with deoxyribonuclease was much stronger than the interaction of aflatoxins B_1 and B_2 with DNA because mixtures of aflatoxins B_{2a} or G_{2a} and deoxyribonuclease could not be separated on Sephadex G25 and G50.

According to equilibrium dialysis, eight molecules of aflatoxins B_{2a} or G_{2a} bind per molecule of deoxyribonuclease. The association constants (K) for these compounds obtained from equilibrium dialysis experiments were 14,500 and 12,000, respectively. Results obtained from equilibrium dialysis experiments were analysed by means of 1/r versus 1/c plots. The slope of the plot is $\dfrac{1}{K \cdot r \, max}$ and the intercept on the 1/r axis is 1/r max

(where r = number of moles of toxin bound per mole of substrate and c = molar concentration of free aflatoxin).

Aflatoxins B_{2a} and G_{2a} were precipitated in the presence of deoxyribonuclease by high concentrations of ammonium sulphate. According to difference spectroscopy, 5 to 10 μM urea could not completely abolish the interaction between these aflatoxins and the enzyme.

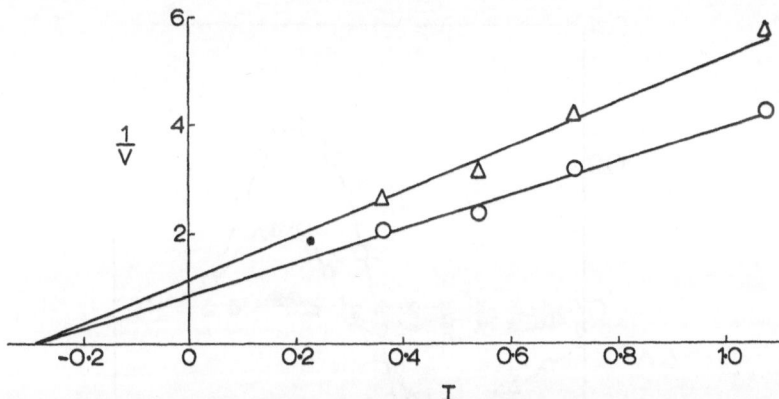

FIG. 4. The inhibition of DNase by aflatoxin G_{2a} at DNA-P concentrations of 0·08 mM ($\triangle$) and 0·16 mM ($\bigcirc$), respectively.

Symbols v and I are similar to those described in the legend to Figure 2.

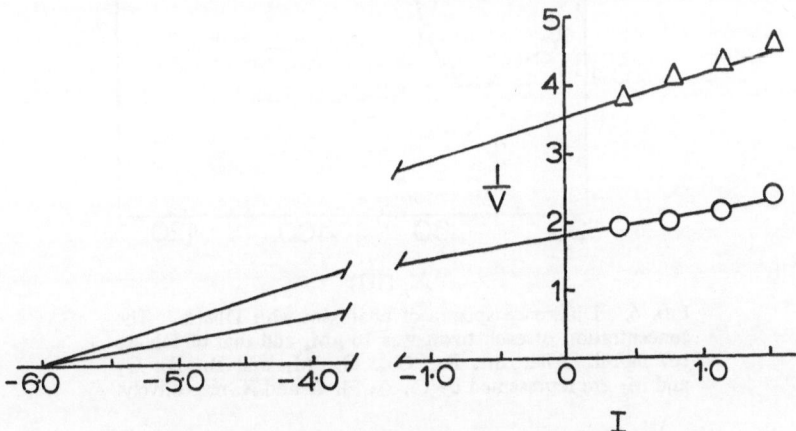

FIG. 5. The inhibition of DNase by aflatoxin M_1 at DNA-P concentrations of 0·08 mM ($\triangle$) and 0·16 mM ($\bigcirc$), respectively.

Symbols v and I are similar to those described in the legend to Figure 2.

According to difference spectroscopy, aflatoxins B_{2a} and G_{2a} interact with certain amino acids. The largest spectral shifts were obtained with lysine and second largest with arginine. It is very likely that these aflatoxins bind to the ε-amino group of lysine in deoxyribonuclease because the value of eight molecules of aflatoxin bound per molecule of enzyme corresponds closely to the lysine content of pancreatic deoxyribonuclease of 9 residues per molecule. Binding probably occurs through Schiff-base formation between the ε-amino group of lysine and keto groups of these toxins (Table 5).

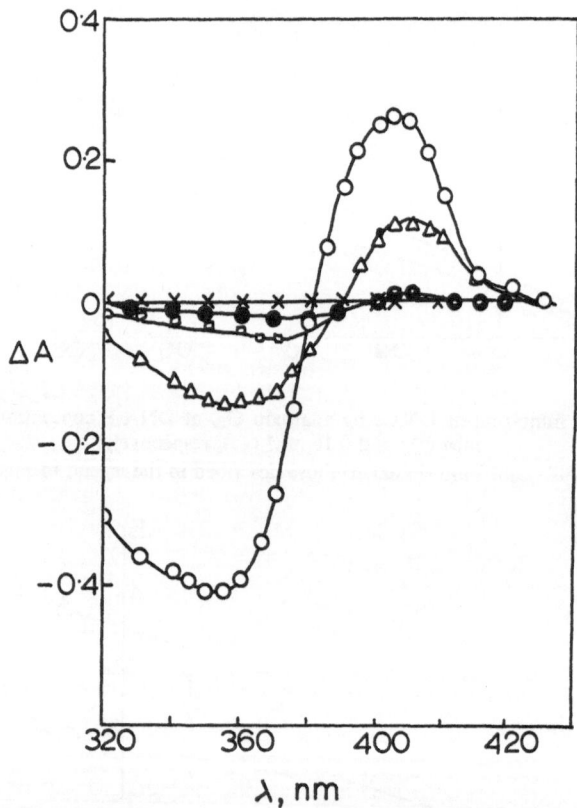

FIG. 6. Difference spectra of aflatoxins with DNase. The concentration of each toxin was 10 μM, and that of DNase 167 μg/ml. Aflatoxins B_{2_a}, G_{2_a}, G_2, M_1 and B_1, B_2, G_1 and M_2 are represented by ○, △, □, ● and X, respectively.

An interesting observation was the time dependence of the spectral shifts obtained during binding studies of aflatoxins B_{2_a} and G_{2_a} with deoxyribonuclease and certain amino acids. A characteristic red shift to about 410 nm has also been obtained which may be related to opening of the first furane ring due to a nucleophilic attack of a basic group in the enzyme molecule.

Aflatoxins, chromosomes and cancer

Certain conclusions can be made about the relationship between the chemical structure of the aflatoxins and their biochemical activity from the

Table 5

Binding Studies of Aflatoxins B_{2a} and G_{2a} to Amino Acids
Employing Difference Spectroscopy

Amino acid	Spectral shift given as A410 nm-A360 nm Aflatoxin B_{2a}	Aflatoxin G_{2a}
lysine	0·225	0·220
arginine	0·180	0·135
glycine	0·135	0·115
cysteine	0·120	0·100
methionine	0·103	0·061
serine	0·120	0·016
phenylalanine	0·050	0·090
valine	0·046	0·050
alanine	0·040	0·021
histidine	0·028	0·040
glutamic acid	0·027	0·062
aspartic acid	0·010	0·016
proline	0·000	0·000
threonine	0·000	0·000
leucine	0·000	0·000
isoleucine	0·000	0·000
tyrosine	0·000	0·000
tryptophan	0·000	0·000

results reported here. In the case of the deoxyribonuclease activating toxins, the absence of a Δ^2-bond in the terminal furane ring seemed to cause an increase in the activating effect at aflatoxin concentrations higher than 80 μM. This is illustrated by the fact that the effect of aflatoxin B_2 was greater than that of aflatoxin B_1 and that aflatoxin M_2 was a reasonably strong activator in comparison with aflatoxin M_1 which was found to be an inhibitor of deoxyribonuclease activity.

A hydroxyl group in position 4 of the terminal furane ring seemed to decrease the activating activity of the aflatoxins, e.g. aflatoxin M_2 is a weaker activator than aflatoxin B_2 and aflatoxin M_1 is an inhibitor in comparison with aflatoxin B_1 which is an activator.

The presence of another lactone ring in the molecular structure of the aflatoxins caused a large decrease in their activating activity, e.g. aflatoxin B_2 is an activator whereas aflatoxin G_2 is an inhibitor and aflatoxin G_1 had no definite effect on the enzyme activity in comparison with aflatoxin B_1 which is an activator.

An hydroxyl group in position 2 of the terminal furane ring and the simultaneous saturation of the Δ^2-bond of this ring caused the aflatoxins to be very strong inhibitors of deoxyribonuclease activity *viz.*, aflatoxins B_{2a} and G_{2a} which are strong inhibitors in comparison with aflatoxin B_2 (a strong activator) and aflatoxin G_2 (a much weaker inhibitor). It also seemed that these toxins (aflatoxins B_{2a} and G_{2a}) bind much more strongly to deoxyribonuclease than the weaker inhibitors like aflatoxins G_2 and M_1 due to the hydroxyl group in position 2 of the terminal furane ring. Preliminary studies revealed that this bond is much stronger than a hydrogen bond.

The most significant results obtained during these studies are that the activation of deoxyribonuclease was related to interaction with DNA and the inhibition to interaction with the enzyme. It is also interesting to note that two of the aflatoxins that showed the weakest binding to DNA *viz.*, aflatoxins B_{2a} and G_{2a}, were reported to be non-toxic. Clifford, Rees and Stevens[6] concluded that there seemed to be a correlation between the interaction of aflatoxins B_1, G_1 and G_2 with DNA, their inhibitory effect on RNA synthesis and most probably their toxicity. The possible role of DNA interactions in the carcinogenicity of the aflatoxins can be deduced from the fact that the carcinogenic dose and LD_{50} of aflatoxins B_1 and G_1 were found to be proportional.[5] T'so[11] stated that when carcinogens enter a living cell the compounds are more likely to interact with DNA than anything else. Strong carcinogens, such as the butter-yellow type of carcinogens increased the activity of deoxyribonuclease *in vivo*[12, 13]. It is known that the butter-yellow type of carcinogens can bind to DNA. It was reported by Melzer[7] that certain strong carcinogens had an activating effect on deoxyribonuclease whereas certain much weaker carcinogens had no effect and other weak carcinogens had an inhibitory effect on the activity of the enzymes *in vitro* most probably due to their interaction with the enzyme molecule. An inhibitory effect on deoxyribonuclease activity due to interaction with DNA was, however, found in the cases of certain antibiotics like actinomycin D, nogalamycin, etc. Their mode of interaction with DNA is, however, much different from that of the aflatoxins and they also bind much more strongly to DNA than the aflatoxins.

In view of our present knowledge on the general effects of the aflatoxins on the cell it is conceivable that they exert their influence at the information-transcription level which is most probably related to the extent of their interaction with DNA. Interaction with proteins in the cases of certain aflatoxins has also been reported. The inhibitory effect of certain aflatoxins on deoxyribonuclease activity seems to be related to their interaction with this enzyme.

In addition, the activating effect of aflatoxin B_1 could indirectly produce chromosomal mutation in somatic cells. It is widely believed (not universally, however) that the basic defect in cancer is a chromosomal mutation in somatic cells. This could allow deletion of genetic information (for instance, that of controlling growth) without affecting the capacity of cells to divide. Allison and Paton[14] introduced DNase (obtained from pancreas and liver lysosomes) into mammalian diploid cells and observed chromosome breakage. They also found that selective inhibitors of DNase, double-stranded polyribonucleotides with anti-parallel chains, inhibited the chromatid-breaking effect. Another point of interest is the uptake of polybenzenoid hydrocarbon carcinogens by lysosomes.[15] If aflatoxin B_1 could penetrate the lysosomes and alter their structure with the ensuing release of activated DNase, this enzyme could invade the nucleus, attack the chromosomal DNA and cause chromosomal aberration.

REFERENCES

1. NESBITT, B. F., O'KELLY, J., SARGEANT, K. and SHERIDAN, A. (1962). *Nature* (Lond.), **195**, 1062.
2. ASAO, T., BUCHI, G., ABDEL-KADAR, M. N., CHANG, S. B., WICK, E. L. and WOGAN, G. N. (1963). *J. Amer. Chem. Soc.*, **85**, 1706.
3. CHEUNG, K. K. and SIM, G. A. (1964). *Nature* (Lond.), **201**, 1185.
4. DICKENS, F. and JONES, H. E. H. (1963). *Brit. J. Cancer*, **17**, 100.
5. DICKENS, F. and JONES, H. E. H. (1963). *Brit. J. Cancer*, **19**, 392.
6. CLIFFORD, J. I., REES, K. R. and STEVENS, M. E. M. (1967). *Biochem. J.*, **103**, 258
7. MELZER, M. S. (1967). *Biochem. Biophys. Acta.*, **138**, 613.
8. KUMITZ, M. (1950). *J. Gen. Physiol.*, **33**, 349.
9. SCHABORT, J. C. (1969). *J. S.Afr. Chem. Inst.*, **22**, 80.
10. DIXON, M. and WEBB, E. C. (1964). In: *Enzymes*, 2nd Edition, p. 436. Longmans, Green and Co. Ltd.
11. T'SO, P. O. P. (1964). In: *The Nucleohistones*, Bonner, J. and T'so, P. O. P., p. 149. Holden-Day Inc., San Francisco.
12. SCHNEIDER, W. C., HOGEBOOM, E., SHELTON, E. and STRIEBACH, W. J. (1953). *Cancer Res.*, **13**, 285.
13. REID, E. (1962). *Cancer Res.*, **22**, 398.
14. ALLISON, A. C. and PATON, G. R. (1965). *Biochem. J.*, **115**, 23P.
15. ALLISON, A. C. and MALLUCCI, L. (1964). *Lancet*, **2**, 1371.

THE EFFECT OF AFLATOXIN B_1, AFLATOXIN B_2 AND STERIGMATOCYSTIN ON NUCLEAR DEOXYRIBONUCLEASES FROM RAT AND MOUSE LIVERS

by

M. J. Pitout and H. A. McGee

Division of Toxicology, National Institute for Nutritional Diseases
South African Medical Research Council

and

J. C. Schabort

Department of Biochemistry, Rand Afrikaans University, Johannesburg

There have been a number of *in vitro* and *in vivo* studies on the effects of various potent carcinogens such as the butter-yellow-type carcinogens, urethane, γ-butyrolactone and diepoxybutane on the activity of pancreatic DNase I. In these studies, considerable increases in activity were found as a result of treatment with the carcinogens.[1, 2] With weak carcinogens no activation of pancreatic DNase I was observed. The potent carcinogens have been found to be devoid of any effect on the activity of spleen DNase II. However, Lesca *et al.*[3] decisively demonstrated a sharp rise in pulmonary DNase II activity when rats were treated with the carcinogen benz-3,4-pyrene.

It is widely, although not universally, believed that the basic defect in cancer is a chromosomal mutation in somatic cells. Evidence suggesting a relationship between lysosomal damage and the occurrence of chromosomal aberrations has been presented and it was, therefore, suggested that the released lysosomal DNase might be able to penetrate the nucleus and attack the chromosomes.[4, 5]

Although the presence of an acid DNase (DNase II), in nuclei from various sources, has been shown by several workers,[6, 7] the enzyme has never been isolated and neither has any function been ascribed to it. Apart from DNase II, alkaline DNases (DNases I) which are associated with the non-histone fraction of chromatin have only recently been described.[8- 11]

In the light of the above-mentioned observations, it was decided to investigate the possible influence of the hepatocarcinogens aflatoxin B_1 and sterigmatocystin on the activities of the two DNases from rat liver. In addition, the effect of aflatoxin B_2 on the activities of the two nuclear DNases from rat liver was also studied. Aflatoxin B_2 has a similar molecular structure to aflatoxin B_1 but it has a relatively weak toxic and carcinogenic action in rats in comparison to aflatoxin B_1, the most potent carcinogen known.[12] For the sake of comparison, the effect of aflatoxin B_1 and sterigmatocystin on the activity of acid and alkaline DNases from mouse liver nuclei was also studied. It is known that the mouse is resistant to aflatoxin B_1 carcinogenesis.[13]

MATERIALS

Animals

Random bred male Wistar-derived rats with an average body weight of 200 ± 10 g and male albino mice (22 ± 2 g body weight) were used. The mice were obtained from Onderstepoort Veterinary Research Institute, Pretoria, which originally obtained them from the Wellcome Bureau of Scientific Research, London, England. Rats and mice were fed a balanced pellet diet, and were provided with tap water *ad libitum*. Rats and mice were divided into 3 groups, i.e. aflatoxin B_1 and sterigmatocystin treated rats and the control group, respectively. Each group consisted of 3 rats or 4 mice. Dimethylsulphoxide (DMSO) was used as solvent for the toxins and the control animals were dosed only with DMSO.

Chemicals

Thymus gland DNA was obtained from Sigma Chemical Co., Ohio, U.S.A. All other chemicals used were of analytical reagent grade. Aflatoxin B_1 and sterigmatocystin was isolated and purified according to Steyn[14] and Holzapfel *et al.*,[15] respectively. Aflatoxin B_2 was prepared from aflatoxin B_1 by means of hydrogenation according to Van Dorp *et al.*[16]

METHODS AND RESULTS

Extraction and isolation of nuclei from mouse and rat liver

All operations were done in the cold (2-5°C). The nuclei were prepared according to the method of Maggio *et al.*[17] with minor alterations.

The livers of each group were pooled and homogenised in 0·88 M sucrose-3 mM $MgCl_2$ solution in the ratio of 10-15 g liver/100 ml sucrose solution. The suspension was filtered through 4 layers of cheesecloth muslin gauze and centrifuged at 1,500 ×g for 10 min. The precipitate was suspended in 2·3 M sucrose-3 mM $MgCl_2$ solution and the supernatant was recentrifuged as described above. The process was repeated twice. To separate the nuclei from contaminants, the 2·3 M sucrose suspension (180 ml/10-15 g liver) was centrifuged at 44,000 ×g for 65 min. The purity of the nuclei was checked by electron and light microscopy.[18]

Extraction and some properties of the acid and alkaline DNases from rat liver nuclei

Since previous studies on the effect of carcinogens on DNases were done *in vitro* (see refs. 1, 2), an attempt was made to isolate and purify these enzymes from rat liver nuclei. The extraction and purification of the acid

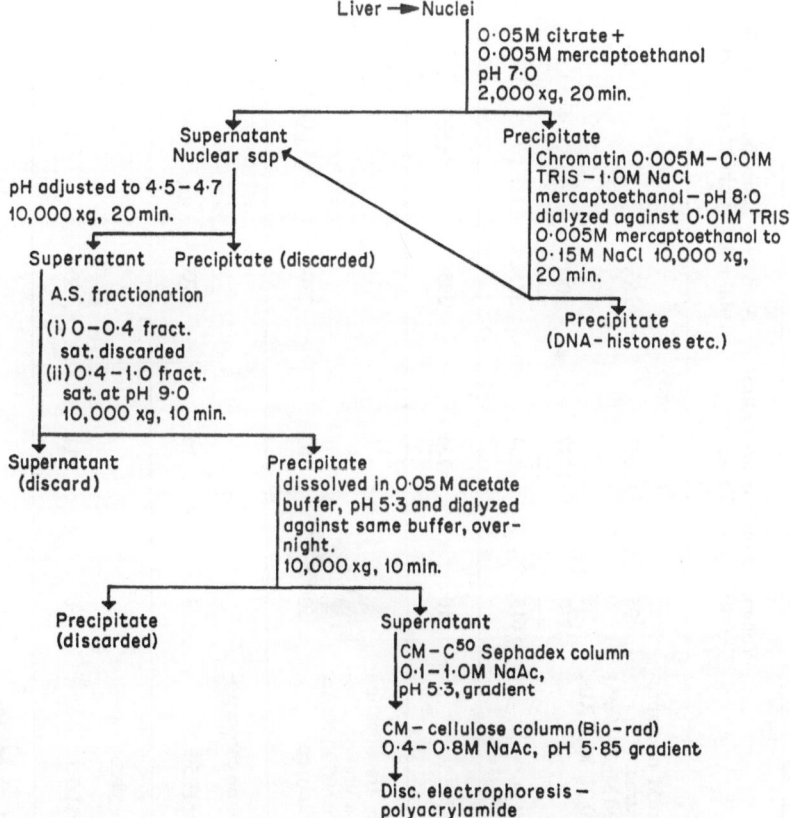

Fig. 1. Flow diagram of DNase II extraction from rat liver nuclei.

and alkaline DNases are illustrated in Figures 1 and 2 and Tables 1 and 2, respectively.

Of the two enzymes, the acid DNase is the more stable enzyme, and was, therefore, purified to a greater extent. Polyacrylamide disc electrophoresis indicated a very heterogeneous preparation (Fig. 3). The enzyme has an optimum activity at pH 4·7, prefers native, double-stranded DNA as substrate (see Figs. 4 and 5), and it is stable up to 55°C. The enzyme is inhibited by Mg^{2+} and SO_4^{2-} ions.

Table 1

Purification Table of DNase II

Step No.	Extractant	Volume (ml)	Protein concentration Total, mg	Activity Total units	Specific activity units/mg protein	Recovery (%)	Purification
2	(i) 0·05 M citrate-5 mM mercapto-ethanol, pH 7·0 extract	405	1077	2550			
	(ii) 0·15 M NaCl-5 mM MgCl$_2$-5mM mercaptoethanol-0·01 M TRIS, pH 8·0 extract	210	1087	1000	1·64	100	1·0
		615	2164	3552			
3	Acidification to pH 4·7	610	754	3230	4·3	93	2·6
4	Ammonium sulphate fractionation 0·4-1·0 fractional saturation. Precipitate dissolved in 0·05 M NaAc, pH 5·3 buffer and dialysed	50	160	2300	14·4	65	8·7
5	CM-C^{50} sephadex column chromatography. Gradient: 0·1-1·0 M NaAc, pH 5·3	78	16	1700	106	48	65
6	CM-cellulose column chromatography. Gradient: 0·1-1·0 M NaAc, pH 5·3	68	11	1600	145	44	88
7	CM-cellulose column chromatography. Gradient: 0·4-1·0 M NaAc, pH 5·85	50·5	7·0	1290	185	37	115

For the *in vitro* experiments, however, crude nuclear DNases from rat and mouse livers were prepared by the following procedure: To lyse the nuclei, they were suspended in 5 ml of 0·05 M citrate-5 mM mercaptoethanol buffer, pH 7·0. Centrifugation at 2,000 ×g for 20 min. yielded a precipitate (chromatin) and the supernatant (nuclear sap). The chromatin

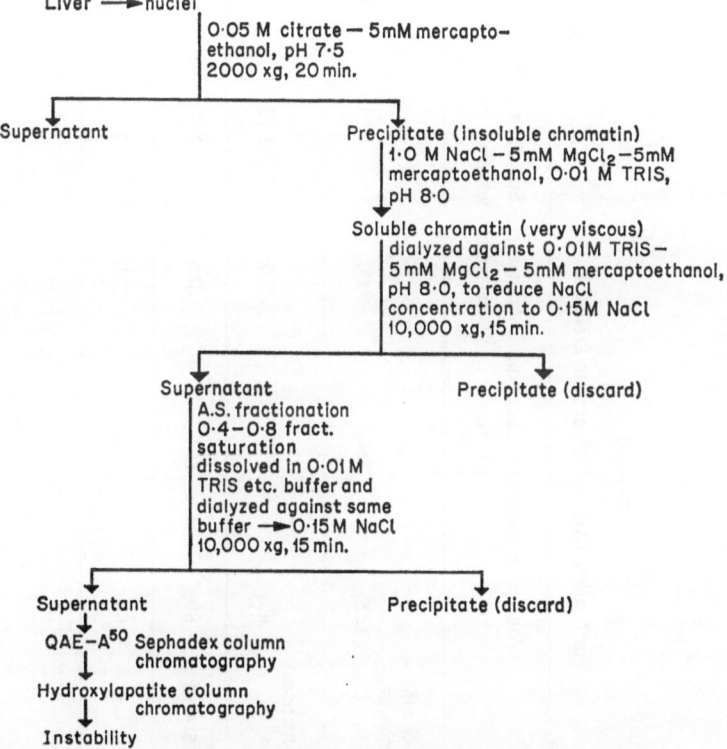

FIG. 2. Flow diagram of DNase I extraction from rat liver nuclei.

acidic proteins were obtained by the procedure of Wang.[19] The pH of the nuclear sap was carefully adjusted to 4·7 by the addition of acetic acid, and the resultant milky suspension was clarified by centrifugation at 10,000 ×g for 20 min. to give a clear, colourless supernatant which contained the acid DNase.

The activities of acid and alkaline DNases were estimated according to Hodes *et al.*[20] and O'Connor,[9] respectively. For both enzymes, one unit of enzyme is that amount of enzyme which produces one ΔA^{260} unit/hr. Specific activity is expressed as units/mg protein.

Protein was determined according to the method of Lowry *et al.*[21]

Table 2

Purification Table of Chromatin DNase I

Step No.	Extractant	Volume (ml)	Protein concentration Total, mg	Activity Total units	Specific activity units/mg protein	Recovery (%)	Purification
2	0·15 M NaCl–0·01 M TRIS–5 mM MgCl₂–5 mM mercaptoethanol, pH 8·0	135	788	1000	1·29	100	1·00
3	Ammonium sulphate fractionation 0·2–0·8 fractional saturation	68	590	802	1·33	80	1·03
4	QAE-A⁵⁰ sephadex chromatography	88	164	440	2·7	44	2·1
5	Hydroxylapatite	60	150	280	1·8	28	1·4

A comparison of the effects of aflatoxin B_1 and sterigmatocystin on the activities of acid and alkaline DNases from rat liver

In vitro investigations could not be done with sterigmatocystin due to its very poor solubility. No definite activating or inhibitory effect of aflatoxin B_1 on the activities of the two DNases under *in vitro* conditions was observed.

Since we could not demonstrate any effect of the toxin with *in vitro*

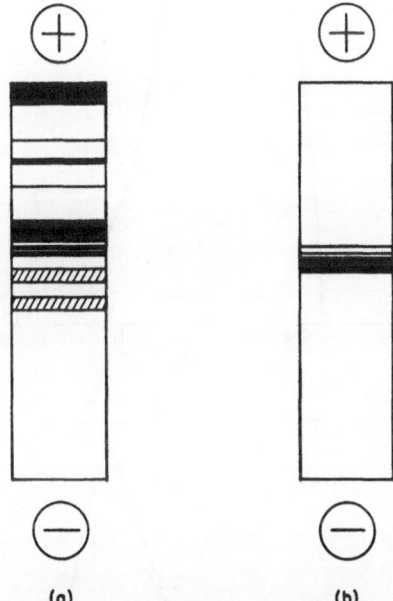

(a)   (b)

FIG. 3. Polyacrylamide disc electrophoresis
(15% gel) of acid DNase preparation (a)
and a standard solution of beef heart cytochrome c (b).

experiments, *in vivo* studies were attempted, as it is possible that aflatoxin B_1 could be converted *in vivo* to the active toxin. In addition, the possible effect of sterigmatocystin on these enzymes could only be investigated *in vivo*.

For *in vivo* investigations, Wistar rats were given a daily *per os* dose over a 30-day period. The daily dose was equivalent to $\frac{1}{5}$ LD_{50} of aflatoxin B_1 and sterigmatocystin, where the LD_{50} values of aflatoxin and sterigmato-cystin were taken as 7 mg/kg and 160 mg/kg body weight, respectively.[13, 22] Rats were killed by decapitation at predetermined time intervals, the livers excised, nuclei isolated, the two enzymes extracted and their activities assayed as described above. The results are illustrated in Figure 6 and Table 3. From these data it seems that the activity of DNase II, when rats

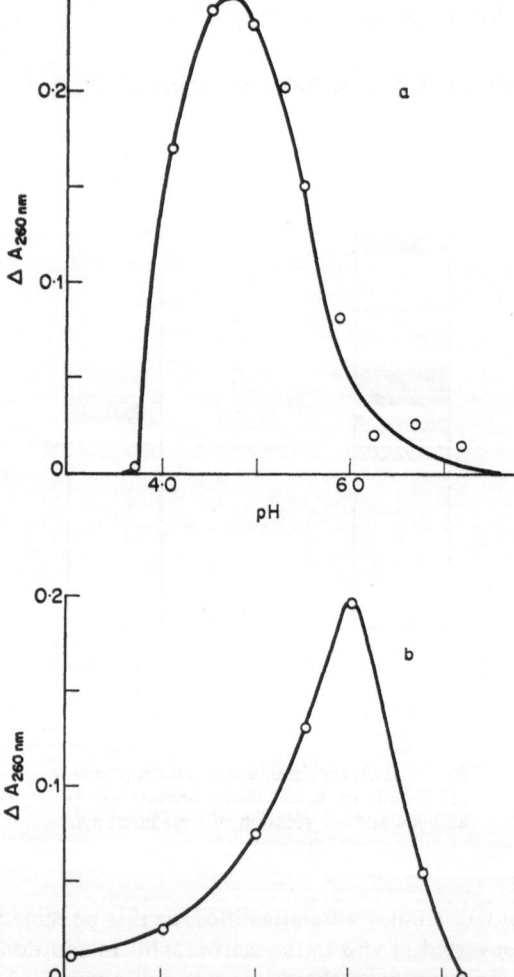

FIG. 4. pH optimum curves of acid DNase (curve *a*) and alkaline DNase (curve *b*) from rat liver nuclei.

were exposed to aflatoxin B_1, increased considerably. No significant effect of sterigmatocystin on the activities of the two nuclear enzymes was observed.

The effect of aflatoxin B_2 on the activities of the two nuclear DNases

The similarity in chemical structure between aflatoxins B_1 and B_2 prompted an *in vivo* study of the effect of aflatoxin B_2 on the activities of the acid and alkaline DNases. Male Wistar rats were dosed with aflatoxins B_1 and B_2 at 1·75 mg/kg daily over a period of 18 days. Rats were killed at predetermined time intervals, nuclei isolation from the livers, the two enzymes extracted and their activities assayed as described above.

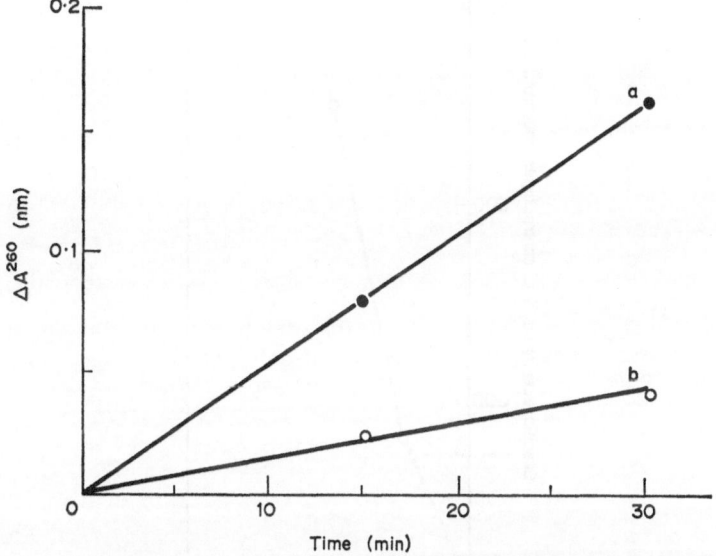

FIG. 5. Hydrolysis of native DNA (curve *a*) and heat-denatured DNA (curve *b*) by rat liver nuclear acid DNase. Alkaline DNase has no preference for native or heat-denatured DNA.

Whereas aflatoxin B_1 caused a substantial elevation in the activity of DNase II, aflatoxin B_2 had no effect on the activities of the two enzymes (see Fig. 7). This difference could be ascribed to the difference in chemical structures of the toxins as the Δ^2-bond of the terminal furane ring of aflatoxin B_2 is saturated (see Fig. 8).

The effect of aflatoxin B_1 and sterigmatocystin on the activities of mouse liver nuclear DNases

Mice were dosed *per os* with toxin every second day for a period of 15 days. Aflatoxin was administered at a rate of 2·5 mg/kg body weight and sterigmatocystin at a rate of 10 mg/kg. Nuclei were prepared, the two enzymes extracted and their activities assayed as described above. In

Figure 9 it can be seen that both aflatoxin B_1 and sterigmatocystin had no effect on the activity of the alkaline and acid DNases from mouse liver

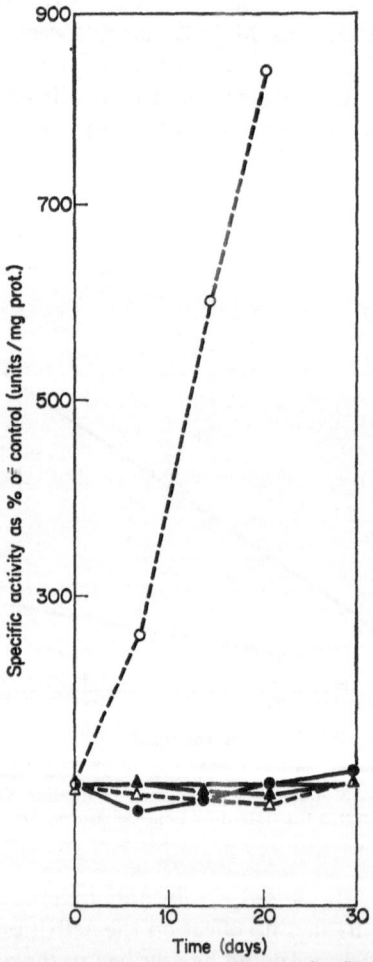

FIG. 6. The *in vivo* effects of aflatoxin B_1 and sterigmatocystin at dosing rates of $\frac{1}{8}$ LD_{50} on the activities of Wistar rat liver nuclear DNases I and II over a period of 30 days. DNase I: ●— aflatoxin B_1, ▲— aflatoxin B_2. DNase II: ○—aflatoxin B_1, △—sterigmatocystin.

nuclei. Since the mouse is resistant to aflatoxin B_1 carcinogenesis,[13] the difference in action of this toxin in the mouse could be attributed to a possible conversion of aflatoxin B_1 to a non-carcinogenic substance(s).

Table 3

The Effects of Aflatoxin B$_1$ and Sterigmatocystin on Acid DNase from Rat Liver Nuclear Sap at $\frac{1}{5}$ LD$_{50}$ dosing over a 30-day period

Treatment	Day	Liver weight (g)	Total nuclear sap protein (mg)	Total units (U)	Spec. activity (U/mg prot.)	Total protein mg/g liver	U/g liver
A*	0	17·2	2·34	13·0	5·6	0·14 (1·0)†	0·76
C*		18·0	2·48	13·0	5·2	0·14 (1·0)	0·72
S*		18·0	2·70	13·6	5·1	0·15 (1·1)	0·76
A	7	13·2	1·60	19·2	12·0	0·12 (0·8)	1·46
C		17·4	2·74	13·2	4·8	0·16 (1·0)	0·76
S		15·4	2·80	13·5	4·8	0·18 (1·1)	0·90
A	14	10·3	1·19	26·4	21·0	0·12 (0·6)	2·64
C		24·2	4·52	15·8	3·5	0·19 (1·0)	0·65
S		21·2	4·24	13·7	3·2	0·20 (1·0)	0·65
A	21	4·8	0·81	18·4	22·7	0·17 (0·7)	3·83
C		20·0	5·14	14·4	3·75	0·26 (1·0)	0·72
S		18·3	4·7	10·9	2·11	0·26 (1·0)	0·60
A	30	—	—	—	—	—	—
C		21·7	4·4	12·4	2·8	0·21	0·57
S		18·0	4·6	13·4	2·9	0·25	0·75

* A, C and S represent aflatoxin B$_1$, control and sterigmatocystin, respectively.
† The values in parentheses indicate the ratio obtained by dividing by C.

DISCUSSION

Relationship between aflatoxin B_1 and the increased DNase II activity

The presence of DNase II in the nucleus raises many issues. In the normal cell the activity of this enzyme must be under rigorous control in order to preserve the integrity of the genetic message. Abnormal circumstances

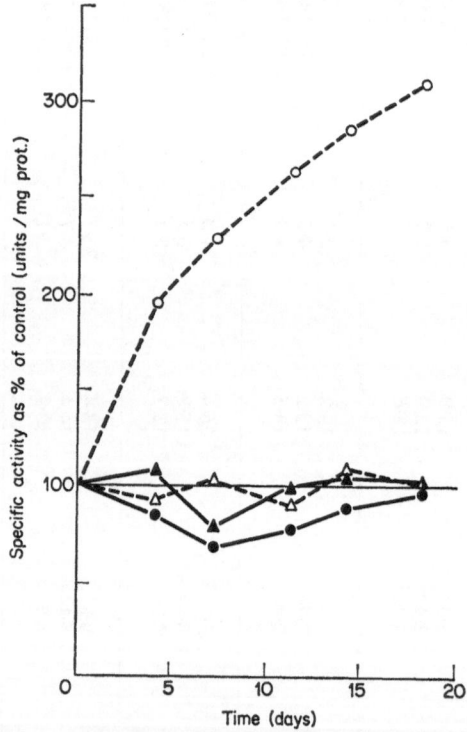

FIG. 7. The *in vivo* effects of aflatoxins B_1 and B_2 on the activities of Wistar rat liver nuclear DNases I and II over a period of 18 days. DNase I: ●—aflatoxin B_1, ▲—aflatoxin B_2. DNase II: ○—aflatoxin B_1, △—aflatoxin B_2.

causing release of activity, might induce anomalies in the genetic expression mechanism.

It is known that mouse liver contains a protein which is capable of inhibiting acid DNase, whether extracted from the same organ or obtained from other sources.[23] At present, our knowledge of the biological functions of this protein is negligible. The possibility exists that aflatoxin B_1, or a converted derivative, could interact in some way with the natural inhibitor to cause an increase in DNase II activity. It is known that aflatoxin B_1

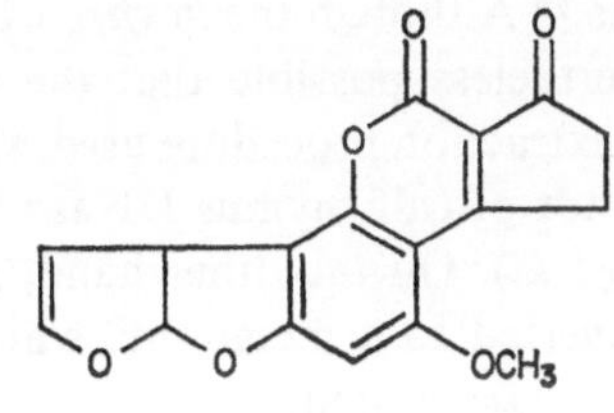

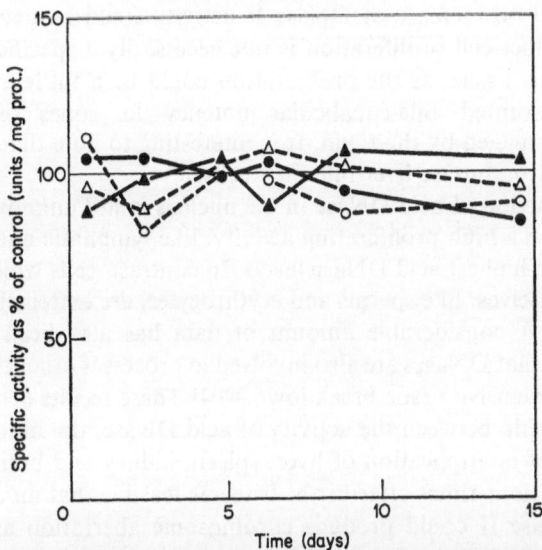

FIG. 8. Chemical formulae of aflatoxins B_1 and B_2 and sterigmatocystin. Aflatoxins B_1 and B_2 and sterigmatocystin are represented by I,
II and III, respectively.

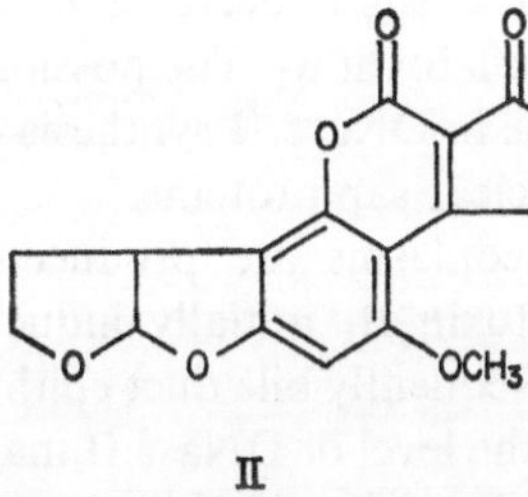

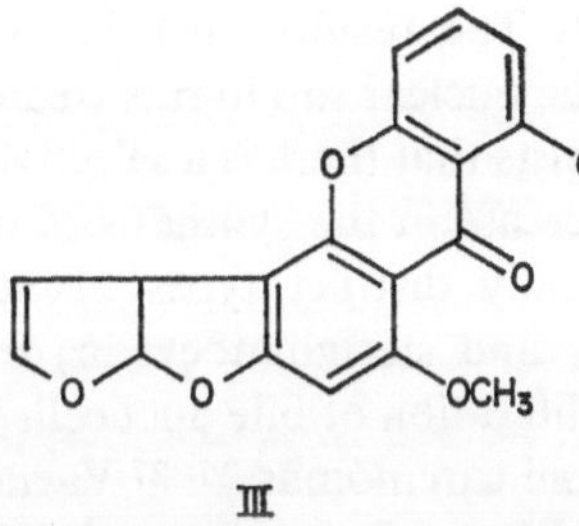

FIG. 9. The *in vivo* effects of aflatoxin B_1 and sterigmatocystin on the activities of mouse liver nuclear DNases
I and II over a period of 15 days. Aflatoxin B_1 was dosed
at a rate of 2·5 mg/kg body weight and sterigmatocystin at a
rate of 10 mg/kg. Dosings were done every second day.
DNase I: ●—aflatoxin B_1, ▲—sterigmatocystin.
DNase II: ○—aflatoxin B_1, △—sterigmatocystin.

interacts with certain proteins.[24] Although the *in vitro* experiments did not confirm this idea, it is nevertheless possible that the inhibitor may be unstable and not survive the extraction procedure used, since it has already been reported that the inhibitor of calf thymus DNase I is very unstable, even at low temperatures ($\pm 5°C$). On the other hand, it is also possible that aflatoxin B_1 is first converted to a metabolite which interferes with the normal DNase II-inhibitor association.

It has been shown that aflatoxin B_1 inhibits only the synthesis of a few specific proteins but total liver protein synthesis appeared to be largely unaffected.[25] The results in Table 1 indicate a slight decrease in total protein of the nuclear sap in rats treated with aflatoxin B_1. The possibility, therefore, exists that there is a selective increase in DNase II synthesis or a selective decrease in the synthesis of other nuclear sap proteins.

Histologically distinct types of hepatic neoplasms are produced by aflatoxin B_1 and sterigmatocystin; only aflatoxin B_1 initially induces a marked proliferation of bile duct cells and subsequently bile duct epithelial adenomas and carcinomas.[26, 27] Variation in the level of DNase II may be associated with the alterations in the amount of proliferating bile duct cells present in the tissue. In contrast, sterigmatocystin does not induce a comparable degree of bile duct cell proliferation or ultimate biliary malignancy and no increase of DNase II activity could be detected. An increased bile duct cell proliferation is not necessarily a specific effect of the toxin on this tissue, as the proliferation could be a futile attempt to re-establish disrupted bile-canalicular potency in zones of hepatic parenchymal damaged by the toxin. It is interesting to note that aflatoxin B_1 has no effect on mouse liver bile duct cells.[28]

The exact function of acid DNase in the nucleus is still unknown. However, tissues with a high proliferating activity, like lymphatic and tumoral tissues, have the highest acid DNase levels. In contrast, cells which do not reproduce themselves, like sperms and erythrocytes, are extremely poor in acid DNase.[29] A considerable amount of data has also been reported which indicates that DNases are also involved in processes other than those which lead to extensive tissue breakdown.[30, 31] These results demonstrate a close relationship between the activity of acid DNase, the mitotic index and the speed of multiplication of liver, spleen, kidney and brain cells of rats killed at various times after birth. It seems feasible that an abnormal activity of DNase II could produce chromosome aberration and hence profound and irreversible changes of the genetic expression mechanism which in turn could lead to the production of neoplastic cells.

It is generally accepted that the mouse is resistant to aflatoxin B_1 carcinogenesis. Therefore, the lack of effect of aflatoxin B_1 on the activities of both nuclear DNases from mouse liver, could be attributed to the conversion of aflatoxin B_1 to noncarcinogens,[32] or to the inability of aflatoxin B_1 to react with the inhibitory protein of DNase II. In either case, the lack of effect tends to confirm that nuclear acid DNases play some role, however minor, in the mechanism by which aflatoxin B_1 produces cancer.

REFERENCES

1. MELZER, M. S. (1967). *Biochim. Biophys. Acta.*, **138**, 613.
2. MELZER, M. S. (1968). *Can. J. Biochem.*, **47**, 987.
3. LESCA, P., TOUTAIN, D. and TRUHAUT, R. (1969). *C.R. Acad. Sci. Paris, Série D*, **t.268**, 1238.
4. ALLISON, A. C. and PATON, G. R. (1965). *Nature* (Lond.), **207**, 1170.
5. ALLISON, A. C. and PATON, G. R. (1969). *Biochem. J.*, **115**, 31P.
6. SWINGLE, K. F. and COLE, L. J. (1964). *J. Histochem. and Cytochem.*, **12**, 442.
7. LESCA, P. (1968). *Nature* (Lond.), **220**, 76.
8. SWINGLE, A. C., COLE, L. J. and BAILEY, J. S. (1967). *Biochim. Biophys. Acta*, **149**, 467.
9. O'CONNOR, P. J. (1969). *Biochem. Biophys. Res. Comm.*, **35**, 805.
10. HAWK, R. and WANG, T. Y. (1970). *Eur. J. Biochem.*, **13**, 455.
11. O'CONNOR, P. J. and AYAD, S. R. (1970). *Biochim. Biophys. Acta.*, **217**, 56.
12. LEGATOR, M. S. (1969). In: *Aflatoxin, Scientific Background, Control and Implications* (Ed.: Goldblatt, L. A.). Academic Press, N.Y.
13. BUTLER, W. H. (1969). In: *Aflatoxin, Scientific Background, Control and Implications* (Ed.: Goldblatt, L. A.). Academic Press, N.Y.
14. STEYN, M. (1970). *J. Ass. Off. Anal. Chem.*, **53**, 619.
15. HOLZAPFEL, C. W., PURCHASE, I. F. H., STEYN, P. S. and GOUWS, L. (1966). *S.A. med. J.*, **40**, 1100.
16. VAN DORP, D. A., VAN DER ZIJDEN, A. S. M., BEERTHUIS, R. K., SPARREBOOM, S., ORD, W. O., DE IONGH, H. and KEUNING, R. (1963). *Rec. Trav. Chim.*, **82**, 587.
17. MAGGIO, R., SIEKEVITZ, P. and PALADE, G. E. (1963). *J. Cell. Biol.*, **18**, 267.
18. BRESNICK, E. and SCHWARTZ, A. (1968). In: *Functional Dynamics of the Cell*. Academic Press, New York.
19. WANG, T. Y. (1967). *J. Biol. Chem.*, **242**, 1220.
20. HODES, M. E., YIP, L. C. and SANTOS, F. R. (1967). *Enzymologia*, **32**, 241.
21. LOWRY, O. H., ROSEBROUGH, N. J., FARR, A. L. and RANDALL, R. J. (1951). *J. Biol. Chem.*, **193**, 265.

22. PURCHASE, I. F. H. and VAN DER WATT, J. J. (1969). *Fd. Cosmet. Toxicol.*, **7**, 135.
23. LESCA, P. and PAOLETTI, C. (1969). *Proc. Natl. Acad. Sci. Wash.*, **64**, 913.
24. BLACK, H. S. and JIRGENSONS, B. (1967). *Plant Physiol.*, **42**, 731.
25. WOGAN, G. N. (1968). *Cancer Res.*, **28**, 2282.
26. PURCHASE, I. F. H. and VAN DER WATT, J. J. (1970). *Fd. Cosmet. Toxicol.*, **8**, 289.
27. BUTLER, W. H. and BARNES, J. M. (1968). *Fd. Cosmet. Toxicol.*, **6**, 135.
28. FERREIRA, M. N. (1968). *Revista de Cliniear Medica*, **1**, 111. Universidade de Lourenço Marques.
29. CORDONNIER, C. and BERNARDI, G. (1968). *Can. J. Biochem.*, **46**, 989.
30. LEHMAN, I. R. (1970). *Ann. Rev. Biochem.*, **36**, 645.
31. HOWARD-FLANDERS, P. (1968). *Ann. Rev. Biochem.*, **37**, 175.
32. STEYN, M., PITOUT, M. J. and PURCHASE, I. F. H. *Brit. J. Cancer.* In press.

AFLATOXIN METABOLISM

by

I. F. H. Purchase

Director, National Institute for Nutritional Diseases
South African Medical Research Council

and

M. Steyn

Division of Toxicology, National Institute for Nutritional Diseases

Aflatoxin B_1, a carcinogenic metabolite of the fungus *Aspergillus flavus*, is acutely toxic to a number of species, including rats. Male rats (LD_{50} 7·2 mg/kg) are more susceptible to the acute oral effects of aflatoxin than are females (LD_{50} 17·9 mg/kg).[1] Aflatoxin B_1 is metabolised to aflatoxin M_1 which is present in the blood and urine of dosed rats,[2] and in the milk of lactating rats, sheep and cows ingesting aflatoxin.[3, 4]

Aflatoxin M_1 is the hydroxylated derivative of aflatoxin B_1[5] and has the same acute toxicity as aflatoxin B_1 in ducklings.[6] The presence of aflatoxin M_1 in the blood of dosed animals indicates that this compound is a metabolic product of aflatoxin B_1.

It has been shown that female rats produce a larger amount of aflatoxin M_1 when given a dose of 10 mg aflatoxin B_1 per kg body weight, indicating that the female's greater resistance is due to a more rapid metabolism of aflatoxin B_1 than is the case in the male.[7] This report describes further investigations into the effects of hormones on metabolism in castrated rats.

METHODS

Comparison of aflatoxin metabolism in male and female rats

Adult male (mean weight 359 g) and adult female (mean weight 220 g) rats (of our own Wistar-derived strain) were distributed into 7 groups of 3 males and 3 females. Each rat was housed in a separate cage and received an oral dose of aflatoxin B_1 (10 mg/kg) dissolved in DMSO (10 mg/ml). Groups of rats were killed with ether at $\frac{1}{2}$, 1, 2, 4, 6 and 8 hours after dosing and their livers, kidneys, stomachs and intestines removed and placed in separate weighed containers. The organs were stored at $-17°C$ until assayed for aflatoxin B_1 and M_1 using the technique described by Purchase and Steyn.[7]

Comparison of aflatoxin metabolism in castrated rats given various hormones

Male and female rats were castrated at 4 weeks of age (± 60 g) and kept for 6 weeks by which time their average weights were: $\male$:223 g and $\female$: 211 g. Rats from each sex were distributed into 5 groups which received the following treatments.

Group 1 received 0·1 ml each of sunflower-seed oil daily for 5 days. Groups 2, 3, 4 and 5 received individual doses of progesterone (500 μg), 17β–oestradiol (10 μg), testosterone acetate (50 μg) and oestrone (50 μg), respectively, dissolved in 0·1 ml sunflower-seed oil daily for 5 days. The progesterone was received as a solution of 10 mg/ml in ethyloleate and this was diluted to 5 mg/ml with sunflower-seed oil.

On day 6 all rats received a dose of aflatoxin B_1 (10 mg/kg) in DMSO (10 mg/ml) and 3 males and 3 females from each group were killed with ether $\frac{1}{2}$, 1, 2 and 4 hours after dosing. The stomachs and intestines, livers and kidneys were removed and placed in separate weighed containers which were treated as described above.

Aflatoxin B_1. The aflatoxin used in this experiment was chromatographically pure and contained 98 % of aflatoxin B_1 on assay by U.V. absorption spectrophotometry.

RESULTS

Comparison of aflatoxin metabolism in male and female rats

The results of this study have been published previously.[7] On inspection there appeared to be no significant difference between the amount of aflatoxin remaining in the stomachs of the male and female rats. It was therefore concluded that there was no difference in the absorption of aflatoxin. Subsequent statistical analysis suggests that the females had more aflatoxin in the stomachs than males and this difference was significant at the 5 % level (Table 1).

The amount of aflatoxin M_1 present in liver, kidney and intestine was significantly greater in females than in males (Table 1).

Comparison of aflatoxin metabolism in castrated rats

The amount of aflatoxin B_1 in the stomachs of the castrated males and females was not significantly different even at the 10 % level of significance (Table 1). In the livers, kidneys and intestines, there was very little difference between the two groups and what difference there was (in the livers) was much less significant, compared with the intact rats.

Comparison of aflatoxin metabolism in castrated rats given various hormones

The figures given in Table 2 indicate that none of the hormone treatments produced consistent alterations in the aflatoxin M_1 levels in all

Table 1

Results obtained from Analysis of Variance of Aflatoxin Values in
Male and Female Rats

	Organ	Hypothesis No difference between sexes
Normal rats	Liver	+ +
	Kidney	+ +
	Intestine (M_1)	+ +
	Stomach (B_1)	+
Castrated rats	Liver	+
	Kidney	−
	Intestine (M_1)	−
	Stomach (B_1)	−

+ Hypothesis rejected at 5 % level of significance
+ + Hypothesis rejected at 1 % level of significance
− Hypothesis cannot be rejected

organs. Some of the differences concerning a particular organ were significant (at the 5 % level) but as these occurred in such diverse treatment
groups and in different organs their importance is open to question.

DISCUSSION

Female Wistar rats are more resistant to the acute toxic effects of aflatoxin than are males. There are many possible reasons for this difference.

Entire female rats absorbed slightly less aflatoxin from their stomachs
than did entire males as judged by the amount of aflatoxin B_1 left in the
stomach after a single dose. Whether this difference was great enough to
account for the difference in susceptibility is open to question. There is a
2·5-fold difference in acute toxicity but only a slight difference in the rate
of absorption. A more likely reason, as deduced from these experiments, is
that the female is capable of metabolising aflatoxin B_1 at a faster rate than
the male. The higher aflatoxin M_1 values in female organs indicates that
metabolism of aflatoxin is indeed greater in females.

The question as to why the female metabolises aflatoxin faster remains.
The fact that castration removes the difference in aflatoxin M levels
indicates that sex hormones play a part in influencing the metabolism of
aflatoxin. Confirmation that this change in aflatoxin metabolism is
accompanied by a change in acute toxicity is not yet available.

Table 2

The results of aflatoxin assays in organs from castrated rats treated with sunflower-seed oil (controls) and various hormones. The figures are the average values obtained from individual analyses of organs from 3 rats killed at the same time after a dose of aflatoxin B_1 (10 mg/kg). The columns marked * indicate a significant difference (5%) from the controls of the same sex.

Treatment	Time hours	Aflatoxin M μg/g Liver		Aflatoxin M μg/g Kidney		Aflatoxin M μg Intestine		Aflatoxin B_1 % of dose Stomach	
		♂	♀	♂	♀	♂	♀	♂	♀
Control	½	4·00	3·50	10·10	2·80	46·20	16·4	14·7	10·5
	1	5·90	2·70	7·90	1·80	79·80	61·9	13·7	15·9
	2	0·83	1·30	2·80	1·70	65·60	136·7	11·8	13·4
	4	0·27	0·35	0	1·00	123·10	101·7	11·9	13·2
Progesterone	½	2·90	5·50	3·60	6·30*	35·40	56·2	14·9	14·6
	1	5·00	4·30	5·40	12·90	196·00	52·6	17·4	15·4
	2	0·66	2·80	0·25	2·10	61·60	147·6	12·8	14·3
	4	0·14	0·36	0·20	0·40	100·50	87·0	12·7	13·4
17β–oestradiol	½	3·10	5·60	3·00	2·90	45·60	90·0	16·6	16·2
	1	3·30	5·50	6·50	10·60	53·70	79·3	13·8	13·8
	2	1·20	3·00	0·50	1·10	74·80	98·5	14·7	14·8
	4	0·60	0·46	0·80	0·42	140·30	118·0	10·8	12·1
Testosterone	½	3·80	6·00*	7·30	6·90	27·60	60·9	8·4	13·3
	1	3·50	6·00	2·60	8·30	59·30	71·7	13·8	11·1
	2	0·94	2·80	3·00	1·20	57·50	84·0	13·9	15·9
	4	0·27	0·24	0·50	0·10	86·70	59·0	9·8	10·2
Oestrone	½	3·30	5·30	3·30	5·90	47·70*	80·0	16·8	16·7
	1	3·10	3·90	1·10	5·40	53·70	50·3	12·8	16·1
	2	1·60	1·40	1·90	2·50	42·70	127·0	14·5	13·4
	4	0·26	0·14	0·10	0·06	67·00	89·3	12·8	12·9

The difference between male and female metabolism could be influenced by hormones due to a specific interaction with a particular hormone. These figures indicate that no single hormone influenced aflatoxin M levels consistently in either castrated male or female rats. The inference that can be drawn is that female hormones (progesterone, oestrogens) did not specifically inhibit metabolism of aflatoxin. The effect must, therefore be non-specific. The female liver has to metabolise a greater quantity of steroid hormones than the male liver and the drug-metabolising enzymes will, therefore, be more active in the females. Aflatoxin is structurally similar to steroids and indications are that the microsomal 'drug metabolising enzymes' are responsible for aflatoxin metabolism. The greater metabolism in females can be attributed to the fact that the microsomal enzymes, which have to handle a larger load of steroids, are more active and can metabolise the aflatoxin more quickly once it is absorbed from the stomach.

ACKNOWLEDGEMENTS

We wish to thank Dr N. Laubscher and Mr T. L. Gilfillan for their help with the statistical analyses.

REFERENCES

1. BUTLER, W. H. (1964). *Brit. J. Cancer*, **18**, 756.
2. BUTLER, W. H. and CLIFFORD, J. I. (1965). *Nature* (Lond.), **206**, 1045.
3. DE IONGH, H., VLES, R. O. and VAN PELT, J. G. (1964). *Nature* (Lond.), **202**, 466.
4. NABNEY, J., BURBAGE, M. B., ALLCROFT, R. and LEWIS, G. (1967). *Fd. Cosmet. Toxic.*, **5**, 11.
5. HOLZAPFEL, C. W., STEYN, P. S. and PURCHASE, I. F. H. (1966). *Tetrahedron Letters*, **25**, 2799.
6. PURCHASE, I. F. H. (1967). *Fd. Cosmet. Toxicol.*, **5**, 339.
7. PURCHASE, I. F. H. and STEYN, M. (1969). *Brit. J. Cancer*, **23**, 800.

BIOCHEMICAL STUDIES ON OCHRATOXIN A

by

M. J. Pitout

Division of Toxicology, National Institute for Nutritional Diseases
South African Medical Research Council

Ochratoxin A is one of three chemically related metabolites isolated from *Aspergillus ochraceus* Wilh.[1] It has been structurally characterised as 7-carboxyl-5-chloro-8-hydroxy-3,4-dihidro-methylisocoumarin linked over its 7-carboxyl group to L-β-phenylalanine.[2] The LD_{50} in rats dosed *per os* is 20 mg/kg and the toxin causes enteritis, renal necrosis and an increase in the quantity of glycogen in rat liver.[3] The route and time course of the

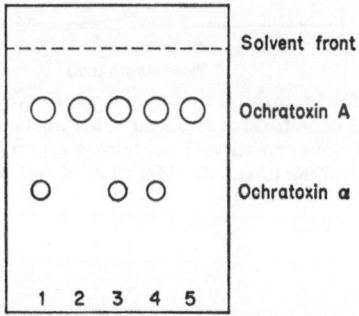

FIG. 1. A chromatogram of ochratoxin A before and after hydrolysis with carboxypeptidase A, α-chymotrypsin and trypsin. A standard mixture of ochratoxins A and α is illustrated by 1, while 2, 3, 4 and 5 represent ochratoxin A before hydrolysis and after reaction with carboxypeptidase, chymotrypsin and trypsin, respectively. Hydrolysis was performed at 25° for 5 min and the concentrations of ochratoxin A, carboxypeptidase, chymotrypsin and trypsin were 1.5×10^{-4} M, 50 μg/ml, 300 μg/ml and 300 μg/ml, respectively (from ref. 6).

metabolism of ochratoxin A was investigated by Nel and Purchase[4] in view of the fact that the increase in glycogen only became evident 4 to 5 days after dosing. They concluded that ochratoxin A is hydrolysed *in vivo* to the isocoumarin moiety (ochratoxin α) most probably by proteolytic enzymes.

In the light of the above-mentioned observations, it was decided to investigate:

(i) the possible hydrolysis of ochratoxin A by proteolytic enzymes, and
(ii) the effect of ochratoxin A on glycogen storage in the rat liver.

Both these studies were conducted under *in vitro* conditions.

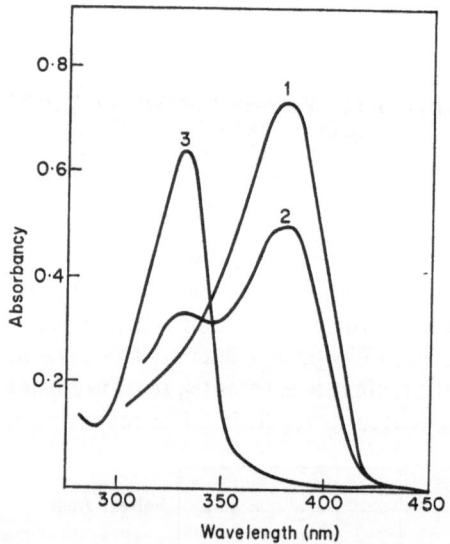

Fig. 2. The hydrolysis of ochratoxin A by proteinases. Curve 1 represents ochratoxin A $(0.5 \times 10^{-4}$ M), curve 2 ochratoxin A $(1.0 \times 10^{-4}$ M) treated with 50 μg/ml carboxy-peptidase A at 25° for 30 min and curve 3 ochratoxin α $(1.0 \times 10^{-4}$ M). Ochratoxin α was prepared according to van der Merwe *et al.* (ref. 2) (from ref. 6).

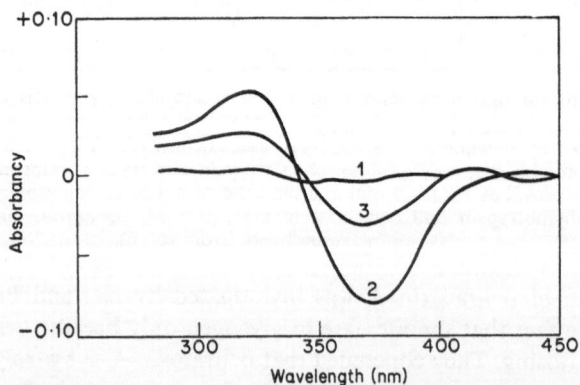

Fig. 3. The difference spectra of hydrolysed and non-hydrolysed ochratoxin A. Curve 1 represents the baseline and curves 2 and 3 represent ochratoxin A treated with carboxy-peptidase and chymotrypsin, respectively. The concentration of ochratoxin A is 1.0×10^{-4} M while the concentration of carboxypeptidase A is 50 μg/ml and that of α-chymotrypsin 300 μg/ml (from ref. 6).

Hydrolysis of ochratoxin A by proteolytic enzymes

Carboxypeptidase A (E.C. 3.4.2.1.) from the pancrease requires a free carboxyl group and the specificity, including stereochemical specificity, of the enzymes is determined primarily by the amino acid bearing the free carboxyl group.[5] Since carboxypeptidase A is most active on substances containing a terminal aromatic amino acid, it was reasoned that ochratoxin A would be hydrolysed by this enzyme. In addition, the activities of two other proteinases, α-chymotrypsin (E.C., 3.4.4.5) and trypsin (E.C. 3.4.4.4) on ochratoxin A were investigated.

By means of thin layer chromatography on silica gel and spectrophotometrical methods such as difference and absorption spectra, it was found that ochratoxin A is hydrolysed by carboxypeptidase A and α-chymotrypsin[6] (see Figs. 1, 2 and 3). The apparent K_m values, determined by the usual methods, for the hydrolyses of ochratoxin A by carboxypeptidase[4] and α-chymotrypsin at 25°C are 1.5×10^{-4} M and 1×10^{-3} M, respectively. These results indicate that ochratoxin A has a much greater affinity for carboxypeptidase A than for α-chymotrypsin. Trypsin does not hydrolyse ochratoxin A since the specificity of this enzyme is dependent on the hydrolysis of peptide bonds of which an L-arginine or L-lysine residue contributes the carbonyl group. Replacement of either of these amino acids prevents enzymic action.[7] Although the specificity of pepsin favours the hydrolysis of peptide linkages in which an aromatic amino acid provides the amino group for the sensitive peptide linkage, this enzyme was not studied since at pH values lower than 4, ochratoxin A is very poorly soluble.

Using liver perfusion experiments, Purchase[8] observed that ochratoxin A is hydrolysed in the liver to ochratoxin α which is excreted in the bile. This could indicate that ochratoxin A, being a toxic substance, is probably absorbed by means of pinocytosis of the lysosomes in the liver and then hydrolysed by the proteolytic enzymes. Lysosomes contain *inter alia* cathepsin C which acts preferentially on peptide linkages in which an L-phenylalanine or L-tyrosine provides the amino group for the peptide bond.[9] The reaction of hydrolyses of ochratoxin A by the proteolytic enzymes would be as follows:

$$\text{ochratoxin A} \rightarrow \text{ochratoxin } \alpha + \text{L-phenylalanine}$$

(see Fig. 4).

The inhibitory effect of certain dipeptides on carboxypeptidase A was investigated by Yanari and Mitz.[10] They concluded that these dipeptides were effective competitive inhibitors of carboxypeptidase A, although their apparent K_m values were substantially lower than that of carbobenzoxy-glycyl-L-phenylalanine (N-CBZ-glyc-phe, 0.03 M). Since the structure of

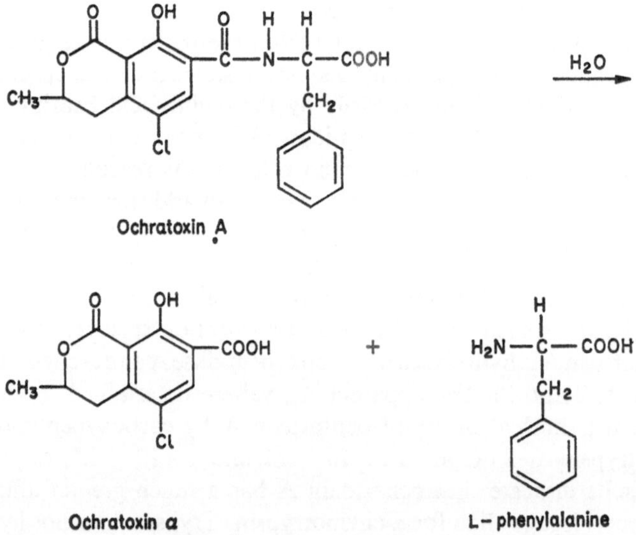

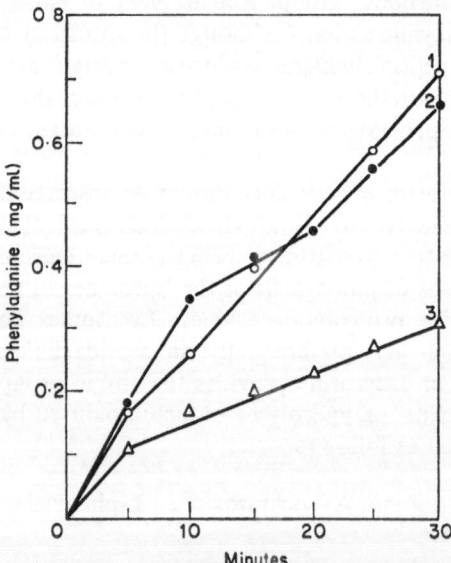

Ochratoxin A

Ochratoxin α   L- phenylalanine

FIG. 4. The hydrolysis of ochratoxin A by carboxypeptidase A and
α-chymotrypsin (from ref. 6).

FIG. 5. The effect of ochratoxins A and α on the rate of hydrolysis of N-carbobenzoxyglycyl-L-phenylalanine by carboxypeptidase A. Curves 1, 2 and 3 represent the
hydrolysis of the substrate in the presence of ochratoxin α, in the absence of both
toxins and in the presence of ochratoxin A, respectively. The concentrations of substrate, ochratoxins A and α were 0·02 M and that of carboxypeptidase A 7 μg/ml
protein solution (from ref. 12).

ochratoxin A resembles that of a dipeptide, this toxin might exert an inhibitory effect on the activity of carboxypeptidase A. In addition, ochratoxin α might also exert an inhibitory effect because the structure of this compound is related to benzoic acid which inhibits the action of carboxypeptidase A.[11] The inhibitory effect of ochratoxins A and α on carboxypeptidase A activity was investigated by Pitout[12] and only ochratoxin A was found to be a competitive inhibitor of carboxypeptidase A (see Fig. 5). The inhibition constant (K_i) is 14·2 mM and the binding energy (B-E) of ochratoxin A to the enzyme was estimated to be 2·5 kcal/ mol (see Fig. 6, Table 1; results in Table 1 were obtained from refs. 11, 14).

It is suggested by Webb[11] that a three-point attachment of the substrate

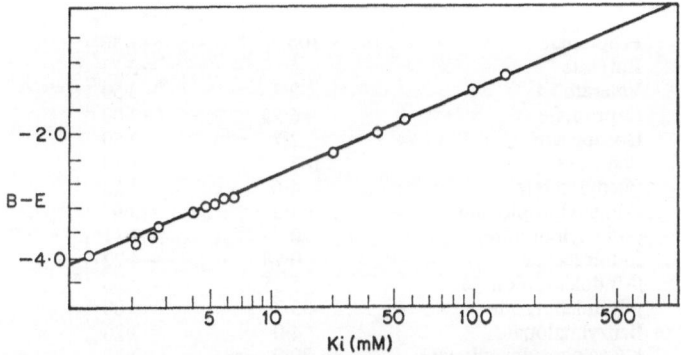

FIG. 6. A plot of relative binding energy against K_i. The values of K_i and relative binding energy were obtained from Table 1 (from ref. 12).

on the surface of carboxypeptidase A is necessary for catalysis. The postulated enzyme sites are indicated in Fig. 7. It is therefore easy to see why D-substrates cannot be hydrolysed since the peptide bonds would not be able to approach the peptidatic site.

Specific competitive inhibitors for carboxypeptidase A require only two interacting groups, and most of which have been studied bind at the cationic and electrokinetic sites. Although the structure of ochratoxin A indicates no inhibition at the peptidatic site, the molecular configuration of the toxin (see Fig. 7) suggests that it exerts an inhibitory effect by binding at the cationic and electrokinetic sites. This is in accordance with the inhibitory effect of L- and D-phenylalanine and β-phenylpropionic acid, although the findings of Elkins-Kaufman and Neurath[13] showed that only the anionic forms, and not the dipolar ions, of the two amino acids are competitive inhibitors.

Ion-ion type interactions are known to be important in the binding of

substrates and inhibitors to peptidases but Smith *et al.*[14] have presented
evidence that Van der Waal's forces are also involved. The inhibition
constants and calculated binding energies for a number of compounds with
carboxypeptidase A are given in Table 1. Smith *et al.*[14] concluded that
Van der Waal's interactions of the side chains of the substrate provide a
significant contribution to the total binding energy.

Table 1

The Relationship Between Relative Binding Energies and K_i of
Various Inhibitors to Carboxypeptidase (from ref. 12)

Inhibition	K_i (mM)	Relative binding energy (kcal/mol)
Propionate	100	−1·36
Butyrate	5	−3·13
Valerate	2·7	−3·50
Caprionate	6·25	−3·00
Isocaproate	2·7	−3·50
Benzoate	143	−1·15
Phenylacetate	4·6	−3·18
β-Phenylpropionate	1·2	−3·97
γ-Phenylbutyrate	20	−2·31
Indoleacetate	0·78	−4·22
β-Indolepropionate	5·55	−3·06
γ-Indolebutyrate	33·3	−2·00
Benzylmalonate	4·0	−3·26
β-Cyclohexylpropionate	20·0	−2·31
β-Naphthaleneacetate	45·5	−1·82
D-Phenylalanine	2·0	−3·82
p-Nitrophenylacetate	2·5	−3·68

The differences in the binding energies of inhibitors may be attributed
mainly to Van der Waal's forces, and particularly to dispersion forces.
Although the relative binding energy of substrate and inhibitors to
carboxypeptidase can easily be calculated from the K_i values according to
Smith *et al.*,[14] an additional method of estimation is afforded by Fig. 6.
Once the K_i value is known, the relative binding energy can be read off the
graph (see Fig. 6).

From Table 1, it is obvious that indoleacetate, indolepropionate and
phenylpropionate are bound more strongly than ochratoxin A, suggesting
that some steric repulsion of the latter analogue occurs. This steric repulsion
is probably due to the presence of the isocoumarin moiety because ochratoxin α has no effect on the enzyme, while benzoate is an inhibitor (see
Figs. 7 and 8 and Table 1).

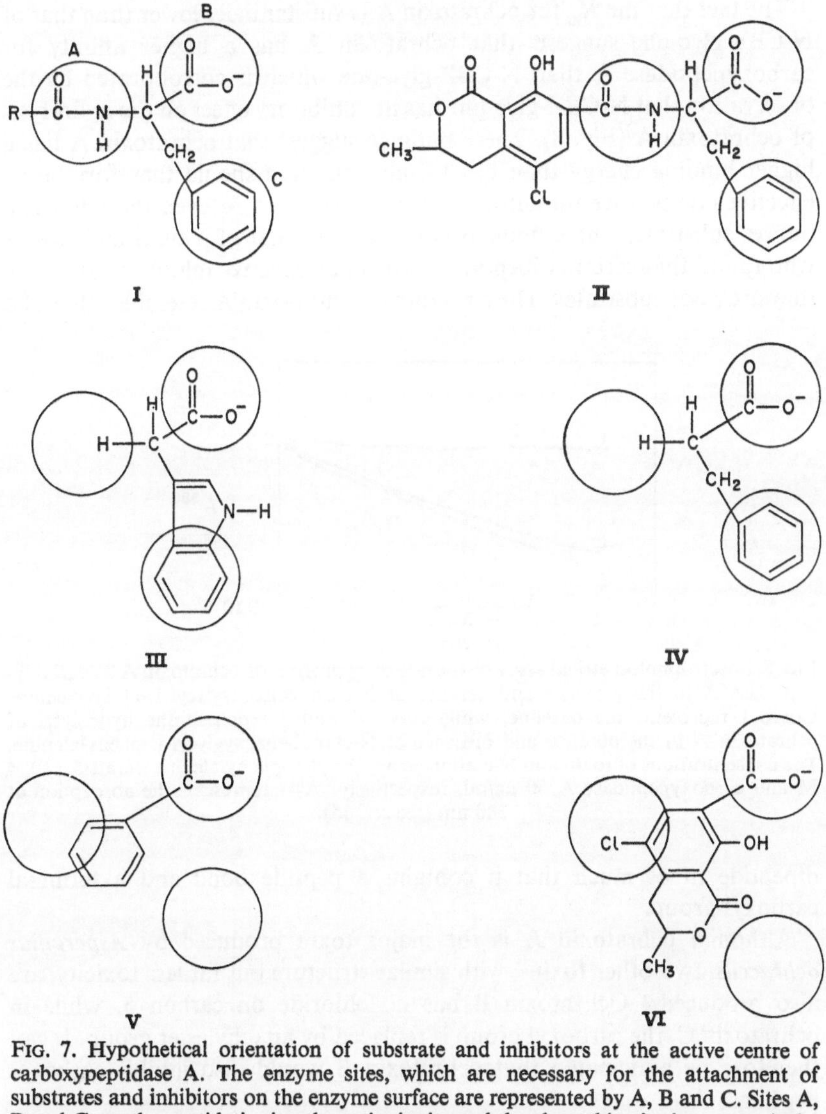

FIG. 7. Hypothetical orientation of substrate and inhibitors at the active centre of carboxypeptidase A. The enzyme sites, which are necessary for the attachment of substrates and inhibitors on the enzyme surface are represented by A, B and C. Sites A, B and C are the peptidatic site, the cationic site and the electrokinetic site, respectively. The latter site is perhaps a lipophilic region capable of reacting with alkyl or phenyl groups by dispersion forces. Configurations I, II, III, IV, V and VI are acyl-L-phenylalanine (substrate), ochratoxin A, 3 indoleacetic acid, β-phenylpropionate, benzoate and ochratoxin α, respectively. The molecular configurations are only approximate (see ref. 12).

The fact that the K_m for ochratoxin A is substantially lower than that of N-CBZ-glyc-phe suggests that ochratoxin A has a higher affinity for carboxypeptidase A than N-CBZ-glyc-phe which is corroborated by the observation that N-CBZ-glyc-phe has no inhibitory effect on the hydrolysis of ochratoxin A (Fig. 8). These findings suggest that ochratoxin A has a higher binding energy than N-CBZ-glyc-phe and should therefore be an effective competitive inhibitor of carboxypeptidase A, even though it is a poorer substrate. These findings coincide with that of Yanari and Mitz[10] who found that certain dipeptides perform as effective inhibitors although they are poor substrates. The structure of ochratoxin A resembles that of a

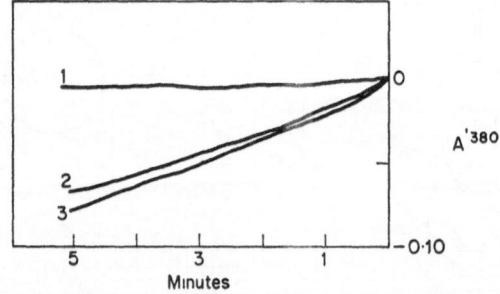

FIG. 8. Spectrophotometrical assay of the rate of hydrolysis of ochratoxin A by carboxypeptidase A in the presence and absence of N-carbobenzoxyglycyl-L-phenylalanine. Curve 1 represents the baseline, while curves 2 and 3 represent the hydrolysis of ochratoxin A in the absence and presence of N-carbobenzoxyglycyl-L-phenylalanine. The concentrations of toxin and N-carbobenzoxyglycyl-L-phenylalanine were 1.5×10^{-4} M and carboxypeptidase A 50 μg/ml, respectively. A[380] represents the absorption at 380 nm (see ref. 15).

dipeptide in as much that it contains a peptide bond and a terminal carboxyl group.

Although ochratoxin A is the major toxin produced by *Aspergillus ochraceus*, two other toxins, with similar structure but far less toxicity, are also produced.[2] Ochratoxin B has no chloride on carbon 5, while in ochratoxin C, the carboxyl group is replaced by an ethylester group. It can therefore be anticipated that ochratoxin B would also inhibit carboxypeptidase A.

Since it was observed that ochratoxin A is hydrolysed by carboxypeptidase A *in vitro* to ochratoxin α,[6] it was decided to investigate this hydrolysis reaction as a possible assay method for the activity of bovine carboxypeptidase A. It is known that ochratoxin A has an absorption peak at 380 nm at pH 7·5 while ochratoxin α has only an absorption peak at 330 nm at the same pH (see ref. 6). When ochratoxin A is hydrolysed by means of HCl or carboxypeptidase A, the absorption peak at 380 nm disappears while a peak at 330 nm appears (see Figs. 2, 3 and 9). Difference and absorption spectra indicate that the decrease at 380 nm is much more

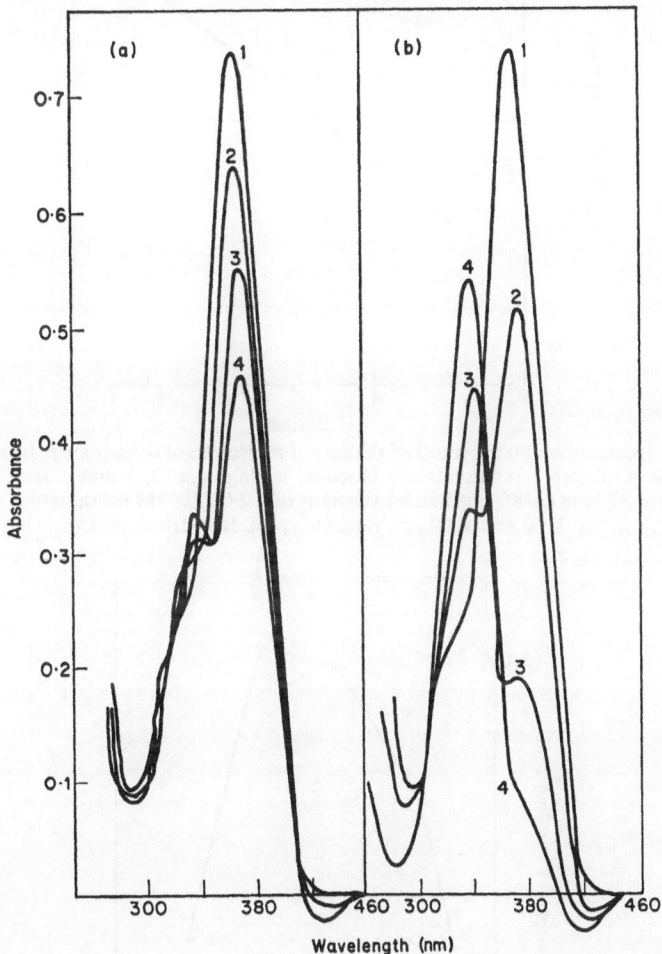

FIG. 9. The hydrolysis of ochratoxin A by three different carboxypeptidase A concentrations. In (a) curve 1 represents ochratoxin A (2 ml of 1.95×10^{-4} M) before hydrolysis, curves 2, 3 and 4 (2.0 ml of 1.0×10^{-4} M) treated with 2, 50 and 1200 μg enzyme/ml for 180 min, respectively. In (b) curve 1 represents an ochratoxin A solution before hydrolysis while curves 2, 3 and 4 represent the rate of hydrolysis at 25° after 120, 1620 and 2880 min, respectively. The concentration of substrate was 1.95×10^{-4} M and enzyme concentration was 1200 μg/ml (from ref. 15).

sensitive than the increase of absorption at 330 nm. A spectrophotometric method is described which could be used for assaying carboxypeptidase A

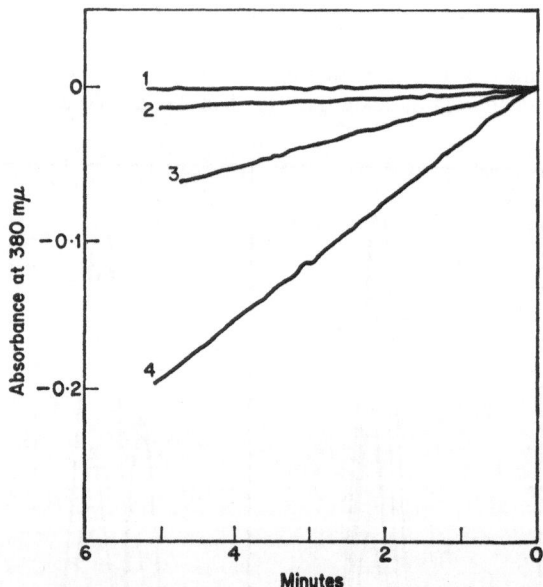

FIG. 10. Spectrophotometric assay of the rate of hydrolysis of ochratoxin A by carboxy-peptidase A. Curve 1 represents the baseline, while curves 2, 3 and 4 represent the decrease at 380 nm (A^{380}) due to the hydrolysis of a $2 \cdot 0 \times 10^{-4}$M ochratoxin A solution by 2, 50 and 1200 μg/ml carboxypeptidase (from ref. 15).

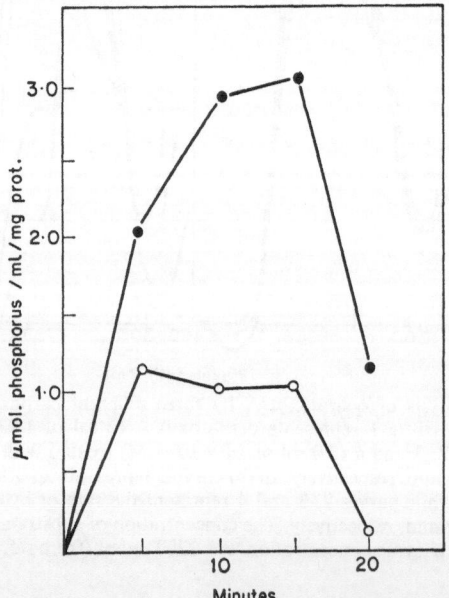

FIG. 11. Inhibitory effect of ochratoxin A on the phosphorylase system. The activity of the enzyme in the absence and presence of the toxin is indicated by ● and ○, respectively (from ref. 17).

which affords certain advantages over the colorimetric methods.[15] The assay method is illustrated in Figure 10.

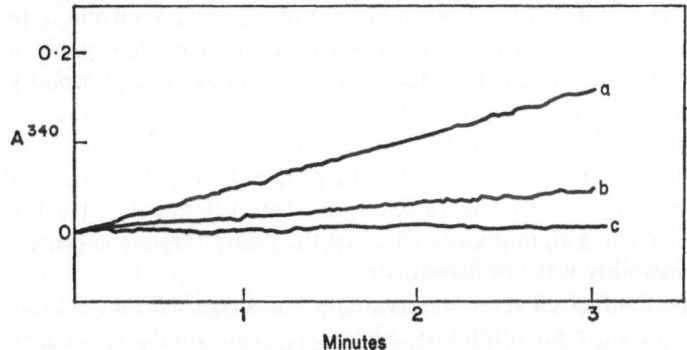

FIG. 12. Inhibitory effect of ochratoxin A on the phosphorylase system. Curves *a* and *b* represent the activity of the phosphorylase system in the absence and presence of ochratoxin A, respectively. Curve *c* is the baseline (from ref. 17).

Table 2

Inhibitory Effect of Ochratoxin A on the Enzymes Phosphorylase *a*, Phosphoglucomutase, Glucose-6-Phosphate Dehydrogenase, Hexokinase and the Phosphorylase Enzyme System (from ref. 17)

Enzyme	% inhibition
Phosphorylase *a*	0
Phosphoglucomutase	0
Glucose-6-phosphate dehydrogenase	0
Hexokinase	0
Phosphorylase system	about 70

Ochratoxin A and glycogen storage in rat liver

A single dose of 10 mg of ochratoxin A per kg of body weight produced accumulation of glycogen in the liver of rats.[3] In man, hereditary glycogen storage disease results in the accumulation of glycogen in various organs.[16] Electron microscope studies showed that the changes induced by ochratoxin A in rat liver closely resemble those seen in type 6 of glycogen storage disease (Hers' disease) where there is a deficiency of phosphorylases a and b in the liver. To initiate the study it was decided to investigate the action of ochratoxin A on the phosphorylase enzyme system because an increase in liver glycogen can result from an inhibition of the various

D

enzymes in the phosphorylase enzyme complex.[17] In addition, the effect of the toxin on other enzymes of carbohydrate metabolism was investigated. The results are given in Figures 11 and 12 and Table 2. Since the phosphorylase enzyme system was affected, but not phosphorylases a and b, the next obvious enzyme in the phosphorylase enzyme system, namely, phosphorylase b kinase could be inhibited by ochratoxin A. The phosphorylase b kinase is activated by a protein kinase, e.g. phosphorylase b kinase kinase, which needs 3'–5' cyclic AMP as a co-factor. It could be that ochratoxin A competes with the cyclic AMP for the protein kinase. Since ochratoxin A could be hydrolysed to ochratoxin α *in vivo*, it is possible that the latter could also exert an inhibitory effect on the phosphorylase enzyme system. This possibility was not investigated.

In the light of all these observations it is suggested that ochratoxin A exerts not only an inhibitory effect on carbohydrate metabolism, but possibly also on protein metabolism.

REFERENCES

1. SCOTT, DE B. (1965). *Mycopathol. Mycol. Appl.*, **25**, 213.
2. VAN DER MERWE, K. J., STEYN, P. S. and FOURIE, L. (1965). *Fd. Cosmet. Toxicol.*, **6**, 479.
3. PURCHASE, I. F. H. and THERON, J. J. (1968). *Fd. Cosmet. Toxicol.*, **6**, 479.
4. NEL, W. and PURCHASE, I. F. H. (1968). *J.S.A. Chem. Inst.*, **XXI**, 87.
5. SMITH, E. L. (1951). *Adv. Enzymol.*, **12**, 191.
6. PITOUT, M. J. (1969). *Biochem. Pharm.*, **18**, 485.
7. HOFFMAN, K. and BERGMANN, J. (1941). *J. Biol. Chem.*, **138**, 243.
8. PURCHASE, I. F. H. (1969). Personal communication.
9. BRUTON, J. S. (1962). In: *The Enzymes* (Eds. Boyer, P. D., Lardy, H. and Mÿrback, K.), Vol. **4**, p. 233. Academic Press.
10. YANARI, S. and MITZ, M. A. (1957). *J. Am. Chem. Soc.*, **79**, 1154.
11. WEBB, J. L. (1963). In: *Enzyme and Metabolic Inhibitors*, Vol. **1**, p. 292. Academic Press, New York.
12. PITOUT, M. J. (1969). *Biochem. Pharm.*, **18**, 1837.
13. ELKINS-KAUFMAN, E. and NEURATH, H. (1948). *J. Biol. Chem.*, **175**, 893.
14. SMITH, E. L., LUMNY, R. and POLGLASE, W. J. (1951). *J. Phys. Chem.*, **55**, 125.
15. PITOUT, M. J. (1969). *Biochem. Pharm.*, **18**, 1829.
16. HUG, G., GARANCIS, J. C., SCHUBERT, W. K. and KAPLAN, S. (1966). *Am. J. Disease Children*, **111**, 437.
17. PITOUT, M. J. (1968). *Toxicol. Applied Pharm.*, **13**, 299.

PORPHYRIN METABOLISM IN
PRIMARY HEPATOMA*

by

J. M. Silva† and C. Manso‡

*Laboratory of Physiological Chemistry, Faculty of Medicine
University of Lourenço Marques, Mozambique*

The cancer cell is characterised by a peculiar metabolism, in which certain pathways have an increased activity, whereas others tend to disappear.[1] A definite absence of the usual controls also seems to be a characteristic of malignancy.[2] Among other metabolic abnormalities is the phenomenon, described by Warburg, of enhanced fermentation, which is not depressed by oxygen. This lack of the Pasteur effect was the basis of Warburg's theory that anoxia is the cause of cancer.[3] Despite all the subsequent studies in different countries, and especially by Weinhouse,[4] no definite conclusions to this problem could be reached.

A definite lowering of iron-containing pigments was demonstrated in animals with several types of experimental tumours and this was attributed to the presence of an abnormal substance, toxohormone.[5] Toxohormone was at first thought to be a polypeptide specific to cancer cells, although, according to Nakahara, it may just be a normal constituent of the cell which has a controlling effect on the formation of iron-containing pigments, and which increases in amount in the malignant cell. Mutant staphylococci with neoplastic characteristics also produce toxohormone and their energy is derived from fermentation.[6]

A correlation between all these facts cannot be obtained until we know more about the mechanisms that control synthesis and degradation of haem pigments, and of their tetrapyrrole precursors. A study of porphyrin metabolism in patients with cancer is therefore justified.

The present study describes the results obtained so far in a group of Bantu subjects with primary hepatoma.

MATERIAL AND METHODS

A group of 28 Bantu patients, affected with primary hepatoma, and admitted to Hospital Miguel, Bombarda, was studied. Their age varied

* This work was supported by a grant from Instituto de Alta Cultura.
† Assistant, Department of Physiological Chemistry.
‡ Director, Department of Physiological Chemistry.

Table 1

Results Obtained in Cases with Hepatoma and Controls

	Faeces		Urine				Blood		
	CP*	PP*	ALA†	PBG†	UP‡	CP‡	CP§	PP§	Hb$_4$¶
Controls									
n_1	10	10	10	10	10	10	10	10	10
$\bar{x}_1$	15·2	24·6	1·1	2·14	0·42	37·2	4·98	29·1	16·74
s_1	9·5	21·6	0·3	0·6	0·7	17·6	5·26	9·5	1·94
Hepatoma									
n_2	28	28	28	28	28	28	22	22	22
$\bar{x}_2$	19·4	50·9	3·37	3·96	16·4	155·35	14·88	54·38	11·05
s_2	20·7	75·7	2·7	1·51	34·3	207·6	68·2	64·6	3·86
$t =$	0·6	81·25	2·55	0·3	1·43	2·8	0·92	3·03	4·28
$p =$	0·05	0·05	0·05	0·05	0·05	0·01	0·05	0·01	0·01

* μg/g dry weight.   † mg/l.   ‡ μg/l.   § μg/100 ml red cells.   ¶ Grams %.
ALA: delta-aminolevulinic acid;   PBG: porphobilinogen;   UP: uroporphyrin;   CP: coproporphyrin;
PP: protoporphyrin;   Hb: haemoglobin.
n_1: number of controls; $\bar{x}_1$: average of controls; s_1: standard deviation of controls.
n_2: number of hepatomas; $\bar{x}_2$: average of hepatomas; s_2: standard deviation of hepatomas.

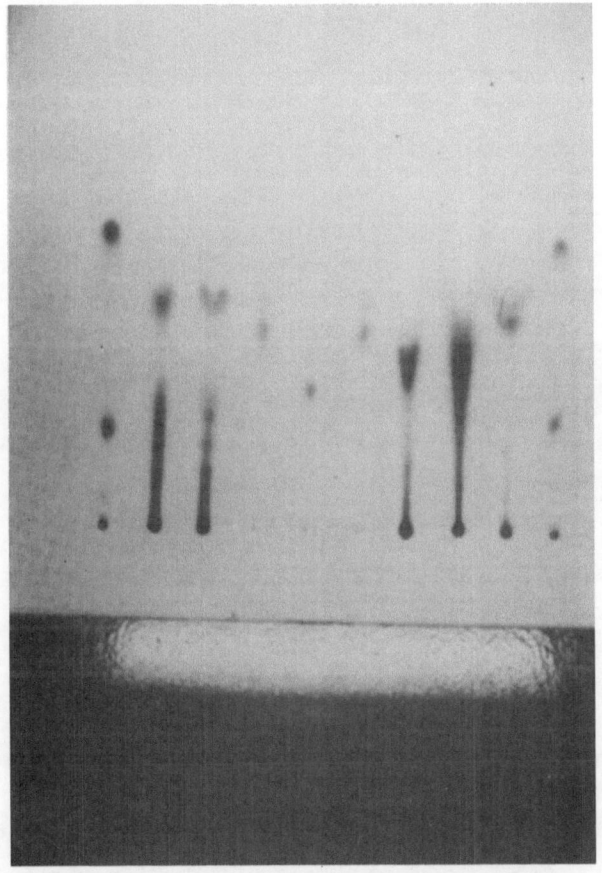

FIG. 1. Thin-layer chromatography of urine of five patients.
From left to right:
Channels 1 and 10: controls (copro-upper, uro-middle,
    initial deposit-bottom);
Channels 2, 3 and 9: patients with viral hepatitis;
Channels 4 and 6: control with five carboxyl groups;
Channel 5: control with six carboxyl groups.

between 20 and 65 years and, in all cases, the diagnosis was confirmed histologically.

Porphyrins were determined in urine, faeces and erythrocytes by the methods of Rimington.[7, 10] Delta-aminolevulinic acid and porphobilinogen in the urine were determined by the techniques of Mauzerall and Granick.[8]

For a better characterisation of urinary porphyrins, we utilised the technique of thin-layer chromatography, as described by Grosser et al.[9]

RESULTS

The results are presented in two parts. In the first part the quantitative results of the determination of porphyrin and of its precursors are presented.

In the second part the qualitative results obtained with thin-layer chromatography are described.

(a) *Quantitative results*

Table 1 summarises the results described in detail in a previous publication.[11] The urinary delta-aminolevulinic acid, urinary coproporphyrins, and erythrocyte protoporphyrin values are definitely elevated, whereas those of haemoglobin are significantly decreased in comparison to normal individuals.

(b) *Qualitative results*

Figure 1 shows the results obtained by thin-layer chromatography. Two cases of hepatoma show much slower migration when compared with the cases of hepatitis.

DISCUSSION

The first part of our study shows definite elevation in the concentration of certain types of porphyrins. The explanation for this fact may be either an increased production of porphyrins, or a block in a subsequent metabolic step, or both.

Figure 2 describes schematically the main pathways related to the synthesis of porphyrins and haem, namely the tricarboxylic acid cycle (A) and the Shemin cycle (B).[12]

By condensation of succinyl-CoA and glycine, delta-aminolevulinic acid is produced, which may be metabolised in two different ways: either towards the synthesis of porphyrins by ALA dehydrase, or by transamination towards alpha-ketoglutaraldehyde, in which case succinate is recovered.

Only porphyrinogens of type III are used for haem synthesis. Porphyrins of type III and porphyrinogens of type I are not used for haem synthesis.[12]

The increased production of ALA in hepatomas may be due to a decreased activity of ALA dehydrase or of ALA transaminase. An increase in activity of ALA synthetase could also be responsible for it, although this is less likely because of Tschudy's observations in other kinds of digestive tumours.

In addition, tumour metabolism is anaerobic. This fact could impair the transformation of succinyl-CoA in the Krebs cycle, and more succinyl-CoA would be available for the synthesis of ALA.

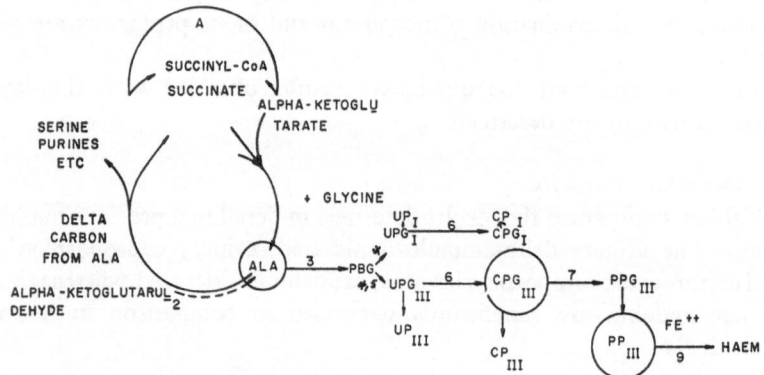

FIG. 2 (Adapted from Shemin, the abnormal values found are circled.)
1—ALA synthetase. 2—ALA transaminase. 3—ALA dehydrase. 4—UPG I synthetase. 5—UPG III cosynthetase. 6—UPG decarboxidase. 7—CPG oxidase. 8—enzyme? 9—haem synthetase. ALA—delta-aminolevulinic acid; PBG—porphobilinogen; UPG—uroporphyrinogen; UP—uroporphyrin; CPG—coproporphyrinogen; CP—coproporphyrin; PPG—protoporphyrinogen; PP—protoporphyrin.

The increased urinary excretion of coproporphyrins may also be explained by the low oxygen content of tumours, since the oxidative de-carboxylation mediated by coproporphyrinogen oxidase requires the presence of oxygen as an electron acceptor.

The increased protoporphyrin levels in the erythrocytes accompanied by decreased haemoglobin, may be explained by the presence of toxohormone, which, among other physiological effects, has the ability to interfere with haem synthesis, lowering the activity of haem synthetase.[5, 14]

Finally the studies using thin-layer chromatography demonstrate a definite slowing of migration of porphyrins from hepatoma patients when compared with those from hepatitis patients, indicating an impaired decarboxylation of uroporphyrin.[9, 15] Two possible explanations are acceptable: either the increased amount of coproporphyrins exceeds the normal capacity for decarboxylation, or a decreased activity of uroporphyrinogen decarboxylase is unable to decarboxylate the uroporphyrin substrate. Since coproporphyrins are produced in increased amounts, we believe that the first hypothesis is the most likely one.

REFERENCES

1. WEBER, G. (1966). *GANN monograph*, **1**, 151.
2. WEBER, G. (1963). *Ad. Enzyme Reg.*, **1**, 321.
3. WARBURG, O. (1956). *Science*, **123**, 309.
4. WEINHOUSE, S. (1956). *Science*, **124**, 267.
5. NAKAHARA, W. and FUKUOKA, F. (1958). *Adv. Can. Res.*, **5**, 157.
6. CALLOA, V. and MONTOYA, E. (1967). *Science*, **157**, 2041.
7. RIMINGTON, C. (1961). *Ass. Clin. Path.*, **36**, 1.
8. MAUZERALL, D. and GRANICK, S. (1956). *J. Biol. Chem.*, **219**, 435.
9. GROSSER, Y., SWEENEY, G. and EALES, L. (1967). *S. Afr. med. J.*, **41**, 460.
10. RIMINGTON, C., MORGAN, P., NICHOLLS, K., EVERALL, J. and DAVIES, R. (1963). *Lancet*, **2**, 318.
11. SILVA, J. and MANSO, C. *S. Afr. med. J.* (in publication).
12. SHEMIN, D. (1955). Ciba Foundation Symposium, pp. 4-26.
13. TSCHUDY, D. and COLLINS, A. (1957). *Cancer Res.*, **17**, 976.
14. ONO, T., UMEDA, M. and SUGIMURA, M. (1956). *GANN*, **47**, 171.
15. SCOTT, R., LABBE, R. and NUTTER, J. (1967). *Clin. Chem.*, **13**, 493.

SURVEYS FOR ALPHA-FETO-PROTEIN AMONG BANTU GOLDMINERS

by

L. R. Purves

South African Institute for Medical Research, Johannesburg

One of the major stumbling-blocks of epidemiology is the difficulty of establishing a relation between two remote events, e.g. childhood ingestion of a hepatotoxic mycotoxin and the development of primary liver cancer in adulthood. Any technique that will shorten the interval between the two events will therefore be of interest to the epidemiologist. The purpose of this communication is to present evidence that such a technique might be possible for primary liver cancer and to report our current progress.

Alpha-feto-protein (AFP) when found in the blood of adults by immuno-diffusion techniques denotes the invariable presence of a primary liver cancer.[1, 2] No false positive result has been documented yet. The range of AFP levels is very wide,[2] extending from nearly 1 g % to low levels that are determined by the sensitivity of the tests used. The lowest practical limit for an Ouchterlony type technique is about 0·1 mg %. We found that 75% of our cases of primary liver cancer were positive at this level.[2] This has been widely confirmed (see Ref. 3 for documentation).

We have developed a radio-immuno assay for AFP that is capable of extending the sensitivity to low levels. Our results when suspected cases of primary liver cancer were tested with an assay limit of 0·03 mg %, are shown in Figure 1. The percentage positivity is increased and cases are found extending to the assay limit. Not all these cases however have been proven but it is highly probable that they have tumours. Sera from suspected cases of primary liver cancer and samples taken from otherwise healthy Bantu mineworkers were tested. Preliminary results indicate that most of the sera caused inhibition at a level equivalent to about 0·001 to 0·002 mg %. In both series results were found extending up to 0·1 mg %. While it is not yet established that 0·001 mg % is the normal adult level of AFP (the author doubts this) it nevertheless appears that otherwise healthy Bantu mineworkers can have discernible amounts of AFP in their serum (Fig. 2).

The sera from the Bantu mineworkers were studied with a prospective study in mind and this is currently in progress with the object of assessing the significance of these AFP results.

The possibility seems to exist that detectable AFP levels might be present in hepatoma-vulnerable populations. Whether this will prove to be

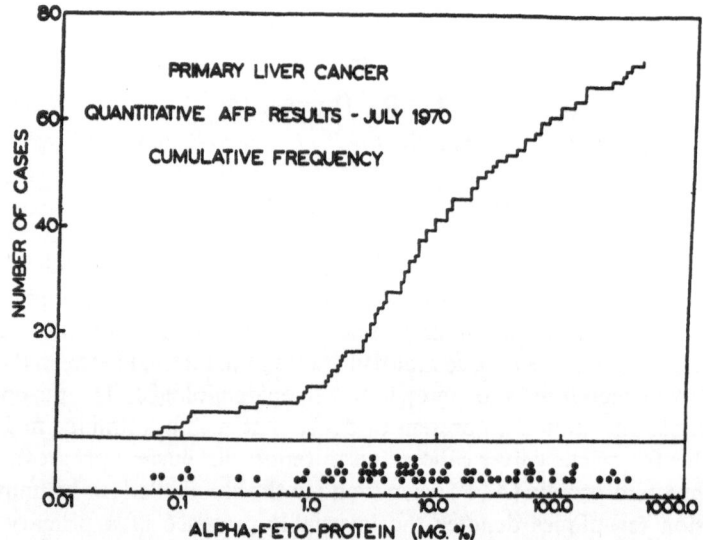

FIG. 1. Radio-immuno assay of AFP levels in the serum of Bantu goldminers with primary liver cancer. Individual results and the cumulative frequency are shown. The lower limit of the assay was 0·03 mg %.

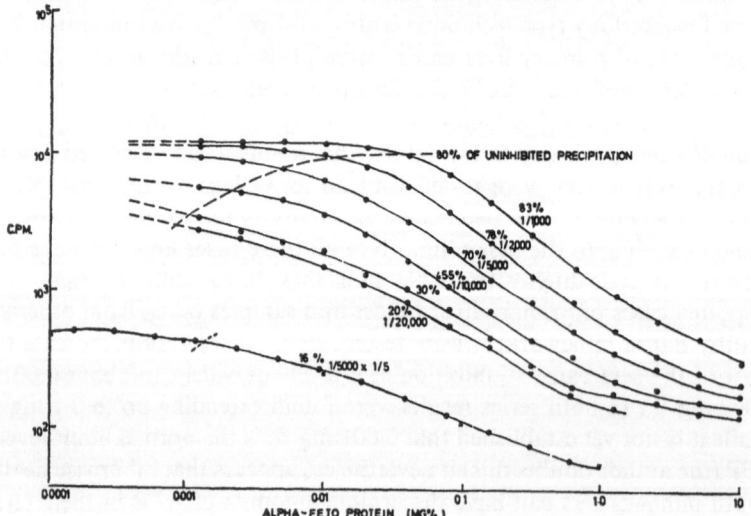

FIG. 2. Radio-immuno assay of alpha-feto-protein. The percentage of the total radio-activity precipitated by a given dilution of rabbit-anti-human-AFP is set beside each graph (e.g. 78%, dilution 1 in 2000). The line connecting the point of 80% of un-inhibited precipitation of I^{125}-AFP by anti-AFP, for each graph, has been drawn in. Results with more than 80% precipitation were considered negative. When the AFP^{125} was diluted 5x and antiserum of strength 1/25,000 was used the slope was not sufficient for reliable results. The 80% limit was introduced to obviate mainly interference by physical factors since the antiserum and I^{125}-AFP were at least 95% pure. The 'normal' level of AFP appeared to be in the region of 0·001 mg % and asymptomatic miners coming from high incidence areas, as well as Ouchterlony-negative primary liver cancer cases, were found to have results extending as high as 0·1 mg %.

associated with the presence of established cancer or merely indicate an hepatotoxic effect (as in rodents[4]) remains to be seen. However, the use of AFP screening at low levels might provide the clue that epidemiologists need for establishing causal relationships between nutritional factors and the development of primary liver cancer.

REFERENCES

1. ABELEV, G. I. (1968). *Cancer Res.*, **28**, 1344.
2. PURVES, L. R., MACNAB, M. and BERSOHN, I. (1968). *S. Afr. med. J.*, **42**, 1138.
3. PURVES, L. R., BERSOHN, I. and GEDDES, E. W. (1970). *Cancer*, **25**, 1261.
4. STANISLAWSKI-BIRENCWAJG, M. (1967). *Cancer Res.*, **27**, 1982.

MYCOLOGIC AND
MYCOTOXIC EXAMINATION OF CYCADS*

by

Joseph Forgacs†

Good Samaritan Hospital, Suffern, New York

Cycads are palm-like plants that have shown very little evolutionary change during the period of their existence since the Mesozoic age. There are several genera in existence today in tropical and subtropical climatic regions of the world. Where plants belonging to these genera are indigenous, starch prepared from the seed, rhizome, or stem is used for human consumption. In addition, dried husks from the seed of *Cycas circinalis* are chewed by natives where this cycad is indigenous. In other areas, young sprouts and leaves of members of the genus *Zamia* are ingested by animals. In the Orient, seeds of *C. revoluta* are processed into fermented food.

Consumption of various species of cycads has caused both acute and chronic toxic manifestations in man and animals. Toxicity in man associated with ingestion of endosperm of *Cycas circinalis* has generally been attributed to cycasin present in improperly prepared cycad starch. Seeds of *Cycas revoluta* are used as an ingredient in miso processing in the Orient, and although extraneous fungi may proliferate on such substrata, the possible role that toxigenic fungi may play in the health of individuals that consume such fermented products has received very little study in the past. Cattle that have grazed portions of plants of *Zamia debilis*, a cycad indigenous to the Dominican Republic and other areas, have developed a locomotor ataxia, the aetiology of which remains to be elucidated. Although it has been established that a toxic factor is present in the *Zamia* plants, the possible role that fungi, either as phytopathogens or saprophytes, may play in this toxicosis has been neglected.

Since natives are cognisant of the inherent toxicity associated with consumption of some cycads, such as *C. circinalis*, special precautions are taken to detoxify the seed before it is used as human food. Although cycasin or its degradation products have been shown to be present in seeds

* Investigations in this report were supported in part under Contract No. PH43-64-606, NINDB, National Institutes of Health, Bethesda, Maryland.

† Present address: Automated Biochemical Laboratories, Inc., Spring Valley, N.Y.

of unwashed cycads, soaking and concurrent leaching in water or fermenting the sliced green endosperm presumably removes these toxic entities. During drying of the processed endosperms, fungi frequently proliferate on and into the endosperms. According to Whiting,[1] fungi frequently are associated with processing of the cycad. Indeed, in some areas fungi appear to be used to detoxify the cycads.

Seeds of *C. revoluta* are often fermented into sake, and when mixed with other substrata, such as rice and soybeans, are fermented into miso. In the Caribbean region, freshly-extracted starch from a species of *Zamia* is made into large loaves which are fermented for several days, after which the loaf is broken and reveals a dark discolouration, presumably due to fungal proliferation. This microbiological process apparently detoxifies the starch. In parts of Australia, the cycad is buried in the ground for a month or longer in a trench lined with grass. In other regions, the cycad is wrapped in skins or leaves and likewise buried. Both steps result in profuse fungal growth, but the mould or moulds have not been isolated and subjected to taxonomic studies. Nishida (cited by Whiting[1]) observed fungi growing on slices of *C. revoluta* endosperm that had been stored in a bag for 20 to 30 days and alternately exposed to drying conditions every 5th day. Following this procedure, the pretreated slices were soaked and leached in water for several days and then thoroughly sun-dried. It was considered that this treatment method detoxified the cycad slices. In Ashima, according to Kobawyashi (cited by Whiting[1]) specimens of the cut stem of *C. revoluta* were stored under a straw mat to promote growth of black fungi. Although in other areas, such as in Guam, fungi *per se* are not included in the detoxifying process, the cycad slices are soaked and leached in water to remove the toxic entities and then dried, and fungi inadvertently may contaminate the treated endosperm.

Since fungi frequently are associated with cycad processing, the possible role that toxigenic fungi may play, either directly or as complementary entities deserves investigation.

METHODS AND RESULTS

The specimens of *C. circinalis* included hulls, sliced endosperms, entire endosperms, crude ground meal, and refined flour, all of which had been stored at room temperatures for some time. Subsequently samples received from other sources which included dried husks and fresh entire mature seed of *C. circinalis* from Guam, and leaves and entire plants of *Zamia floridiana* (from Florida) and *Z. debilis* (from the Dominican Republic) were tested. In addition, samples of endosperms of *C. revoluta* were also studied.

1. General methods

The cycadaceous substrata were subjected to mycologic examination, and, in some cases, the fungal isolates were screened for peracute toxicity in white Swiss mice. Mycological examination consisted of examining the substrata macroscopically (with a dissecting microscope) for apparent defects, such as lesions and areas of discolouration, typical of fungal origin; microscopically for fungal bodies at 100 and 400 magnifications before and/or after digestion with 20% KOH and before and after staining with lactol phenol blue; and culturally on several mycologic agars. Plating media included carrot-potato agar, Czapek's solution agar, Czapek's solution agar containing 20% sucrose, Littman's oxgall medium, potato-dextrose agar, and Sabouroud's dextrose agar. In addition, each specimen was plated aseptically on to filter paper overlying a layer of absorbent cotton in Petri plates and to which Czapek's solution broth was added as a source of moisture and supplementary nutriment. The original procedure was described by Sarkisov and Orshanskaiya[2] for isolating cellulose-decomposing fungi such as *Stachybotrys alternans* (*S. atra*) especially when in the presence of less fastidious fungi such as Mucors, Fusaria, and other luxuriant fungi.

The inoculated media in at least 3 replications were incubated for 3 to 6 weeks at ordinary room temperatures (*ca.* 24°C) and observed daily with a dissecting microscope for fungal proliferation. When good growth with aerial fructifications occurred, the relative distribution of various fungi was recorded, subcultures made for purification studies, and subsequently on to appropriate mycologic agars for stock cultures. In most cases, isolates were subjected to taxonomic studies on media generally used for taxonomy of species within a given genus. Based on relative prevalence of fungi as determined primarily by initial microscopic findings of the various samples and to a lesser extent on cultural studies, certain fungal isolates were subjected to additional cultural studies before toxicity testing in mice.

2. Mycologic examination of C. circinalis substrata

Initially, 25 specimens comprising various portions of the seed were received in one shipment and subjected to mycologic studies. Subsequently samples of fresh and dried husks also were studied. Studies of the husks are presented in the section to follow. Of the original 25 specimens, 21 were dried samples; the remaining ones consisted of fresh entire seeds. Of the first 12 specimens, only the surface layers were cultured. The succeeding samples received a more thorough examination, each subsequent specimen, in general, being subjected to a more detailed study. In some specimens, scrapings were made of the surface and subsurface layers, diluted serially in 1% peptone water containing a non-toxic surfactant, and plated on to the mycologic agars. In all cases, scrapings of surface and subsurface areas showing macroscopic abnormalities were plated directly on to the agars. For determining presence of fungal structures within the endosperms, the surface of the specimen was sterilised by swabbing with 5% aqueous phenol, and placing the specimen for 5 minutes in a Petri dish on paper towelling saturated with the phenolic solution. Thereafter, the surface layer of the

Table 1

Microscopic Fungal Findings in *C. circinalis* Substrata
(Summarised Data)

Fungal morphologic structures	No. specimens containing fungal structures indicated at left/No. specimens examined			
	Outside, dried, whole and sliced endosperm (specimens 1-20)	Inside, dried, whole and sliced endosperm (specimens 12-18, 20)	Fresh, green nut: absciss and pulpy layers (specimens 22-25)	*Summary* Total specimens (1-25)
Hyaline conidia as in *A. flavus*, etc.	14/20		2/4	16/25
Brown conidia as in *A. niger*	9/20		4/4	13/25
Pycnidia and/or pycnidiospores as in *Phoma*	5/20		1/4	6/25
Phragmospores as in *C. lunata*	14/20	1/8	1/4	16/25
Hyaline mycelia as in *A. flavus*, etc.		6/8	4/4	10/25
Dematiaceous mycelia as in *C. lunata*, *Phoma*, etc.		6/8	2/4	8/25
Sporophores of *A. niger*			2/4	2/25

specimen was aseptically scraped with a surgical blade, the specimen then broken, and scrapings from the interior plated on to the various media. Summarised microscopic and cultural findings are presented in Tables 1 and 2.

Practically all of the dried specimens examined with the dissecting microscope contained superficial lesions and areas of discolouration typical of past or current fungal proliferation. Lesions on the dried hull or dried endosperm coat of the cycads varied from minute, buff spots to large, black irregular, confluent areas. Most of the dried sliced endosperms contained

Table 2

Cultural Fungal Findings in *C. circinalis* Substrata
(Summarised Data)

Fungal species	Description of specimen below							
	Outside, dried, whole and sliced endosperm (specimens 4-18, 20)	Inside, dried, whole and sliced endosperm (specimens 12-18, 20)	Hull, shell of dried nut (specimens 1-3*, 17, 18)	Absciss and pulpy layers, fresh green nut † (specimens 22-25)	Crude cycad meal; lot no. Ci632-4A-18 ‡ (specimen 19)	Refined cycad flour § (specimen 21)	*Summary* All specimens (1-25)	Total aggregate sites tested from all specimens
	Fungal distribution in specimens indicated above							
Aspergillus flavus	11	0	2	2	0	1	16	18
Aspergillus niger	6	0	4	4	1	1	16	20
Aspergillus tamarii	3	0	2	0	0	1	6	5
Curvularia lunata	13	6	2	1	0	0	15	26
Macrosporium spp.	7	0	2	0	0	0	8	9
Mucor spp.	0	0	0	0	0	1	1	1
Penicillium spp.	1	0	1	0	0	1	3	3
Phoma spp.	8	6	3	1	0	0	10	20
Total specimens examined	16	8 ¶	5	4	1	1	25 ¶	35 ‖

* Where applicable, numbers in series are inclusive.

† No fungi were detected microscopically or isolated from the endosperm of the fresh, green, intact seed.

‡ Microscopic examination revealed numerous conidia and fungal mycelia characteristic of more than one fungal species, although *A. niger* only was isolated.

§ On microscopic examination, specimen was heavily laden with conidia and other fungal bodies. On culture, *A. flavus*, Link and *A. niger* predominated.

¶ Two specimens contained no fungi.

‖ No fungi were isolated from 6 sites.

stria which varied from a light brown to a blue-black colour. In some instances of the sliced and entire endosperms, these penetrated deep into the sub-epidermal layers and, in one specimen subjected to more detailed studies, the stria were particularly visible along vacuolations within the megasporangium.

Conidia, mycelia, and/or other fungal morphologic structures were observed in most areas of all dried specimens examined microscopically (Table 1).

In 14 of 20 specimens the exterior surfaces of the dried cycads contained fruiting bodies representative of *Curvularia lunata*, and *Aspergillus flavus*, or structurally similar fungi. Conidia characteristic of the *A. niger* group were observed in 9 specimens, and pycnidia or pycnidiospores representative of the *Phoma* group in 5 samples.

Within the dried endosperm of 8 specimens examined, 6 contained dematiaceous mycelia and one also contained phragmospores characteristic of *C. lunata*. Six also contained hyaline mycelia, but no conidia, commonly observed in the Aspergilli, Penicillia, or other structurally similar fungi. Two samples contained neither conidia nor mycelia.

In the freshly-collected green cycad nut all contained, on the absciss layer, dark brown-barred, echinulate conidia, and 2 even contained complete sporophores characteristic of the *A. niger* group of fungi. On the absciss layer, 2 contained dematiaceous mycelia and/or phragmospores typical of *C. lunata* and, similarly, 2 contained hyaline conidia, and all contained hyaline mycelia representative of such structural fungi as the Aspergilli or Penicillia. Pycnidia or pycnidiospores, as commonly observed in such fungi as *Phoma*, were detected in 1 specimen in the same area. Of 3 sound, green, fresh nuts examined one sample contained only morphologic structures characteristic of *A. niger* in all areas tested; whereas, a second sample contained morphologic structures typical of *A. niger* and *C. lunata* in the absciss layer and within the pulp. The third sample, whose absciss layer only was examined, showed predominantly conidia characteristic of the *A. niger* group and some conidia characteristic of other Aspergilli or structurally related fungi. The fourth specimen, a partly-decomposed green nut, showed numerous dark brown-barred, echinulate conidia and complete sporophores of *A. niger*, together with brown pycnidia and hyaline pycnidiospores resembling those observed in the genus *Phoma*. In addition, hyaline conidia and mycelia were observed and resembled those observed in such fungi as the Aspergilli.

In the crude cycad meal and in refined cycad flour were observed dark brown-barred, echinulate conidia, characteristic of *A. niger*, and hyaline conidia and mycelia typical of such fungi as the Penicillia and certain Aspergilli, or other structurally related fungi.

Cultural findings. As indicated in Table 2 several genera of fungi were isolated from the various samples. The dried cycad samples of Guamanian origin, were obtained from Dr Marjorie G. Whiting from the National Institutes of Health, but the history of these specimens, particularly the time interval between original collection and receipt of the specimens for mycologic examination, and conditions of storage is not complete. This may be important mycologically, because sequential fungal growth and, particularly, survival time under various conditions varies among fungi. This phenomenon has been illustrated by results from Specimen 25 (fresh green nut). Immediately upon receipt and microscopic examination, this specimen revealed numerous dark brown-barred, echinulate conidia, characteristic of fungi in the *A. niger* group, and hyaline conidia and mycelia typical of nondematiaceous fungi. Correspondingly, on culture, *A. niger* and *A. flavus* were isolated. After 4 months' storage at room temperature, microscopic examination, particularly of the pulpy layer, revealed a pre-dominance of dematiaceous mycelia and numerous dematiaceous phrag-mospores, characteristic of *C. lunata*, and numerous pycnidia and pycnidio-spores as observed in such fungi as *Phoma* species. Yet, on cultural exami-nation, *A. niger* predominated, and a few colonies of *A. flavus* and a *Penicil-lium* species were found. No *C. lunata* or other similar dematiaceous fungi could be isolated, and only an occasional *Phoma* was found. These observa-tions indicate a sequential change in the mycologic flora during the storage period with a resultant death, or perhaps, dormancy of the *Curvul-aria* and *Phoma* during storage at room temperatures. Therefore, on casual examination, the results obtained from the culture of the dried specimens might not represent the true flora. The microscopic findings of these speci-mens, however, indicate a good correlation between the colour and fungal structures observed microscopically, and the fungi actually isolated on culture. As an illustration in Specimen 1 (hull of dried seed), the dark brown-barred, echinulate conidia detected microscopically, generally would be considered common to members of the *A. niger* group of fungi. Similarly, hyaline conidia would be typical of such fungi as some of the Aspergilli, Penicillia, or other structurally similar, nondematiaceous fungi. Dematiaceous phragmospores, although resembling, structurally, a *Helminthosporium*, has 3 septa and 4 cells, and the spore generally was curved with the penultimate cell distinctly larger and darker than the other 3. These characteristics are found in the genus *Curvularia*. Presence of black pycnidia and hyaline pycnidiospores would suggest a member of the order Phomales. In this case, cultural results confirmed the microscopic observations in that an *A. niger*, a species of *Penicillium*, a *C. lunata*, and a species of *Phoma* were actually isolated. Thus the cultural findings correlated very well with the microscopic observations.

In general, the Aspergilli and the Penicillia were relatively simple to isolate; however, the *Phoma* and, particularly, the *C. lunata* and *Macro-sporium* were somewhat more difficult to grow, since the latter fungi grew very slowly and were readily overgrown by the former less fastidious moulds. The filter paper-mineral-salts technique mentioned in the materials and methods section was used successfully, but with considerable manipulation for isolating the more fastidious, dematiaceous fungi.

The distribution of fungi in the various samples of *C. circinalis* as determined by culturing is summarised in Table 2. All of the 25 samples examined contained fungi, *A. flavus*, *A. niger* and *C. lunata* prevailing. The *Phoma* was somewhat less prevalent and was followed, in decreasing order, by a species of *Macrosporium*, an *A. tamarii*, a species of *Penicillium* and a species of *Mucor*. The order of prevalence, however, was somewhat different in the 35 total aggregate sites examined among the various samples. The *C. lunata* was isolated from 26 sites; the *A. niger* and *Phoma* from 20 sites, and the *A. flavus* from 18. The remaining fungi prevailed in the same order and in essentially the same numerical values as in the total samples. It is noteworthy that of the 35 sites tested, only 6 were devoid of fungi and only 2 of these were the interior of dried, sliced endosperms and 4 were endosperm covering and/or interior of the endosperm of the fresh, green nut.

3. *Peracute toxicity of selected fungi isolated from* C. circinalis

Fungi listed in Table 3 were cultured at room temperatures (*ca.* 24°C) on Czapek's or Mycophil agars, preparatory to testing for peracute toxicity in white Swiss Webster mice (Rockland Strain). Initially all 6 fungi were grown on both agars; however, during incubation, the *Phoma* spp. on Czapek's agar and the *A. tamarii* on Mycophil agar became contaminated and were discarded. The fungi were cultured in Petri plates for 28 days on Czapek's agar and for 13 days on Mycophil agar (15 ml of medium per plate) since it has been determined in previous studies that at least some of similar fungi formed toxins under these conditions. The optima for toxic production by the fungi isolated in these studies, of course, remains to be determined. The cultured substrata were stored in a deep freeze at −30°C until needed. At the time of toxicity testing, one Petri plate of a respective agar-fungus culture was thawed at room temperature, cut into thin sections, mixed with 30 ml of sterile distilled water, and mechanically homogenised in a Ten Broeck tissue grinder. The homogenate was stored at 4°C during feeding studies, but storage length did not exceed 7 days. Thereafter, another Petri plate of fungus culture was treated likewise. This procedure was repeated for each fungus culture, and after one fungus culture was homogenised, the Ten Broeck apparatus was washed under a stream of tap water and finally rinsed with sterile distilled water to prevent carry-over to the next homogenate. A Petri plate of each sterilised, noninoculated agar medium that had been stored in a frozen state was homogenised and used as a control.

Five, male, white Swiss Webster mice weighing approximately 19 g were

Table 3

Body Weight (g) of Mice Subjected to Force-feeding of Fungal Substrata

	Days				
	0	7	14	21	28
Group no. and fungal substratum	Av. wt.	Av. wt.	Av. wt.	Av. wt.	Av. wt.
1. *A. flavus*, Czapek Agar	19·2	24·0 (2)*	20·0 (2)*	20·5 (1)*	Animal dead
2. *A. niger*, Czapek Agar	18·6	20·6	19·8	21·2	21·7
3. *A. tamarii*, Czapek Agar	18·8	21·2	19·5	20·4 (4)*	23·7 (3)*
4. *C. lunata*, Czapek Agar	18·8	20·4	21·0	21·4	22·6 (4)*
5. *Macrosporium* sp., Czapek Agar	18·8	20·8 (4)*	23·5 (4)*	25·0 (4)*	27·5 (4)*
6. *A. flavus*, Mycophil Agar	19·0	20·4	20·4	22·5	23·3
7. *A. niger*, Mycophil Agar	18·8	21·2	22·2	24·5 (3)*	24·7 (3)*
8. *C. lunata*, Mycophil Agar	18·8	23·0	22·4	21·6 (4)*	21·3 (4)*
9. *Phoma* sp., Mycophil Agar	18·8	21·2	23·8	21·0	22·6
10. *Macrosporium* sp., Mycophil Agar	19·0	22·8	23·0	25·3 (3)*	28·0 (3)*
11. Medium control, Czapek	19·0	23·0	24·8	26·0	27·6
12. Medium control, Mycophil	18·8	22·4	23·4	25·6	26·8
13. Normal food control	18·8	22·6	25·2	26·3	30·4

* Five mice were present in each group at the beginning of the experiment. The asterisk indicates number of surviving animals on the days of body weight indicated at the top of table.

used for testing a fungal homogenate for toxicity. Each mouse was force-fed by gavage 1·0 ml daily of a fungal homogenate. Similarly, each mouse in one control group received 1·0 ml of a respective noninoculated agar homogenate. A second control group received no homogenate. All mice were maintained on 'Milk-Bone' (product of National Biscuit Company, New York, N.Y.) dog biscuits (*ca.* 4·0 g each) and supplemented with fresh leafy vegetables and carrots. For each group of 5 mice, 6 biscuits were fed daily, plus a $\frac{1}{4}$ of an average size carrot and one large lettuce leaf. It was previously determined that 5 normal mice weighing initially 20 to 21 g each, under our experimental conditions, consumed, over a 24-hour period, approximately 4 biscuits when tested for a period of 2 weeks. Thus the amount of biscuits consumed over a 24-hour period served as a convenient measure for determining anorexia in any given group. All mice had a constant source of

Table 4

Clinical Observations in Mice Fed Fungal Homogenates (Czapek's Solution Agar)

Toxic effects* induced by fungi indicated

Day of test	A. flavus					A. niger				A. tamarii				C. lunata				Macrosporium				Medium & normal feed controls			
	Anorexia	Hypotonia	Cachexia	Depression	Subcue. Hem.	Anorexia	Hypotonia	Cachexia	Depression	Anorexia	Hypotonia	Cachexia	Depression	Anorexia	Hypotonia	Cachexia	Depression	Anorexia	Hypotonia	Cachexia	Depression	Anorexia	Hypotonia	Cachexia	Depression
1	1	—	—	1	1	—	1	—	—	—	—	—	—	—	—	—	—	1	1	—	—				
2	1	—	—	2	1	1	1	—	1	—	—	—	—	—	—	—	—	1	1	—	—				
3	2	—	—	2	3	1	1	2	2	—	1	—	2	—	—	—	—	1	1/5 DEAD	—	2				
4	3	1	1	3	3	1	1	2	2	1	2	—	2	—	—	—	2	1	1	—	2				
5	3	2	2	3	3	2	2	2	2	2	2	—	2	—	1	—	2	1	1	—	2				
6	3	3/5 DEAD	3	3	3	2	2	2	2	2	2	—	3	1	1	1	3	1	1	—	2				
7	3/5 DEAD	3	3	3		2	2	2	2	2	2	1	1	1	1	1	1	1	1	—	2				
8	3	3	3	3	3	2	2	2	2	3	3	3	2	2	2	2	2	1	1	—	1				
9	3	3	3	3	3	2	2	2	1	1/5 DEAD	3	3	3	2	2	1/5 DEAD	1	1	1	—	1				
10	4/5 DEAD	4/5 DEAD	3	3	3	2	2	2	1	3	3	3	3	2	2	2	2	1	1	—	1				
15	3	3	3	3	—	1	1	1	1	3	3	3	3	2	2	2	2	1	1	—	1				
17	3	3	3	3	—	2	2	2	2	3	3	3	3	2	2	1/5 DEAD	2	1	1	—	1				
18	3	3	3	3	—	1	1	1	1	3	3	3	3	2	2	2	2	1	1	—	1				
19	3	3	3	3	—	1	1	1	1	3	2	3	2	1	1	1	1	1	1	—	1				
20	3	3	3	3	—	2	2	2	2	3	2	3	—	—	—	—	—	1	1	—	1				
21	3	3	3	3	—	1	1	1	1	3	1	—	1	1	1	1	1	1	1	—	1				
22	3	3	3	3	—	2	2	2	2	2/5 DEAD	2/5 DEAD	—	—	1	—	—	—	1	1	—	1				
23	3	3	3	3	—	1	1	1	1	3	3	3	—	1	—	—	—								
24	3	3	3	3	—	2	2	2	2	—	—	—	—	1	—	—	—								
25	3	3	3	3	—	2	1	1	1	3	3	3	—	1	1	—	—								
26	MORIBUND	—	—	—	—	2	1	1	1	—	—	—	—	—	—	—	—								
27	5/5 DEAD	—	—	—	—	2	1	1	—	—	—	—	—	—	—	—	—								
28	—	—	—	—	—	2	—	—	—	—	—	—	—	—	—	—	—								
29	—	—	—	—	—	2	—	—	—	—	—	—	—	—	—	—	—								

NORMAL THROUGHOUT STUDY *(Medium & normal feed controls)*

Table 5

Clinical Observations in Mice Fed Fungal Homogenates (Mycophil Agar)

Day of test	*Toxic effects induced by fungi indicated																									
	A. flavus					*A. niger*				*C. lunata*				*Phoma*				*Macrosporium*				Medium & normal feed controls			
	Anorexia	Hypotonia	Cachexia	Depression	Subcue. Hem.	Anorexia	Hypotonia	Cachexia	Depression	Anorexia	Hypotonia	Cachexia	Depression	Anorexia	Hypotonia	Cachexia	Depression	Anorexia	Hypotonia	Cachexia	Depression	Anorexia	Hypotonia	Cachexia	Depression
2	1	1	—	1	1	1	1	—	—	—	—	—	—	—	—	—	—	—	—	—	—				
3	1	1	—	1	2	1	1	—	1	—	—	—	—	—	—	—	—	—	—	—	—				
4	2	1	—	2	3	1	1	—	1	—	—	—	—	—	—	—	—	—	—	—	—		NORMAL		
5	2	2	2	3	3	1	1	—	1	—	—	—	—	—	—	—	—	1	1	—	1		THROUGHOUT		
6	2	3	3	3	3	1	1	—	1	—	1	—	—	—	—	—	—	1	1	—	1		STUDY		
7	2	3	3	3	3	1	1	—	2	—	1	—	1	1	1	—	—	1	1	—	1				
8	2	3	3	3	1	1	3	—	2	—	1	—	1	1	1	—	—	1	1	—	1				
10	2	3	3	3	—	2	3	—	2	1	1	—	1	1	1	1	—	1	1	—	1				
11	2	2	2	3	—	2	3	—	2	3	2	1	2	1	1	1	—	3	—	—	1				
12	2	2	2	3	—	2	3	—	2	3	3	3	3	2	2	2	3	3	—	—	—				
15	2	2	2	3	—	2	3	1	2	3	3	3	3	2	2	2	3	3	—	—	—				
16	2	2	2	3	—	2	2	1	1	3 (1/5 DEAD)	2	2	2	2	2	2	1	3	—	—	—				
18	2	2	2	3	—	2 (2/5 DEAD)	2	1	1	2	2	3	2	2	2	2	—	3	—	—	1				
20	2	2	2	3	—	2	—	—	1	2	2	3	2	2	2	3	—	3	—	—	—				
22	2	2	2	3	—	2	—	—	—	2	2	3	2	2	2	3	—	3	—	—	—				
24	2	2	2	3	—	2	—	—	1	2	2	2	2	2	2	3	—	3	—	—	—				
29	2	2	2	3	—	2	—	—	—	2	2	3	—	2	2	3	—	3	—	—	—				

* Relative degree of toxic effects indicated as: 1, slight; 2, moderate; 3, pronounced.

fresh tap water. The mice were observed daily over 29 days for clinical manifestations of toxicity, and weighed at the start of the experiment and at weekly intervals thereafter, just prior to the next daily oral feeding. Mice dying during the course of the experiment, as well as the survivors that were necropsied on the last day (29th day) were observed for gross changes in various tissues, and sections were taken for histopathologic examination. The pathological findings have been reported.[3] On the 29th day, 2 mice from each group were anaesthetised with ethyl ether, and a sample of blood was taken by cardiac puncture for haematology before death occurred. (Where possible, clinically abnormal mice were selected.) Initial plans did not include blood-clotting time determinations; however, in the first group of mice (Group 8) (Table 6) the blood-clotting time appeared to be unusually long. Based on this observation, clotting time was included in the remaining groups. A simple method for determining clotting time was used *in lieu* of more elaborate and more reproducible methods. A clean, sterile, 1 ml tuberculin syringe with a 25-gauge needle was rinsed in sterile, isotonic saline. Blood was drawn from the heart and 3 to 4 drops were ejected slowly on to a clean watch glass. At every 5 second interval, a clean sterile needle was drawn through the blood. The time between blood first appearing in the syringe and fibrin strands forming on the watch glass was tentatively established as the clotting time. Cognisance is made of the many deficiencies of this procedure; however, the technique did provide a method of observing unusually long clotting times. Haemoglobin, total leucocyte, and differential white cell counts were also performed.

The results of these studies are presented in Tables 3-6. Further comments for each test are as follows:

i. A. flavus, Czapek's Agar. The main symptoms were anorexia, subcutaneous haemorrhage and atonia. All 5 mice had died by the 27th day. At necropsy, the paramount lesion in the 5 mice was pronounced haemorrhage and congestion in many tissues particularly in the mice dying within the first 15 days.

ii. A. niger, Czapek's Agar. Anorexia, depression, atonia and cachexia persisted in all mice for the first 16 days and then decreased in intensity. No mortality occurred. At necropsy, gross lesions were present in liver and kidneys.

iii. A. tamarii, Czapek's Agar. Anorexia and atonia were first observed on the 4th day. By the 9th day anorexia, atonia, cachexia and depression were marked. Two mice died and there was a poor weight gain. The clotting time increased. At necropsy, congestion and paleness of the liver was observed.

iv. C. lunata, Czapek's Agar. The symptoms were milder in this group, and occurred between the 5th and 23rd day. One mouse died. There was

Table 6   Haematologic Studies of Mice Fed Fungal Substrata for 28 Days

Group No. and substratum	Animal No.	Clotting time sec	Haemoglobin (g/100 ml)	Leucocytes/cu/mm	Differential count[a] Poly.	Bands	Myel.	Lymph.	Mono.
1. A. flavus, Czapek Agar	(All animals died in this group before termination of experiment, when haematologic studies were made)								
2. A. niger, Czapek Agar	Ci-31	65	13·2	53,000	25	55	2	13	5
A. niger, Czapek Agar	Ci-32	12	14·4	12,400	39	10	—	45	6
3. A. tamarii, Czapek Agar	Ci-38	205	16·9	19,800	18	4	—	63	15
A. tamarii, Czapek Agar	Ci-39	85	16·9	15,300	10	2	—	86	2
4. C. lunata, Czapek Agar	Ci-42	280	15·6	14,300	11	2	—	84	3
C. lunata, Czapek Agar	Ci-43	140	15·6	15,900	32	7[b]	—	58	3
5. Macrosporium, Czapek Agar	Ci-47	185	16·9	14,200	28	2	—	67	3
Macrosporium, Czapek Agar	Ci-48	12	15·4	21,300	25	1	—	74	0
6. A. flavus, Mycophil Agar	Ci-51	20	19·4	21,000	22	0	—	77	1
A. flavus, Mycophil Agar	Ci-52	20	20·2	16,400	20	2	—	73	5
7. A. niger, Mycophil Agar	Ci-58	25	13·1	5,800	13	3	—	83	1
A. niger, Mycophil Agar	Ci-59	14	14·4	10,200	14	1	—	74	11
8. C. lunata, Mycophil Agar	Ci-62	—[c]	17·4	26,000	40	6	—	53	1
C. lunata, Mycophil Agar	Ci-63	—	17·4	18,000	36	5	—	58	1
9. Phoma, Mycophil Agar	Ci-66	240	12·9[d]	31,800	34	31 (Norm. 1)	—	32	3
Phoma, Mycophil Agar	Ci-67	576	4·8[e]	9,600	50	15 (Norm. 2)	—	28	7
10. Macrosporium, Mycophil Agar	Ci-73	60	15·1	25,300	7	0	—	87	6
Macrosporium, Mycophil Agar	Ci-74	205	13·6	18,700	8[f]	2	—	85	5
11. Medium control, Czapek	Ci-82	40	12·6	9,250	8	0	—	89	3
Medium control, Czapek	Ci-83	12	16·0	6,200	20	3	—	75	2
12. Medium control, Mycophil	Ci-87	12	9·1	9,000	9	2[g]	—	89	0
Medium control, Mycophil	Ci-88	12	13·1	10,000	18	2	—	74	6
13. Normal food control	Ci-91	12	14·4[h]	13,000	8	0	—	87	5
Normal food control	Ci-92	12	14·7	5,500	15	1	—	82	2

a Abbreviations denote: Poly., polymorphonuclearneutrophile; Myel., myelocyte; Lymph., Lymphocyte; Mono., monocyte; Norm., normoblast.   b Platelets appeared to be slightly decreased.
c This group of mice was the first to be necropsied. Casual observation revealed that the apparent clotting time was unusually long. Based on this observation, clotting time was determined on mice in subsequent groups.   d Blood from this animal had a haematocrit of 43%.
e Blood from this animal had a haematocrit of 21% and the red blood cells showed anisocytosis, poikilocytosis, and hypochromia.
f Red blood cells showed rare basophilic stippling and platelets appeared to be decreased.
g Red blood cells showed slight hypochromia, anisocytosis and poikilocytosis.   h Haematocrit was 51%.

an increase in clotting time and at necropsy, haemorrhage and congestion in most tissues.

v. Macrosporium sp., *Czapek's Agar*. The symptoms in this group were mild depression, anorexia and hypotonia. Gross lesions at necropsy were observed in the liver.

vi. A. flavus, Mycophil Agar. The symptoms in this group were similar to Group 1 (*A. flavus*, Czapek's Agar) but less severe. No mortality occurred.

vii. A. niger, Mycophil Agar. Moderate depression and anorexia and pronounced atonia were observed. Two mice died on the 19th and 20th day respectively. At necropsy, congestion in the lungs and mild changes in other organs were observed.

viii. C. lunata, Mycophil Agar. Symptoms of depression, anorexia, cachexia and atonia developed from the 16th day. There appeared to be an unusually prolonged clotting time in this group which prompted measurement of clotting time in subsequent groups. Haemorrhage and congestion in various tissues was seen at necropsy.

ix. Phoma sp., *Mycophil Agar*. Apart from the symptoms depicted in Table 5, haemorrhage occurred from the tail from the 14th to 20th day. Serum encrustations formed which flaked off on the 21st day, leaving indurated areas in the dermis. At necropsy, lesions were observed in the lungs and liver.

x. Macrosporium sp., *Mycophil Agar*. Anorexia was marked, but other symptoms were mild.

xi-xiii. All control groups were normal clinically and at necropsy.

4. *Mycologic examination of husks of* C. circinalis

As indicated earlier, the husk of *C. circinalis*, either green or in a dehydrated form, is chewed by natives of the South Pacific, particularly in Guam. Thus, samples of cycad husks were examined mycologically for prevailing fungal types, some of which were screened for toxicity. Of the first 6 specimens, 4 consisted of husks removed from fresh, green seeds obtained from Guam; specimens 7 to 12 were obtained from Dr O. Mickelsen (Michigan State University, East Lansing, Michigan), and specimens 13 to 18 were obtained from Dr J. Keresztesy (Laboratory of Nutrition and Endocrinology, NIAMS, National Institutes of Health, Bethesda, Maryland), all of which consisted of milled, dried husks. Mycological findings are in Table 7.

On microscopic examination, all specimens contained fungal morphologic structures indicative of past or current fungal growth. Structures included hyaline to brown conidia, and dematiaceous phragmospores and black pycnidia, depending on the sample examined and indicated presence of several genera of fungi which was confirmed on culture. Hyaline mycelia, and hyaline and brown conidia were present in the 6 samples of fresh husks. In the dried, milled husks, brown conidia, characteristic of the *A. niger* group of fungi, were present in all 12 samples.

Table 7

Mycologic Findings in Husks of *Cycas circinalis* L.
(Summary)

	(MICROSCOPIC FINDINGS)	
	Description of specimen	
Fungal bodies	Fresh husk	Dried, milled husk
Hyaline mycelia	6	8
Dematiaceous mycelia	3	5
Hyaline conidia	6	8
Brown conidia	6	12
Dematiaceous phragmospores	2	1
Pycnidiospores	3	–
Pycnidia	3	–
Sporophores of *A. niger*	2	2
No. specimens examined	6	12
	(CULTURAL FINDINGS)	
A. candidus	–	1
A. flavus	3	7
A. glaucus	–	1
A. niger	6 (6*)	12 (8*)
A. ochraceus	–	3
C. lunata	2	–
Fusarium spp.	–	1
Mucor spp.	–	2
Pae. varioti	–	2
P. purpurogenum	1	11 (4*)
Penicillium spp.	1	1
Phoma spp.	3	–
Rhizopus spp.	–	2

* Figure in parentheses indicates number of samples in which the respective fungus predominated.

On culture, *A. niger* prevailed in the 6 samples of fresh husks and in 8 of 12 of the dried, milled husks. *Penicillium purpurogenum* prevailed in the remaining 4 specimens of the dried husks. Other fungi, though less prevalent, were also isolated from the fresh and milled husks.

There appeared to be a closer correlation between microscopic findings and cultural results of dematiaceous fungi in the fresh husks than in the dried, milled husks. In the former, 3 samples on microscopic examination showed dematiaceous mycelia representative of such fungi as *C. lunata* and *Phoma*, and 2 showed pycnidia and pycnidiospores as observed in species of *Phoma*. Upon culturing, a species of *Phoma* was isolated from 3 samples, and *C. lunata* from 2. On the other hand, in the dried, milled husks, even though dematiaceous mycelia were observed microscopically in 5 samples, no corresponding dematiaceous fungi were isolated on subsequent culture of the respective husks. Presumably, drying and/or storage resulted in death of these fungi.

Although none of the fungal isolates from the dried, milled husks were tested for toxicity, all of the isolates from the fresh husks were subjected to preliminary toxicity tests in mice, and most were toxic. The *A. flavus* was highly toxic, causing haemorrhage and death in mice.

5. *Mycologic examination of seeds of* Cycas revoluta

As indicated previously, the endosperm of *C. revoluta* frequently is used as an ingredient in miso processing in the Orient. Since mycologic studies on *C. circinalis* indicated that various substrata of this cycad contained a variety of fungi, some of which were toxigenic, samples of *C. revoluta* were examined mycologically. The specimens which included 10 samples of seed and/or endosperm during various stages of miso processing and one of bark were collected by Dr M. G. Whiting of the National Institutes of Health and shipped by air. Methods used for mycologic examination, for the most part, were similar to those used with the *C. circinalis*. Although the fungal isolates were screened for toxicity, infection in the treated mice rendered the results inconclusive. The distribution of various fungi is summarised in Table 8.

Macroscopic examination of the seeds of *C. revoluta*, even when freshly picked, showed a black discolouration typical of fungal proliferation at the absciss layer. Entire seeds from the factory supply were very mouldy, showing a brown to black fungal growth. When the seeds were incised, moulding extended from the absciss layer into the sub-epidermal tissues. Sliced seeds obtained from the factory supply likewise were badly discoloured and contained fungi which not only covered the surface layers, but penetrated deep into the underlying tissues. The endosperms of seeds ready for grinding likewise were heavily moulded, and even seeds that were subjected to vigorous washing also were heavily laden with fungal discolourations.

The freshly-picked seeds contained numerous hyaline and dark conidia, entire fructifications of a *Penicillium* species on the surface, and mycelial proliferation which extended into the sub-epidermal layers. Seeds from the factory supply superficially revealed an abundance of brown, echinulate conidia and fructifications of *Aspergillus niger*, and on some specimens, hyaline conidia and fructifications of Penicillia, as well as fuseaux, hyaline macroconidia typical of the genus *Fusarium*. Proliferative, septate mycelia were observed in the underlying tissues. Seeds ready for grinding showed primarily hyaline and brown conidia, and fructifications of *A. niger*. Although two samples of seeds were subjected to vigorous washing, this procedure did not remove fungal bodies. Both specimens superficially contained numerous fructifications of *A. niger*, and one in

Table 8

Distribution of Fungi in Seeds of *C. revoluta*

Fungus	Present/10 specimens
A. candidus	1
A. flavus	8
A. niger # 1	10
A. niger # 2	2
A. ochraceus	4
A. parasiticus	1
Fusarium spp.	2
P. purpurogenum	9
Penicillium spp.	1
Phoma spp.	2
Trichoderma spp.	1

addition showed fructifications of Aspergilli and Penicillia. Both samples contained hyaline, septate mycelia within the endosperms.

Cultural examination revealed that all seeds contained several unrelated fungi, practically all being representative of known toxigenic groups. This was particularly true of seeds that were washed and ready for grinding. As summarised in Table 8, a member of the *A. niger* group was present in all 10 samples of seeds, *P. purpurogenum* in 9, and *A. flavus* in 8.

6. *Mycologic examination of Zamia species*

Cattle in the Dominican Republic that have ingested leaves of *Zamia debilis*, develop an apparent neurologic syndrome called derringue, manifested clinically chiefly as a locomotor ataxia. Although various causes of derringue have been studied, the role of mycotoxins has not been investigated. Accordingly, leaves, stems, and rhizomes of *Zamia* spp. collected in

Florida and in the Dominican Republic were examined to determine whether these cycads might harbour a common fungus, hopefully toxigenic. Initially 6 samples of entire plant of *Zamia floridiana* were collected in Florida, shipped by air and upon receipt immediately subjected to detailed mycologic examination. Subsequently, 3 samples of fresh leaves and one of rhizome of *Z. debilis* collected in the Dominican Republic, and 6 samples of herbarium species of the same cycad were examined.

As with the other cycads, the specimens of *Zamia* were examined macroscopically, microscopically, and culturally. Two samples of rhizome of *Z. floridiana* were stored with the leaves and stem intact at room temperatures for 3 months and then examined mycologically. The various areas of the specimens listed in Table 9 were cultured in Petri plates on mycologic agars used in preceding studies as well as on an agar in which the rhizome of *Z. floridiana* was the sole source of nutriment. For the most part, cultural studies were performed before and after surface sterilisation. Surface sterilisation consisted of placing the specimen in 5% aqueous phenol for 5 minutes, and rinsing with 95% ethanol, and sterile distilled water, respectively. Mycologic findings are summarised in Table 9. The prevailing fungus, a species of *Mycosphaerella*, was cultured on Czapek's solution agar at room temperature for 28 days, and homogenates prepared and tested for toxicity in white Swiss mice. Preparation of homogenate and method of testing were the same as used in preceding studies; however, duration of the experiment was 35 days.

Upon stereo-microscopic examination, all 15 samples of leaves showed evidence of past or active fungal growth, and particularly presence of lesions containing perithecia. Upon compound microscopic examination, sections of all samples of leaves showed perithecia, together with proliferated hyaline mycelia within the sub-epidermal layers. These observations would suggest that the associated fungus is phytopathogenic. Furthermore, presence of perithecia within the fresh stems and presence of proliferative mycelia within the tissues further suggests phytopathogenicity of the fungus. The exterior surface of 7 rhizomes examined contained fungal structures indicative of a mixed flora. The interior of 6 fresh rhizomes collected from Florida contained no fungal bodies, but one collected from the Dominican Republic had mycelia indicative of more than one fungus species.

Culturally, although several fungal types were isolated before surface sterilisation from all of the specimens (except 5 samples of leaves of herbarium specimens which previously had been fixed in formalin and thus sterilised) after surface sterilisation of the remaining specimens, the *Mycosphaerella* species predominated in the specimens examined. As summarised in Table 9, this fungus predominated in 8 of 8 leaves, 6 of 8 stems, 7 of 7 rhizomes samples slightly below the epidermal layer, and in 1 rhizome sample from deep within the sub-epidermal layer. A species of

Table 9

Mycologic Findings in Specimens of *Zamia* Species
(Summary)

	(MICROSCOPIC FINDINGS)			
			Description of specimen	
			rhizome,	rhizome,
	Section of	Section of	shallow	deep
Fungal bodies present in	leaves	stem	subsurface	subsurface
Hyaline mycelia	15	6	–	1
Subhyaline mycelia	15	6	1	1
Dematiaceous mycelia	7	–	1	1
Fusiform macroconidia	2	–	1	–
Heavy-walled, 2-sectored				
conidia (ascospores)	2	–	1	–
Perithecia	15	6	1	1
No. of specimens examined	15	6	1	7

	(CULTURAL FINDINGS)			
			Rhizome,	Rhizome,
			shallow	deep
Fungi isolated from	Leaves*	Stem*	subsurface	subsurface
Fusarium spp.	7	6	7	–
Helminthosporium spp.	–	6	1	–
Mycosphaerella spp.	8†	6†	7†	1†
P. purpurogenum	6	–	6	–
Phoma spp.	1	–	1	–
No. of specimens examined	8	8	7	7

* Cultural findings after surface sterilisation.
† Fungus predominated.

Fusarium was isolated from 7 of 8 leaves, 6 of 8 stems, and 7 of 7 rhizomes.

The interior of 2 rhizomes of *Z. floridiana* after 3 months storage at room temperatures, macroscopically appeared dark grey with numerous black, sclerotial-like areas throughout the tissues, and upon microscopic examination numerous heavy-walled, dark brown mycelia and few hyaline mycelia were detected. After surface sterilisation, and upon culture the *Mycosphaerella* species predominated although a species of *Fusarium* and *Penicillium purpurogenum* were isolated.

Mice that were fed the *Mycosphaerella* sp. agar homogenate showed severe manifestations of a toxicosis. Anorexia and hypotonia which were slight on the 9th day, increased in intensity, and together with depression and apparent cachexia, were severe in intensity from the 11th day to the end of the study. Pronounced body weight losses occurred during the 2nd and 3rd weeks. Deaths began to occur during the 2nd week. Four mice died by the end of the 4th week, and all were dead by the 35th day. Grossly at necropsy, the paramount lesion was haemorrhage in various tissues.

DISCUSSION

It has long been known that various parts of the plant of members of the family Cycadaceae are toxic to man and animals. A comprehensive review of the chemical, ecological, and biological properties of various cycads has been compiled by Whiting.[1] According to various workers as cited by Whiting, cycad toxicosis occurs in both the acute and chronic form. In man, acute cycad poisoning develops soon after ingestion of large amounts of toxic cycad substratum. Symptoms of this form vary from minor discomfort to severe disturbances and frequently terminate fatally. The chronic form is characterised primarily by a 'neurologic' syndrome, involving an incapacitating paralysis. In animals, the acute form is characterised clinically, primarily by gastro-intestinal disturbances and, in some instances, intermittent tremors are observed in various muscles. The chronic form is characterised clinically by a neurologic syndrome which appears to manifest itself by locomotor difficulties in the form of a progressive, but irreversible, paralysis of the hind limbs. This neurological syndrome is observed only after the animal consumes leaves from cycads such as *Zamia debilis*.

The clinical and pathological manifestations observed in animals from field cases have been produced experimentally in animals in the past by feeding various parts of certain cycads and by feeding cycasin and/or its degradation products, as reported by Whiting[1] and Laquer *et al.*[4]. The latter described the clinical and pathological changes in rats fed a meal prepared from unwashed endosperm of *C. circinalis*. Rats that consumed sublethal amounts of the crude meal over prolonged periods of time developed benign and malignant neoplasms, chiefly in the liver and kidneys, but also in the lungs and intestines. Matsumoto[5] fractionated nuts of

C. *circinalis* and isolated methylazoxymethanol (MAM), a degradation product of cycasin, which was toxic when administered intravenously to animals. Cycasin at the same dose and by the same route was nontoxic, and thus differs biologically from the MAM.

Although cycasin and/or its toxic degradation products are present in unwashed cycads, and soaking and concurrent leaching in water or fermenting the sliced green endosperms apparently removes these toxic entities, examination of the literature[1, 6, 7] indicates that in some areas nonspecific fungi are frequently associated with processing of the cycad or inadvertently contaminate the endosperms. However, the cycadaceous substrata have not been subjected to mycologic and mycotoxic studies. That such substrata do indeed contain toxigenic fungi has been verified by this study. Of some 25 specimens of C. *circinalis* examined in Section 2 of this report, all contained lesions or other discoloured areas which contained fungal bodies indicative of past or current fungal proliferation. Cultural examination of 7 samples of washed, sliced endosperms revealed toxigenic fungi in all specimens. Of more importance, the washed cycad starch, when examined microscopically also contained fungal bodies, and on cultural examination a toxic strain each of A. *niger* and A. *flavus* predominated. Although many of the cycad slices showed areas of discolouration indicative of past or current fungal growth, there were some specimens which grossly appeared normal or showed slight discolouration, yet on microscopic and cultural examination revealed an abundance of toxigenic fungi. Examination of endosperms of C. *revoluta* used in miso processing showed that this cycad also contained toxigenic fungi. Of 9 samples of sliced endosperms examined, all were heavily contaminated with a wide variety of fungi, some of which were toxic to mice. Similarly, husks of C. *circinalis* which frequently are chewed by natives were found to be heavily laden with proliferative fungal structures and upon culture toxigenic fungi were isolated.

Although fungi have been observed on the cycads, both in the field and in the studies reported here, their implication to the health of man or animals consuming the cycad or its processed by-products has not been studied. Indeed, there appears to be some difference of opinion regarding the role of fungi in cycad toxicosis.[6] Whereas some individuals speculate that toxigenic fungi might indeed play a role in cycad toxicosis, there are others that maintain that fungi are unimportant in this toxicosis.

Fungi are used to detoxify the cycasin present in cycad endosperm, and although there are no quantitative data indicating the degree of detoxification following the fungal treatment, it is reasonable to assume that fungi, because of their highly complex biochemical potentialities, are capable of breaking down cycasin and other highly complex compounds. The question arises, however, whether these fungi, during their detoxification of cycasin,

E

may synthesise other substances of varying toxicity and physiological activity, not only from the cycasin but also from other cycad components. The possibility also exists that the fungi may convert the cycasin into another toxic component.

As indicated earlier, the chronic form of cycad toxicosis in animals is characterised by a neurologic syndrome. It is interesting to note that mice fed fungal substrata have shown neurologic disturbances, but the relationship of these to the neurologic abnormalities observed in chronic cycad toxicosis is obscure.

The following fungi produced the neurologic syndrome in mice: *A. niger* isolated from various specimens of *C. circinalis*, a similar strain of *A. niger* isolated from seeds of *C. revoluta*, as well as 2 strains of *Penicillium purpurogenum* and a species of *Fusarium* also isolated from the *C. revoluta*, and a species of *Mycosphaerella* isolated from the leaves, stem and rhizome of *Zamia debilis*.

Although toxigenic fungi have been isolated from the cycad specimens, the results do not indicate the presence of mycotoxins in cycads. It is, however, reasonable to speculate that mycotoxins could have been present. This assumption is based on the fact that mycotoxins have been found in toxigenic fungal spores and mycelia.[8-16] Microscopic examination of the cycad specimens in this study indicated presence of spores and mycelia characteristic of toxigenic fungi. It is interesting to note that the *A. flavus* isolated was the most toxic clinically. Most workers indicate that the mouse is, relatively speaking, not very sensitive to toxic strains of *A. flavus* isolated from peanuts and peanut products, or other natural substrata.[17] The strain of this fungus isolated from the cycad is highly toxic to the mouse. The difference in results obtained above may be due to production of a high titre of aflatoxin(s) by the cycad strain, or perhaps due to formation of another more toxic metabolite.

The haematological findings in the peripheral blood in mice obtained after 28 days of force-feeding of the fungal substrata are typical of mycotoxicity. Practically all fungal substrata induced a leucocytosis, with an increase in the neutrophilic series. In the *A. niger* groups of mice, in particular, there was a marked shift to the left with a concurrent appearance of myelocytes. These changes clearly indicate stimulation of the blood-forming elements in the haematopoietic centres. In addition to the above blood dyscrasias, mice in the *Phoma* group revealed a hypochromic anaemia. Interestingly, mice in some fungal groups appeared more or less normal clinically, but on haematologic examination of the peripheral blood showed dyscrasias. This observation indicates the importance of performing such studies on the peripheral blood before declaring a fungal isolate as nontoxic. In some of the well-established mycotoxicoses, particularly stachybotryotoxicosis and alimentary toxic aleukia, the only discrepancies in the clinically quiescent stage are found in the blood picture. These changes are frequently detected in the peripheral blood picture even before the toxin(s) has exerted damage to the bone marrow which can be detected histopathologically.

Fungi, some of which are toxigenic, are present in the cycad nut not only at the time it is picked, but also during various stages of processing. Examination of the fresh green entire nut of *C. circinalis* reveals that fungi appear early after the seed has been removed from the tree and are readily demonstrable at the absciss layer. These fungi readily proliferate and subsequently grow throughout the pulpy layer, forming complete fungal sporophores. As growth progresses, the entire pulpy layer disintegrates and on the adjacent endosperm covering, the fungi likewise proliferate. Although heavily moulded specimens would not be used for starch processing, they certainly serve as an excellent source of inoculum for the sliced endosperms during processing and subsequent drying and storage. Fungal contamination does occur during some stage(s) of processing as shown in results of this study.

Fungal bodies were also found in the refined cycad flour. Since the flour was finely ground, it was impossible to determine whether the fungal bodies were the result of surface contamination or of subsurface growth on the washed sliced endosperm.

According to Whiting[1] the husk of *C. circinalis* frequently is dried and chewed by natives. Four samples of fresh husk and 12 of milled husks showed, upon microscopic examination, conidia and fungal hyphae and, upon culture, several fungi representative of known toxigenic groups. Some samples of husk were extremely heavily laden with fungal bodies. The implications of these findings may be far reaching.

Some of the fungi isolated in this study, particularly the *C. lunata*, and the species each of *Phoma* and *Mycosphaerella*, are known phytopathogens to some plant species. Since it appears that cattle or sheep that graze certain cycad species leaves develop a 'neurologic' syndrome, and since some mycotoxins give rise to neurologic disturbances, phytotoxins may play a role in this cycad toxicosis. Examination of fresh, green leaves of *Zamia floridiana* and *Z. debilis* showed that all contained perithecia embedded within the tissues, and microscopically such areas revealed numerous, proliferative, subhyaline to dark mycelia particularly along the conducting tissues. From the infected tissues, a fungus was isolated which fell within the taxonomic limits of *M. tulasnei*.[18, 19] *M. tulasnei* is said to cause death of leaves of cycads,[20] when the grey spots are very numerous. This statement would imply that, unless the infection by this fungus were severe, casual examination alone would leave the fungus unnoticed. Thus, in the case of *Zamia* species, it appears justifiable to evaluate the possible role of phytotoxic fungi in cycad toxicosis.

In conclusion, the primary objective of this study, which indicated a need to determine whether toxigenic fungi are present in cycad substrata, has been attained. Moreover, fungi that have never been suspected of being toxic have been found highly toxic to mice when cultured on selected media. This is particularly true of the *Aspergillus tamarii, Curvularia lunata*, and the *Macrosporium* and *Phoma* species.

Although it has been established unequivocably that toxigenic fungi do exist in the cycad throughout all stages of handling, the exact significance of the findings reported here in cycad toxicosis as it exists in the field and under experimental conditions remains to be determined.

REFERENCES

1. WHITING, M. G. (1963). *Economic Botany*, **17**, (4) 271.
2. SARKISOV, A. KH. and ORSHANSKAIYA, V. N. (1944). *Veterinariya*, **21**, (2-3) 38.
3. FORGACS, J. and CARLL, W. T. (1964). *Fed. Proc.*, **23**, 1370.
4. LAQUER, G. L., MICKELSEN, O., WHITING, M. G. and KURLAND, L. T. (1963). *Nat. Cancer Inst.*, **31**, 919.
5. MATSUMOTO, H. and STRONG, F. G. (1963). *Arch. of Biochem. and Biophysics*, **101**, 299.
6. Conference on the Identification of Toxic Elements of Cycads—Plant Family, Cycadaceae. Transcript of Proceedings, Feb. 28, 1962 (National Institutes of Health, Bethesda, Md.), pp. 1-68.
7. Second Conference on the Identification of Toxic Elements of Cycads —Plant Family, Cycadaceae. Transcript of Proceedings, Aug. 17, 1962 (National Institutes of Health, Bethesda, Md.), pp. 1-109.
8. Anonymous (1958). *Lancet*, **2**, 701.
9. CARLL, W. T., FORGACS, J., HERRING, A. S. and MAHLANDT, B. G. (1955). *Vet. Med.*, **50**, 210.
10. SALIKOV, M. I. (1940). *Sovyet, Botan.*, **6**, 53.
11. VYSHELESSKI, S. N. (1948). In: *Special Epizootiology*, pp. 374-482. *Ogiz-Selskhozgiz*, Moskva.
12. JOFFE, A. Z. (1960). *Bull. Res. Council of Israel*, **9D**, 101.
13. THORNTON, R. H. and PERCIVAL, J. C. (1959). *Nature* (Lond.), **183**, 63.
14. THORNTON, R. H. and ROSS, D. J. (1959). *New Zealand J. Agr. Research*, **2**, 1002.
15. THORNTON, R. H. and SINCLAIR, D. P. (1960). *New Zealand J. Agr. Research*, **3**, 300.

16. PERCIVAL, J. C. (1959).   *New Zealand J. Agr. Research*, **2**, 1041.
17. ALLCROFT, R. and CARNAGHAN, R. B. A. (1963). *Chemistry and Industry* (Jan. 12), p. 50.
18. CLEMENTS, F. E. and SHEAR, C. L. (1954).   In: *The Genera of Fungi*. Hafner, New York.
19. STEVENS, F. L. (1913).   In: *The Fungi which Cause Plant Disease*.   The Macmillan Company, New York.
20. DODGE, B. O. and RICKETT, H. W. (1948).   In: *Diseases and Pests of Ornamental Plants*.   The Ronald Press, New York, N.Y.

FIELD SURVEY OF MYCOTOXIN-PRODUCING FUNGI CONTAMINATING HUMAN FOODSTUFFS IN JAPAN, WITH EPIDEMIOLOGICAL BACKGROUND

(I) Mycological and chemical aspects of the detection of mycotoxin producers

by

Hiroshi Kurata, Shun-ichi Udagawa, Masakatsu Ichinoe, Shinsaku Natori and Setsuko Sakaki

National Institute of Hygienic Sciences
Tokyo, Japan

Studies on mycotoxin-producing fungi contaminating foodstuffs have been carried out with the aim of disclosing the possible causative agents of human diseases, particularly of human cancer, in Japan. Several areas showing relatively high incidence of liver and stomach cancers were selected for this project, including one rural city in central Japan (Honshu district) and three towns or villages in southern Japan (Kyushu district). Nutritional and epidemiological investigations were also performed in addition to the collection of the foodstuffs in these areas. Final conclusions concerning this mycotoxin-epidemiological study have not yet been obtained but the mycological examination and some of the chemical assays for mycotoxins are nearly completed. The results of these studies will be presented here as the first report.

Localities of the survey and their background
Following the findings from the preliminary epidemiological investigation, four localities have been selected for this survey: Saku City, Nagano Prefecture (located in the central part of Honshu district) where the highest incidence of hypertension and gastric cancer have been estimated. Most of the inhabitants consist of farm families with highland surroundings. The other two localities, i.e. Minamikushiyama village and Tomie-cho, both in Nagasaki Prefecture, have been incriminated with the high incidence of liver diseases following a clinical survey by the research group of the Medical School, University of Nagasaki. Setouchi-machi, Amaniôshima, is situated about 300 km away from Kyushu district, but it belongs to Kagoshima Prefecture. Tomie-cho is also located on a small island named Goto, and the people are the coastal families of fishermen and those engaged in agriculture combined with fishery production. Among the localities

surveyed, no obvious case of human mycotoxicosis has been reported so far. From the nutritional surveys there was no characteristic food habit among the four localities except in Setouchi, Amami-island, where the people are known to eat cycad-starch as material for miso production. All the inhabitants investigated daily eat rice, wheat and some kinds of flour similar to the staple food generally used in Japan. It appeared, if anything, that the Minamikushiyam people consume more fish products than the people from other areas. This was not seen in the Tomie people although they are living in a coastal area. Collecting trips took place on the following dates: Saka, July in 1967 and June in 1968; Minamikushiyama, September in 1967; Setouchi, July in 1968; and Tomie, August in 1968.

Sampling procedure and mycological examination for foodstuffs

For the sampling of foodstuffs, families with cancer cases were taken into consideration. The families were selected by random sampling for this

Table 1

Number of Foodstuffs Examined for their Mycoflora

Kinds of foodstuffs:	Localities surveyed					
	Saku (I) 1967	Saku (II) 1968	Minami-kushiyama 1967	Setouchi 1968	Tomie 1968	Total
Rice	16	11	12	13	24	76
Wheat	—	—	—	—	5	5
Wheat flour	—	5	5	5	15	30
Other flours	—	—	10	—	—	10
Legumes	—	15	4	—	8	27
Miso (Soybean paste)	52	13	9	14	20	108
Moromi (mash)	3	8	—	—	—	11
Soysauce	17	3	2	—	5	27
Dried small sardines	—	—	10	—	8	18
Katsuobushi	—	—	—	—	6	6
Cycas starch	—	—	—	3	—	3
Vegetable pickles	13	11	5	—	—	29
Nukamiso*	3	—	—	—	—	3
Miscellaneous	—	6	9	8	9	32
Total	104	72	66	43	100	385

* Nukamiso (pickled vegetables in a mixture of rice grain, salt and water) is a kind of fermented pickle.

investigation and the families showing a high incidence of cancer mortality were also investigated. A total of 240 families were visited for sampling throughout the surveys and 1057 food samples were collected for mycological examination. As our laboratory facilities are limited, composite samples were made from the original samples. The sampling was performed under good sanitary conditions and the samples, except starch foods, were placed into the cold-container with dry ice and brought immediately to the laboratory for examination. The number and kinds of samples examined are listed in Table 1.

Mycological examination was conducted in the following manner: For grain examination the grain culture method which had been established in our laboratory was employed.[1] Semi-solid or powdered types of foodstuffs were tested by the dilution plate method recommended by the USDA.[2] For examination of miso and other salted foods the MY20 and 40 agar were used for the detection of osmophylic fungi.

METHOD

Preparation for biological assay and chemical assay for mycotoxin-producing fungi

For biological assay[3] conducted by the research group of the Institute of Medical Sciences, University of Tokyo, culture filtrate and chloroform extracts were prepared in our laboratory. The fungi tested were cultured with modified Czapek-Dox, 20% glucose-Czapek, MY20, and potato dextrose for 3 weeks at 25°C, in a stationary condition. The cultures (160 ml) were extracted with chloroform, which was then evaporated. They were stored at 4°C for 1 to 3 weeks before toxicity tests were carried out. Fungal cultures showing toxic effects by biological assay were examined chemically for mycotoxin content by a suitable mycotoxin assay.[4-6]

RESULTS

A total of 2940 strains of fungi have been isolated as food contaminants. Mycoflora of the food samples comprised the two common genera of *Aspergillus* and *Penicillium* which are generally called storage fungi. Generally no mixed fungal contamination was found among the foodstuffs examined. From a view of frequency of occurrence of fungi, it was apparent that the starch foods such as rice, cereals, flour and so on, showed relatively higher fungal contamination than fish products. On the other hand, fermented and salted or brined foods harboured a small number of fungi. During the course of the surveys, we often encountered aged miso, the surface of which were covered with various kinds of fungal colonies. Detailed examination of these fungi indicated that most of the isolates were *Aspergillus oryzae*, *Mucor* spp., but some other genera, and yeasts were also isolated. It is of interest that yeasts were commonly found in miso as one of the components of its mycoflora. Legumes and their products were mainly affected by plant pathogenic fungi belonging to the fungi imperfecti.

The following genera and species of fungi were found to be dominant species:

Rice grain: *Penicillium phoeniceum, Aspergillus repens, Aspergillus versicolor.*
Wheat grain: *A. glaucus* group, *P. citrinum, P. cyclopium.*
Flours: *P. waksmani, P. citrinum, P. viridicatum, A. ochraceus.*
Miso: *A. flavus, A. ochraceus, P. waksmani, Mucor, Rhizopus.*
Moromi: *A. sydowi, A. flavus, Mucor.*
Legumes: *A. ochraceus, Fusarium, Phoma, Cladosporium.*
Vegetable pickles: *Yeasts, Geotrichum, Candida, A. flavus.*

Table 2

Distribution of Mycotoxin-producing Fungi in Foodstuffs Collected
from Four Localities Surveyed

Mycotoxin-producing fungi	Possible production of mycotoxin	Saku	Saku	Minami-kushiyama	Setouchi	Tomie
A. clavatus	patulin, ascladiol		+	+		+
A. flavus	aflatoxins	+	+	+	+	+
A. ochraceus	ochratoxin A, penicillic acid		+	+	+	+
A. fumigatus	fumigatin	+	+	+	+	+
A. versicolor	sterigmatocystin	+	+	+	+	+
Chaetomium globosum	—		+	+	+	+
P. citreo-viride, *P. ochrasalmoneum*	citreoviridin	+	+	+	+	
P. citrinum	citrinin	+	+	+	+	+
P. cyclopium ⎫ *P. puberulum* ⎬	cyclopiazonic acid	+	+	+	+	+
P. implicatum	citrinin	+			+	+
P. islandicum	cyclochlorotine luteoskyrin		+	+		
P. roqueforti			+			+
P. rugulosum	rugulosin	+	+	+		+
P. viridicatum	—	+	+	+		+
P. urticae	patulin					+
Fusarium spp.	butenolide scirpenols		+	+	+	+
Pithomyces chartarum	sporidesmin			+		+
P. purpurogenum	rubratoxin B	+	+	+	+	

Dried fishes: *A. ochraceus, A. glaucus* group, *A. restrictus.*

Katsuobushi: *A. glaucus* group, *A. ochraceus, P. cyclopium, A. flavus,*
                        Phoma.

Cycad starch: *A. niger, A. flavus.*

There were some minor differences in the dominant species from similar kinds of foodstuffs collected from different localities. This is not a significant finding when the relationship between human mycotoxicosis and their geographical occurrence is considered.

Distribution of possible mycotoxin-producing fungi

Distribution of possible mycotoxin-producing fungi in the four localities is shown in Table 2. Of the fungi listed in this table, ten strains of *Aspergillus flavus*, two strains of *Aspergillus ochraceus*, 28 strains of *Aspergillus* and *Penicillium*, and one strain of *Penicillium purpurogenum* were proved to have the ability to produce aflatoxins, ochratoxin A, penicillic acid and rubratoxin B, respectively. Although actual distribution of mycotoxin-producing fungi has not been determined yet, it was of interest that fungi suspected of mycotoxin production were widely distributed in the localities. We would point out that our joint research group has made the first discovery of ochratoxin A and rubratoxin-producing fungi from foodstuffs in Japan in the past few years. Work on the biological assay method will be described in the second part of this report.

DISCUSSION

Our study is concentrating on obtaining clearer information about the relation of mycotoxin contamination in foodstuffs to human diseases. Therefore, final conclusions cannot be drawn as only the mycoflora and some of the distribution of foodborne fungi have been reported.

From the results of our investigation, it is apparent that possible and real mycotoxin-producing fungi are widely distributed in the foodstuffs which were sampled from the four localities. Moreover, it is well known that such contaminating fungi sometimes appear as the dominant species. These facts seem to suggest that, as long as rice, or some other starch foods are the staple foods, the possibility of mycotoxin poisoning in humans cannot be ruled out. We would emphasise here again the significance of the mycotoxin hazard in the field of food hygiene in Japan. A survey for natural mycotoxin contamination in the starch foods by chemical assay should be undertaken in the next phase of our study. Finally, judging from the mycological study, the following mycotoxins and their producing fungi will be marked for future study: Aflatoxins, ochratoxin, sterigmatocystin, citrinin, *Fusarium*-toxins and penicillic acid.

REFERENCES

1. KURATA, H., UDAGAWA, S., ICHINOE, M., KAWASAKI, Y., TAKADA, M., TAZAWA, M., KOIZUM, A. and TANABE, H. (1968). *J. Food Hyg. Soc. of Japan*, **9**, 23.
2. HESSELTINE, C. W., GRAVES, R. R., ROGERS, RUTH and BURMEISTER, H. R. (1969). *Appl. Microbiol.*, **18**, 848.
3. SAITO, M., UMEDA, M., OHTSUBO, K., KURATA, H., UDAGAWA, S. and NATORI, S. Proc. Japan. Cancer Assoc., the 27th Ann. Meeting, p. 59 (October, 1968, Tokyo).
4. KURATA, H., TANABE, H., KANOTA, K., UDAGAWA, S. and ICHINOE, M. (1968). *J. Food Hyg. Soc. of Japan*, **9**, 29.
5. NATORI, S., SAKAKI, S., KURATA, H., UDAGAWA, S., ICHINOE, M. SAITO, M., UMEDA, M. and OHTSUBO, K. (1970). *Appl. Microbiol.*, **19**, 613.
6. NATORI, S., SAKAKI, S., KURATA, H., UDAGAWA, S., ICHINOE, M., SAITO, M. and UMEDA, M. In preparation.

ISOLATION OF
ASPERGILLUS OCHRACEUS PRODUCING
OCHRATOXINS FROM JAPANESE RICE

by

Mikio Yamazaki

Institute of Food Microbiology, Chiba University, Chiba, Japan

Ochratoxin A, first investigated by van der Merwe *et al.*,[1] is a toxic metabolite of certain strains of *Aspergillus ochraceus* Wilh., which is found on African cereals and legume products. The fungi belonging to the group of *Aspergillus ochraceus* are widely distributed in various agricultural products and have been studied as they frequently produce biologically active compounds.

In the course of our investigation on the survey and isolation of toxigenic fungi on rice in this country during 1968-1969, 457 strains of *Aspergillus ochraceus* out of a total of 1721 Aspergilli were isolated (Table 1).

We would like to describe the isolation of the ochratoxin-producing strains and the production of the toxin under various nutritional conditions.

Isolation of ochratoxin-producing strains

A total of 634 samples of polished and unpolished rice from Chiba and Miyagi Prefectures were collected. Ten grams from each sample were weighed in Erlenmeyer flasks and washed with ten successive volumes of sterilised distilled water to remove the surface contamination. Fifty grains from each sample were placed on peptoné-glucose agar plates containing 100 mg per litre of chloramphenicol (five grains into each of 10 Petri dishes). The plates were incubated at 25°C for 5 to 6 days and inspected daily. The colonies which had developed on grains were counted and transferred to potato-dextrose agar (PDA) slants and the isolates were maintained on PDA or Czapek agar containing 20% sucrose.

The genera found on rice are listed in Table 1. Twenty-one species of Aspergillus and 36 species of Penicillium were identified. Among the species of Aspergillus, *Aspergillus ochraceus* and *Aspergillus versicolor* were found to be dominant as shown in Table 2.

To prepare the samples for toxicity tests, 58 strains of *Aspergillus ochraceus* were selected randomly and each cultured on 200 g of rice. Fifty grams of rice and 25 ml of water were dispensed into each of four Erlenmeyer flasks, which were autoclaved for 20 minutes at 120°C and then

Table 1

The Fungi found growing on the Mouldy Rice in Japan

Numbers of grains examined	31700
Numbers of *Aspergillus* found	1721
Numbers of *A. ochraceus* found	457

PHYCOMYCETES
 Cunninghamella   *Rhizopus*
 Mucor   *Syncephalastrum*

ASCOMYCETES
 Chaetomium   *Aspergillus*
 Neurospora   *Penicillium*

ASPERGILLUS
 A. clavatus   *A. niger*
 repens   *candidus*
 ruber   *flavus*
 chevalieri   *oryzae*
 amstelodami   *tamarii*
 montevidensis   *versicolor*
 mangini   *sydowi*
 umbrosus   *nidulans*
 restrictus   *ustus*
 fumigatus   *terreus*
 ochraceus

PENICILLIUM
 P. adametzii   *P. namyslowskii*
 charlesii   *notatum*
 chrysogenum   *ochraceum*
 citreo-viride   *oxalicum*
 citrinum   *palitans*
 claviforme   *paxilli*
 corymbiferum   *phoeniceum*
 cyaneo-fulvum   *puberulum*
 cyclopium   *restrictum*
 decumbens   *roqueforti*
 fellutanum   *roseo-purpureum*
 frequentans   *rugulosum*
 funiculosum   *steckii*
 herquei   *tardum*
 implicatum   *urticae*
 islandicum   *vinaceum*
 meleagrinum   *viridicatum*
 multicolor   *waksmani*

FUNGI IMPERFECTI
 Acrotheca   *Cladosporium*
 Alternaria   *Curvularia*
 Arthrinium   *Cylindrocarpon*
 Candida   *Epicoccum*
 Cephalosporium   *Fumago*
 Chaetomella   *Fusarium*

Table 1—*contd.*

FUNGI IMPERFECTI—*contd.*

Fusidium	*Phoma*
Geotrichum	*Piricauda*
Gliocladium	*Piricularia*
Gliomastix	*Sclerotinia*
Helminthosporium	*Scopulariopsis*
Hemispora	*Stemphylium*
Hormiscium	*Trichoderma*
Monilia	*Trichothecium*
Myrothecium	*Verticillium*
Nigrospora	*Zygosporium*
Paecilomyces	

Table 2

Species of Aspergillus isolated from the Rice Grains

	Numbers of grains contaminated		Numbers of grains contaminated
A. clavatus	5	*A. niger*	10
repens	203	*candidus*	168
ruber	9	*flavus-oryzae*	47
chevalieri	91	*tamarii*	66
amstelodami	88	*versicolor*	525
montevidensis	1	*sydowi*	11
mangini	11	*nidulans*	3
umbrosus	1	*ustus*	1
restrictus	4	*terreus*	8
fumigatus	9	sp.	3
ochraceus	457	Total	1721

seeded with each strain. The flasks were incubated in dark for nine days at 27°C with occasional shaking.

The mycelia grown on rice were extracted repeatedly with ethyl acetate (EtOAc). The solvent was evaporated *in vacuo*. The extracts thus prepared were weighed and dissolved in a given volume of propylene glycol (PG). This solution was injected intraperitoneally into mice, or into the yolk sac of chick embryos through the air cell.

At 24 and 48 hours, and seven days after administration of the sample the mortality in the mice and chick embryos was observed. As a result, two strains, MR 31-1 and MTR 26-1 out of 22 toxigenic strains, were found to be strongly toxic for both mice and chick embryos. The mortality of 100% at 24 hours was observed in administration of the sample extract at 10 mg/0·1 ml PG to the mouse and 1 mg/0·2 ml to the chick embryo.

The two strongly toxic strains obtained were further cultured in a semi-synthetic medium containing 4% sucrose and 2% yeast extract[2] to examine their ability to produce ochratoxins. The culture filtrate was adjusted to pH 3.0 with dilute HCl and extracted with $CHCl_3$. The $NaHCO_3$-soluble part of the extract was then fractionated by silica-gel column chromatography. The crude ochratoxin A in the eluted fraction was crystallised from benzene. The crystalline ochratoxin A, m.p. 92°C, proved to possess chemical and physical properties completely identical to those reported by van der Merwe et al.[1] The production of ochratoxin A by the two strains was thus confirmed.

The production of ochratoxin A on rice and liquid media

Ochratoxin A, like aflatoxin B_1, has the property of being fluorescent, so that a spot of ochratoxin A developed by thin-layer chromatography (TLC) can easily be detected by its strong fluorescence under ultraviolet light. Steyn and van der Merwe[3] used TLC to estimate the amounts of ochratoxin A contained in the mouldy materials. In their method the size of the fluorescent spots was compared with that of a standard ochratoxin A spot when both were developed together. Scott and Hand[4] also described a TLC method for estimating the contents of ochratoxin A. Using a similar method, Ferreira[5] and Davis et al.[2] studied the effect of various carbon and nitrogen sources added to a semi-synthetic medium upon ochratoxin A production by Aspergillus ochraceus.

Ferreira[5] obtained a maximal yield of ochratoxin A (100 mg/l) when a basal medium containing 3% sucrose was supplemented with 1% glutamic acid as a nitrogen source. Davis et al.[2] found further that the addition of 4% sucrose and 2% yeast extract to the basal medium enhanced the production of the toxin in a stationary culture, attaining a yield of 290 mg/l.

A TLC method has been adapted for estimating the ochratoxin A content of mouldy materials in this laboratory, and a simple TLC-fluorodensitrometric method was developed. Each sample solution was spotted on silica-gel plate and developed with benzene-methanol-ethylacetate (15:3:1) solvent system. The greenish-blue fluorescent spot (R_f 0.31) of ochratoxin A was located under ultraviolet light. The developed plate was placed on the stage of a fluorodensitometer, Ozumor SD-91 (Asuka Kogyo Co., Tokyo), at such position that the spot of ochratoxin A would be in the light path. The plate was scanned at a wavelength of 333 mμ for excitation to read the intensity of fluorescence of each spot and the intensity was recorded on a chart by the integrator attached to the densitometer.

Densitometric readings in response to various quantities of ochratoxin A on a TLC plate are illustrated in Figure 1. A linear correlation is observed between 0 and 5 μg of the toxin. Since the smallest quantity of the toxin that the densitometer detects was approximately 0·17 μg/spot, the amounts of the toxin to be spotted on a TLC plate should be in a range between 0·17 and 5 μg. The reading did not change, on the other hand, after the plate was allowed to stand for 1, 2 or 3 hours or even for 4 days in dark at room temperature.

The amounts of ochratoxin A produced on rice by the two toxigenic strains, determined by the present method are shown in Table 3.

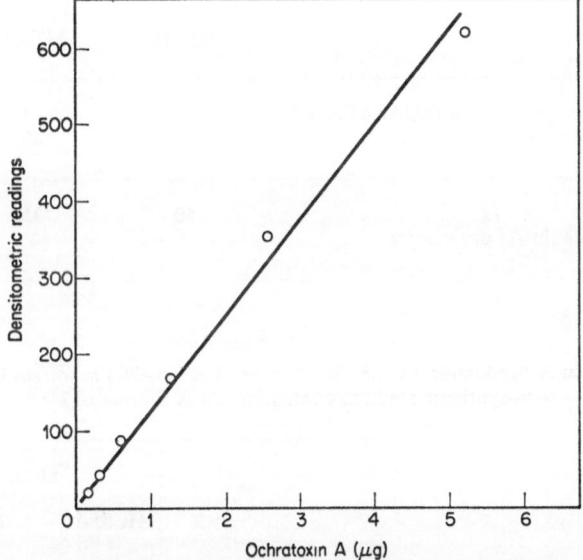

FIG. 1. Relation of fluorodensitometric readings to the amount of ochratoxin A on TLC.

The strain MR 31-1 produced the toxin in quantity approximately three times larger than that produced by the strain MTR 26-1; the amounts of the toxin per gram of gummy solid that was prepared by evaporation of the solvent from ethyl acetate extract were, however, calculated to be 50 and 35 mg, respectively.

The results of similar experiments with culture in semi-synthetic liquid media are shown in Table 4. The strain MR 31-1 produced a larger amount of ochratoxin A than did the strain MTR 26-1 in the liquid media.

In the experiment in which some nutritional factors affecting the toxin production by *Aspergillus ochraceus* were examined, the effect of the addition of various nitrogen sources or growth factors such as yeast extract, polypeptone and malt extract to the basal medium was investigated. From the result shown in Table 5, it is apparent that polypeptone is as effective

MIKIO YAMAZAKI

as yeast extract in stimulating toxin production. However, no effect after addition of malt extract was observed. A marked increase in the yield of the toxin was observed by the addition of 1 % L-phenylalanine to a semi-

Table 3

Ochratoxin A Production by the Two Strains of
Aspergillus ochraceus on Rice

| | | Strain | |
		MR 31-1	MTR 26-1
Residual solid from EtOAc extr. g		2·70	1·15
Ochratoxin A	mg	135	40·3
mg / g Ochratoxin A / dry extract		50	35

Table 4

Ochratoxin A Production by the Two Strains of *Aspergillus ochraceus* in a
semi-synthetic medium containing Yeast Extract of 2%

| | | Strain | |
		MR 31-1	MTR 26-1
pH—Initial		5·9	5·9
Final		6·8	6·2
Dry weight of mycelium	g*	20·2	25·4
Residual solid from CHCl₂ extr. of mycelium	mg*	366	585
Ochratoxin A from mycelium	mg*	30	10
Ochratoxin A from culture filtrate	mg*	240	190

* All figures indicating weight show the yield per litre.

synthetic medium. As large amount as 600 mg of ochratoxin A, for example, was produced by the fungi in 1 litre of a medium containing 2% yeast extract and 1% L-phenylalanine (Table 5). The result of Ferreira's experiment[5] showed that the production was not affected by the addition

Table 5

Ochratoxin A Production by *Aspergillus ochraceus* MR 31-1 in
Response to the Different Nitrogen Sources

		Growth factor added		
		2% Yeast extract	2% Poly-peptone	2% Malt extract	2% Yeast extract +L-Phe
pH—Initial		5·9	6·0	4·8	6·2
Final		7·6	7·8	4·8	7·5
Dry weight of mycelium	g*	19	19	4	25·4
Residual solid from CHCl₃ extr. of mycelium	mg*	345	279	115	484
Ochratoxin A from mycelium	mg*	32	32	trace	44
Ochratoxin A from culture filtrate	mg*	240	384	trace	608

* All figures indicating weight show the yield per litre.
L-Phe—γ-phenylalanine.

of phenylalanine as a sole source of nitrogen. However, phenylalanine appears to increase the yield of the toxin, as ochratoxin contains this amino acid as a structural component.

It seems very plausible, from the result obtained in the present experiment, that L-phenylalanine actually takes part in biosynthesis of ochratoxin A by *Aspergillus ochraceus*. In fact, the incorporation of phenylalanine-1-14C into the amino acid moiety of ochratoxin A was observed in an isotopic tracer experiment by Searcy et al.[6]

Metabolites of *Aspergillus ochraceus* other than ochratoxin A were isolated and found toxigenic in this laboratory; secalonic acid A, a yellow phenolic compound, ergosterol, a neutral metabolite, emodin, a colouring matter and erythritol, a sugar alcohol, were isolated. The final identification of these compounds was performed by mixed fusion and comparing their chemical and spectral properties with those of the authentic samples. Although the isolation of secalonic acid from *Aspergillus ochraceus* has not been reported so far, this compound is generally detected from all of the rice cultures of 58 strains examined.

REFERENCES

1. VAN DER MERWE, K. J., STEYN, P. S., FOURIE, L., SCOTT, DE B. and THERON, J. J. (1965). *Nature* (Lond.), **205**, 1112.
   VAN DER MERWE, K. J., STEYN, P. S. and FOURIE, L. (1965). *J. Chem. Soc.*, 7083.
2. DAVIS, N. D., SEARCY, J. W. and DIENER, U. L. (1969). *Appl. Microbiol.*, **17**, 742-744.
3. STEYN, P. S. and VAN DER MERWE, K. J. (1966). *Nature* (Lond.), **211**, 418.
4. SCOTT, P. M. and HAND, T. B. (1967). *J. Ass. Offic. Anal. Chem.*, **50**, 366.
5. FERREIRA, N. P. (1967). Recent advances in research on ochratoxin. Part 2. Microbiological aspects, 157-168. In: *Biochemistry of some Foodborne Microbial Toxins* (Eds. Mateles, R. I. and Wogan, G. N.). MIT Press, Cambridge, Mass.
6. SEARCY, J. W., DAVIS, N. D. and DIENER, U. L. (1969). *Appl. Microbiol.*, **18**, 622.

PRODUCTION OF CITREOVIRIDIN, A NEUROTOXIC MYCOTOXIN OF *PENICILLIUM CITREO-VIRIDE* BIOURGE*

by

Yoshio Ueno

*Microbial Chemistry, Faculty of Pharmaceutical Sciences,
Science University of Tokyo, Ichigaya, Tokyo, Japan*

In 1940, Miyake *et al.*[1] discovered toxic yellowed rice infected with a *Penicillium* sp. which was designated as *P. toxicarium* Miyake sp.var.[2] and later was identified as *P. citreo-viride* Biourge. Uraguchi[3, 4, 5, 6] has carried out extensive toxicological and epidemiological investigations on the mouldy rice as a causative factor in acute cardiac beriberi (Shoshin-kakke) which was prevalent in Japan in the past. He demonstrated that:

(1) the ethanol extract of *P. citreo-viride* Biourge was actually neurotoxic to several animals, causing the same symptoms as those noted in acute cardiac beriberi;

(2) a marked drop in the high incidence of 'Shoshin-kakke' in Japan occurred in 1910 although the discovery of vitamins occurred 1 year later and their usage in practical medicine only a further 10 years later, indicating that avitaminosis is not acceptable as a reasonable theory for the cause of 'Shoshin-kakke';

(3) when rice inspection conducted by the Ministry of Agriculture was introduced in major rice-producing districts in about 1910 the high incidence of 'Shoshin-kakke' also decreased. Thus, intake of ungraded rice or mouldy rice is presumably a suspected causative factor in the disease.[6] For these reasons Dr Uraguchi,[6, 7, 8] has stressed that acute cardiac beriberi is caused by mycotoxic intoxication originating from the metabolite(s) of *P. citreo-viride* Biourge.

In the present paper, the author attempted to isolate and purify the neurotoxic agent from rice grains polluted by *P. citreo-viride* Biourge, and the results obtained indicated that *P. citreo-viride* Biourge actually produced a neurotoxic mycotoxin on rice and that the isolate was chemically identical with citreoviridin which was isolated by Sakabe *et al.*[9] Environmental factors influencing the production of the mycotoxin were also investigated.

* This investigation was partly aided by the Grant for Cancer Research (1968-1969) from the Ministry of Welfare.

MATERIALS AND METHODS

Culture and inoculum

Penicillium citreo-viride Biourge, strain 4091, which was kindly supplied by Dr Tsunoda (from the Food Research Institute of the Ministry of Agriculture and Forestry), was utilised throughout these experiments. Inoculum was grown on Czapek agar and incubated at 20°C for at least 7 days before use. A spore suspension was prepared by adding 5 ml of sterile de-ionised water per slant, gently scraping the surface of the agar with a sterile loop and then vigorously shaking the slant by hand. Spore suspensions thus obtained were filtered over sterile glass wool to eliminate contaminating fungal hyphae and small pieces of agar.

Fermentation on rice

The substrate was polished rice grains used at the rate of 200 g per petri dish (21 cm in diameter). The rice grains were allowed to stand for 30 min in tap water and autoclaved for 20 min at 15 p.s.i. After cooling, the rice was inoculated with 1·0 ml spore suspension per dish and incubated in a dark room for 3 weeks at 20-24°C. After incubation, the yellowed rice was dried at 52-53°C for 2 days, crushed in a mortar and stored in a dark desiccator until used.

Liquid culture of the fungus

Erlenmeyer flasks (500 ml) containing 100-150 ml of a liquid medium were sterilised for 20 min, and 10^4-10^5 conidia were inoculated in duplicate and incubated in stationary flasks for various intervals at different temperatures. For mass production of the toxin, petri dishes (21 cm in diameter), each containing 200 ml of medium, were used. After the cultivation, the mycelium were first washed with the de-ionised water, then dried at 60-70°C overnight, and powdered in a mortar.

Chemical analysis

Plates for thin-layer chromatography were coated with Kieselgel G to a thickness of 0·25 mm, developed with 1:1 (v/v) *n*-hexane-acetone or 3:1 (v/v) ethylacetate-toluene, and inspected under ultraviolet light (365 mμ).

Toxicity test

The crude or purified toxins were dissolved in olive oil and administered intraperitoneally or subcutaneously to mice, and the mortality and time of death of the mice were recorded.

RESULTS

Isolation of the neurotoxin from the mouldy rice

Using mortality in mice as an index of toxicity, the isolation and purifi-

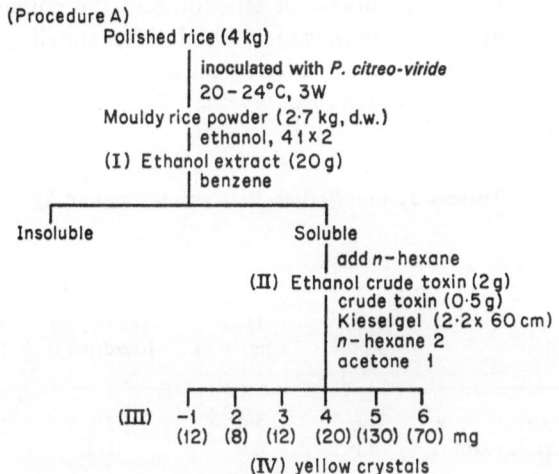

FIG. 1. Isolation of the neurotoxin from *P. citreo-viride*-moulded rice.

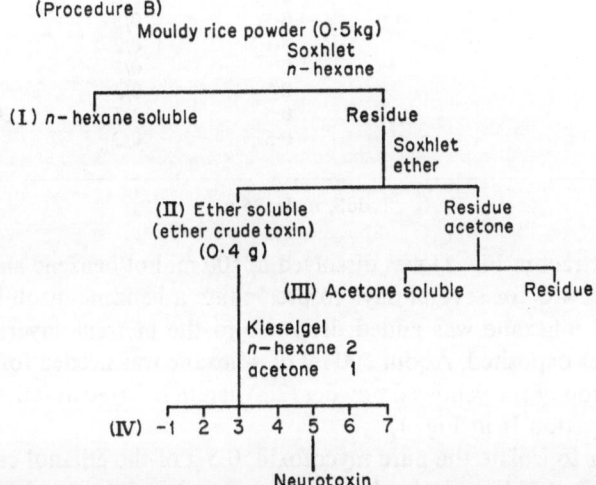

FIG. 2. Isolation of the neurotoxin from *P. citreo-viride*-moulded rice.

cation of the neurotoxin from the mouldy rice were carried out, as illustrated in Figures 1, 2 and Tables 1, 4.

Procedure A :

(a) *Isolation.* The mouldy rice powder, 2·7 kg, was mixed with two volumes of ethanol (about 5 l) and after four hours with occasional shaking a deeply yellowed supernatant was decanted. The residue was then extracted with the same volume of ethanol, and the combined ethanol solution was concentrated *in vacuo* to 200 ml. After standing at 4°C overnight, the white precipitate was filtered off and the yellow solution was further condensed almost to dryness *in vacuo*. The oily residue (Fraction 1,

Table 1

Toxicity Test on Various Fractions (Procedure A)

SAMPLE (*a*)

Fraction	Route	Dose (mg/10 g)	Death rate (dead/used)	Time of death (min)
(1) Ethanol extract	i.p.	5·0	3/3	
(2) Ethanol crude toxin	i.p.	2·0	2/2	8, 26
		1·0	2/2	12, 20
		0·5	2/2	30, 30
		0·25	2/2	50, 60
		0·125	1/2	60
		0·06	0/2	
(3)—1	i.p.	0·5	0/3	
2		0·5	0/2	
3		0·5	0/3	
4		0·5	0/3	
5		0·5	3/3	20, 25, 40
6		0·5	0/3	

ddS, male, 25 g

ethanol extract in Fig. 1) was dissolved in 100 ml hot benzene and allowed to stand at 4°C for several days to precipitate a benzene-insoluble brown oil. When *n*-hexane was added dropwise to the benzene layer, yellowed precipitates deposited. About 300 ml of *n*-hexane was needed for complete precipitation of the yellowed powder (2 g) herein referred as 'ethanol crude toxin' (Fraction II in Fig. 1).

In order to isolate the pure mycotoxin, 0·5 g of the ethanol crude toxin was applied on a Kieselgel column (2·2 × 60 cm) and the development was carried out with 2 litres of 2:1 (v/v) *n*-hexane-acetone with 50 ml fractions. When the yellow powder (130 mg) of the Fraction III-5 was dissolved in 1 ml of methanol and stood at 4°C for several days, yellow needles (25 mg) were obtained.

(b) *Toxicity*. Each fraction and the isolate were dissolved in olive oil and administered to mice. As illustrated in Table 1, the ethanol extract (Fraction I) and ethanol crude toxin (Fraction II) were lethal to mice at the intraperitoneal dose of 5·0 and 0·2-0·5 mg/10 g, respectively.

Table 2

Acute Toxicity of 'Ethanol Crude Toxin' on Mice

SAMPLE (*b*)

Route	Dose (mg/10 g)	Death rate (dead/used)	Time of death (min)
s.c.	2·0	3/3	70, 182, 200
	1·0	0/3	
i.p.	2·0	3/3	17, 18, 20
	1·3	3/3	26, 30, 30
	1·0	2/3	37, 40
	0·67	3/3	34, 53, 55

ddS, female, 30 g

SAMPLE (*c*)

Route	Dose (mg/10 g)	Death rate (dead/used)	Time of death (min)
s.c.	1·0	3/3	44, 68, 52
	0·5	3/3	65, 43, 70
i.p.	1·0	3/3	14, 16, 23
	0·5	3/3	34, 22, 25
	0·25	3/3	35, 40, 45
	0·10	0/3	

ddS, male, 15 g

Further purification by chromatography revealed that 0·5 mg/10 g of fraction III-5 was fatal to mice within 20-40 min of injection. Using the other lots of the crude toxin, the lethal toxicity was examined by different routes of administration. As shown in Table 2, the s.c. LD_{100} was around 0·5-1·0 mg/10 g, and the i.p. LD_{100} was around 0·25-0·7. These results indicated that the s.c. LD of the neurotoxin was about twice as high as that of the i.p. LD.

In Table 3, the lethal toxicity of the pure mycotoxin (Fraction IV) is listed, and the subcutaneous lethal dose is about 0·2 mg/10 g or 20 mg/kg. The first symptom in the mice administered the fractions was a paralysis

Table 3

Acute Toxicity of the Pure Neurotoxin to Mice

Route	Dose (mg/10 g)	Death rate (dead/used)	Time of death (min)
s.c.	1·0	1/1	42
	0·5	2/2	88, 230
	0·3	2/2	229, 80
	0·2	2/2	174, 225
	0·1	0/2	

ddS, male, 26-27 g

appearing in the lower legs and tail within several minutes of the i.p. injection. This paralysis was then observed in the forelegs and neck, and the mice lay on the floor and died with respiratory arrest. In the mice injected subcutaneously with the crude or pure toxin, a marked convulsion was noted. This ascending type of paralysis and convulsion were similar to those observed by Uraguchi who used an ethanol extract of *P. toxicarium* Miyake-moulded rice.[4]

Procedure B:

(a) *Isolation*. The mouldy rice powder (0·5 kg) was extracted continuously first with 200 ml of *n*-hexane for 2 days in a large Soxhlet extractor (12 × 70 cm), then with the same volume of ether, and finally with acetone. The ether soluble fraction (0·7 g) was dissolved in 50 ml of hot methanol and allowed to stand at 4°C overnight, and the clear supernatant was concentrated to dryness. The yellow powder (0·4 g) thus obtained was referred to as 'ether crude toxin' (Fraction II), which in many cases was hygroscopic in contrast to the ethanol crude toxin. The ether crude toxin was subjected to column chromatography with Kieselgel and *n*-hexane-acetone as described above (Fig. 2).

(b) *Toxicity*. Lethal toxicity to mice was investigated. As shown in Table 4, the *n*-hexane-soluble fraction (I) and the acetone-soluble material (III) did not exhibit the lethal effect to mice at an i.p. dose of 5·0 and 2·0 mg/10 g, respectively, while 0·25 mg/10 g of the ether soluble fraction (Fraction II) was lethal to mice causing ascending paralysis. Further

Table 4

Toxicity Test on Various Fractions (Procedure B)

Fraction	Route	Dose (mg/10 g)	Death rate (dead/used)	Time of death (min)
(1) *n*-hexane-soluble	i.p.	5·0	0/2	
(2) ether-soluble	i.p.	0·5	2/2	
		0·25	2/2	
		0·125	0/2	
(3) acetone-soluble	i.p.	2·0	0/2	
(4)—1	s.c.	1·0	0/2	
2	s.c.	1·0	0/2	
3	s.c.	1·0	0/2	
4	s.c.	1·0	0/2	
5	i.p.	0·5	2/2	47, 47
6	s.c.	1·0	0/2	
		2·0	0/2	
7	s.c.	1·0	0/1	
		2·0	0/2	

ddS, male, 25 g

fractionation by chromatography showed that only the fraction IV-5 was lethal to mice at the i.p. dose of 0·5 mg/10 g and the time of death of both mice was 47 min.

Orange-yellow needles

$C_{23}H_{30}O_6$.

m.p. 110-111°C

UV (Ethanol)   388 mμ (ϵ48000)
294 mμ (ϵ27100)
234 mμ (ϵ10200)

TLC (Kieselgel G 20°C)
Acetone:*n*-hexane   (1:1) Rf. 0·55
Ethylacetate:toluene   (1:1) Rf. 0·40
Chloroform:methanol   (9:1) Rf. 0·35

Fluorescence: Brilliant yellow

Solubility: Soluble in benzene, ethanol, acetone, chloroform
Insoluble in *n*-hexane, water

FIG. 3. Chemical properties of the neurotoxin.

Chemical properties of the isolated mycotoxin

The chemical properties of the neurotoxin isolated from the mouldy rice are summarised in Figure 3. Irrespective of the isolation procedure, the isolate formed yellow needles with m.p. 110-111°C, and an ethanol

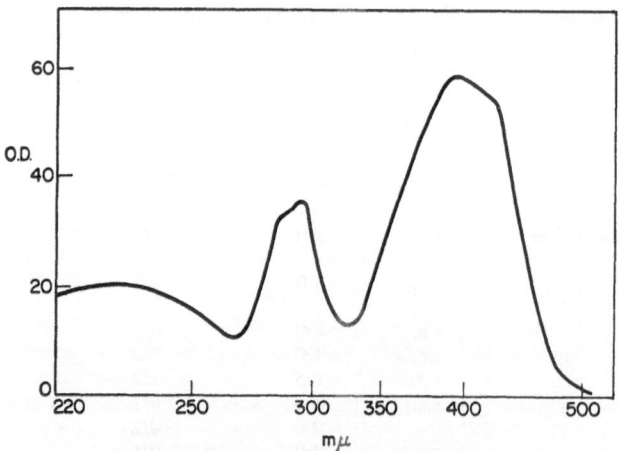

FIG. 4. UV-spectrum of the neurotoxin.
5 μg/ml citreoviridin in ethanol.

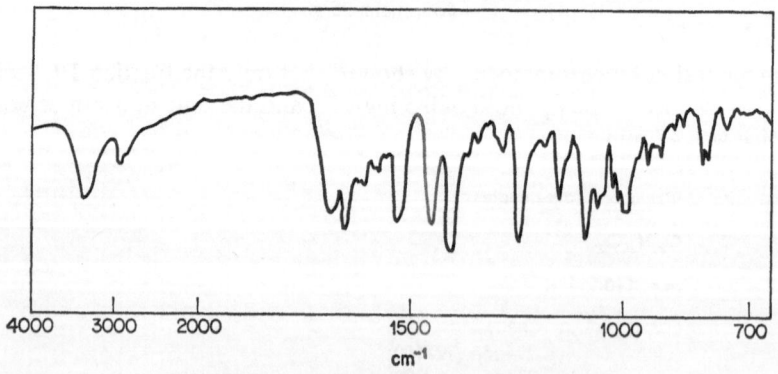

FIG. 5. IR-spectrum of the neurotoxin (KBr).

solution exhibited adsorption peaks at 388, 294, 286 and 234 mμ (Fig. 4), and IR spectra (KBr) gave 3500, 1689, 1654, 1531, 1452, 1405, 1249, 1150, 1094, 1069, 999, 821, 811 cm $^{-1}$ (Fig. 5). The neurotoxin was soluble in benzene, ethanol, acetone, chloroform, and insoluble in n-hexane and water.

Thin-layer chromatography with Kieselgel G revealed a single spot at Rf. 0·55 (acetone-n-hexane, 1:1), 0·40 (ethylacetate-toluene, 1:1) and

0·35 (chloroform, 9:1). Under a UV-lamp, it showed a brilliant yellow fluorescence.

From the chemical properties such as m.p., UV, IR and also from the

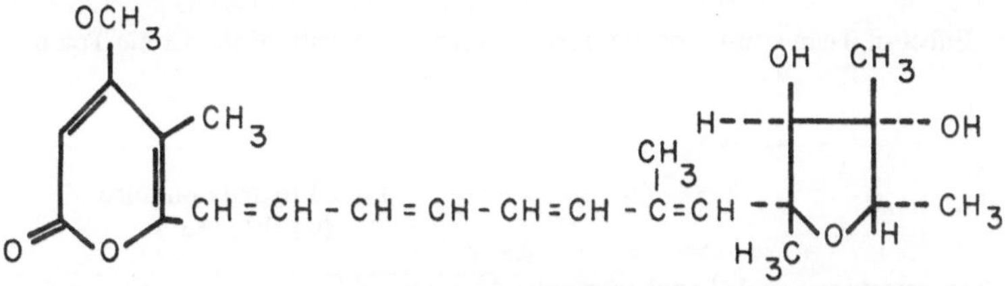

FIG. 6. Citreoviridin.

behaviour on chromatography which was conducted with citreoviridin (kindly given by Dr Hirata, University of Nagoya, Nagoya), the isolated neurotoxin was identified as citreoviridin (Fig. 6) which was previously isolated from the mouldy rice of *P. citreo-viride* Biourge without any description of its toxicity.

Table 5

Recovery of Citreoviridin from Chromatoplate

0·01 μl (10 μg) or 0·02 μl (20 μg) of citreoviridin solution (1000 μl/ml in ethanol) was spotted on Kieselgel G plates and developed with ethylacetate-toluene (3:1). After development, the mycotoxin was eluted with 2 ml of ethanol and the optical density was estimated at 388 mμ

Citreoviridin (μg)	Plate No.	O.D.$_{388}$ after chromatography	Recovery (%)
10	1	0·472	
	2	0·470	
	3	0·494	
	4	0·478	
	5	0·452	
	6	0·460	
	7	0·500 (Av. 0·475)	95
20	1	0·950	
	2	0·925	
	3	0·930	
	4	0·970	
	5	0·950	
	6	0·955	
	7	0·895 (Av. 0·946)	95

Photometric determination of citreoviridin

The neurotoxic citreoviridin is yellow in colour, and by TLC analysis, this chemical is easily separated from other pigments and fluorescent

Table 6

Effect of Temperature on the Production and Toxicity of the Crude Toxin

EXP. (*a*)

Temperature (°C)	Ethanol extract (g/100 g)	Lethal toxicity on mice (mg/10 g, s.c.)	
		5	10
12	0·935	2/2 (88, 55)*	2/2 (39, 46)
18	2·030	2/2 (60, 66)	2/2 (40, 60)
24	2·035	1/2 (120)	2/2 (71, 89)
27	2·567	0/2	2/2 (80, 100)
36	0·962	0/2	0/2

*Time of death in minutes.
The fungus was cultivated on polished rice grains (100 g) at different temperatures. The yield and lethal toxicity of the ethanol-soluble extract and the time of death of the injected mice were determined.

EXP. (*b*)

Temperature (°C)	Ethanol extract (g/100 g)	Lethal toxicity on mice (mg/10 g, s.c.)	
		0·25	1·0
12	0·07	2/2	2/2 (43, 50)
20	0·15	3/3	3/3
24	0·20	2/3	3/3
27	0·18	0/3	2/3
36	0·10	0/3	0/3

The fungus was cultivated on polished rice (100 g) for three weeks, and the ethanol crude toxin was prepared, according to the procedure (*a*).

compounds produced by *P. citreo-viride*. These chemical properties were successfully used for photometric determination of the mycotoxin. As shown in Figure 4, the toxin exhibited UV maximum at 388 mμ in ethanol and the optical density of citreoviridin solution at this maximum was linearly proportional to the concentration of toxin up to 15 μg/ml. Based on this, the recovery of the pure citreoviridin from TLC plates was examined. As shown in Table 5, the agent was easily recovered from the silicagel plate by ethanol extraction. Therefore, as a standard procedure

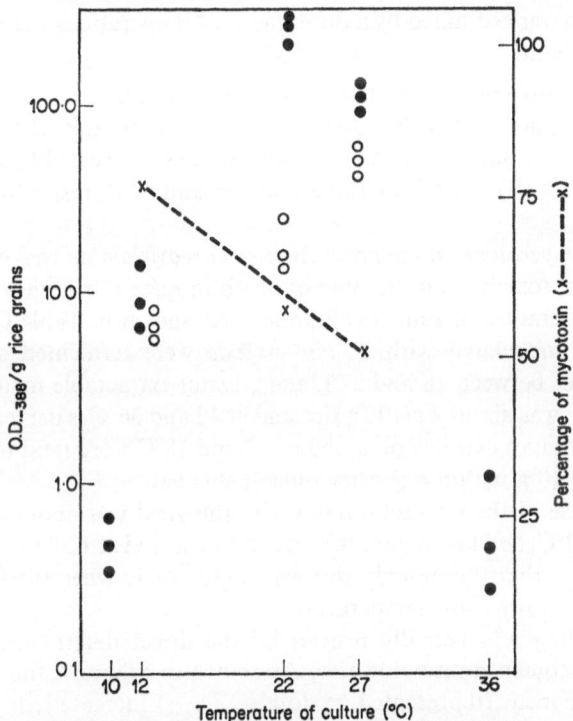

FIG. 7. Effect of culture temperature to the production of citreoviridin on rice grain.

A test-tube containing 5 g of polished rice grains, which were previously immersed in de-ionised water for 30 minutes and autoclaved, was inoculated with the fungus and incubated for 2 weeks at different temperatures listed in Figure. After the cultivation, 5 ml of ethanol was added to the culture tube, and a part of the ethanol extract was chromatographed on TLC with ethylacetate-n-hexane. The optical densities of the first ethanol extract (total) and of the mycotoxin solution were estimated at 388 mμ.

● first ethanol extract   ○ mycotoxin.

for chemical determination of citreoviridin in mouldy rice or fungal contaminated products, the author employed the following procedure:

(1) one g of dried rice grains or fungal material was powdered in a mortar and 1 ml of ethanol was added to the powder;

(2) after standing overnight in a dark room, the ethanol extract was evaporated to dryness, and a known quantity was applied to chromatoplates (5 × 20 cm), which were developed in ethylacetate-toluene (3:1);

(3) after inspecting the position of citreoviridin, the silica gel containing the toxin was scraped from the plate and mixed with 1 ml of ethanol in a small test tube;

(4) after 30 min the tube was centrifuged, and $O.D._{388}$ of the ethanol solution was estimated by a photometer. All operations were conducted in dim light.

Using this simple procedure, a few micrograms of the toxin were able to be determined photometrically. Actual application of this chemical assay method to the ethanol crude toxin described above revealed that the purity of the samples (B) and (C) in Table 2 was 25 and 54%, respectively.

Effect of temperature on the production of citreoviridin on rice grains

The lethal toxicity and the time of death in mice was largely influenced by the temperature of fungal cultivation. As shown in Table 6, when the rice grains inoculated with *P. citreo-viride* were fermented at different temperatures between 18 and 27°C the ethanol-extractable material in the mouldy rice was about 2 g/100 g rice and at 12 and 36°C is decreased to one half. The ethanol extracts obtained at 12 and 18°C were fatal to mice at a dose of 2 g/10 g within a shorter time (Table 6a).

In the case of the ethanol crude toxin, the yield was about 0·2 g/100 g rice at 20-27°C, and the highest toxicity was observed at 12-24°C (Table 6b). This suggests that the mouldy rice was highly toxic when the fungus was cultured at a rather low temperature.

This finding was actually proved by the direct determination of the mycotoxin content in mouldy rice. As shown in Figure 7, the content of the total pigment (represented by total $O.D._{388}$) increased in parallel to the culture temperature and decreased over 27°C, whereas the content of citreoviridin (represented by $O.D._{388}$ after TLC) was 77, 55 and 45% of the total $O.D._{388}$ at 12, 22 and 27°C, respectively. From these results it is very likely that the fungus produces the neurotoxin effectively at lower temperatures.

Production of citreoviridin on liquid media

Production of citreoviridin was examined with five kinds of liquid culture media, namely, (a) Mannit's, (b) Czapek's, (c) Glycerin-supplemented Czapek's, (d) Waksman's and (e) Ushinsky's. Their chemical composition is listed in Table 7 and initial pH of all the media was adjusted to 7·0.

Of the five media (Table 8) the Ushinsky medium gave the greatest mycelial weight and yield of neurotoxin. The toxin content of the dry mycelium reached 2·2% and this yield did not increase in a shaking culture. In order to isolate the pure toxin from the mycelia, the fungus was cultivated on a large scale with 50 dishes (21 cm in diameter) each containing 200 ml of Ushinsky liquid medium (10 litres in total). After cultivation at 20°C for 3 weeks in a dark room, the mycelia were dried at 50°C for 2 days. The dried mycelium (127 g) was subjected to isolation procedure (a), and from 1·1 g of the ethanol crude toxin, 420 mg of the pure mycotoxin was obtained. TLC analysis, m.p., UV and IR spectra coincide with the data noted above.

Table 7

Composition of the Culture Medium

A. Mannit Medium

Mannit	30 g	
Glycerine	10 ml	
Glutamate-Na	2 g	
KCl	0·5 g	
MgSO$_4$	0·5 g	
Water	1 litre	(pH 7·0)

B. Czapek Medium

Sucrose	30 g	
NaNO$_3$	2 g	
K$_2$HPO$_4$	1 g	
KCl	0·5 g	
MgSO$_4$	0·5 g	
Water	1 litre	(pH 7·0)

C. Glycerine-Czapek Medium

(B) Czapek medium	1 litre	
Glycerine	10 ml	
Lactic acid	1 g	(pH 7·0)

D. Waksman Medium

Glucose	10 g	
Peptone	5 g	
KH$_2$PO$_4$	1 g	
MgSO$_4$	0·5 g	
Water	1 litre	(pH 7·0)

E. Ushinsky Medium

Glycerine	40 g	
Ammonium lactate	10 g	
NaCl	5 g	
Asparatate-Na	4 g	
K$_2$HPO$_4$	2·5 g	
MgSO$_4$	0·4 g	
CaCl$_2$	0·1 g	
Water	1 litre	(pH 7·0)

Using Ushinsky liquid medium the correlation between the fungal growth (Fig. 8), the production of citreoviridin (Fig. 9) and pH change in the medium (Fig. 10) was investigated at different temperatures and different culture times.

F

Table 8

Production of Citreoviridin in Different culture Media

Culture	Final pH	Mycelia (g, d.w.)	Citreoviridin (mg)	
			in broth	in mycelia
(A) Mannit's	4·4	0·79	7·56	7·72 (0·98)*
(B) Czapek's	5·3	0·60	1·80	2·30 (0·38)
(C) Glycerin-Czapek's	5·5	0·32	4·35	1·77 (0·54)
(D) Waksman's	8·2	0·72	4·85	1·22 (0·16)
(E) Ushinsky's	8·6	2·22	7·63	49·36 (2·20)

* Percentage of the mycotoxin in the mycelium.

P. citreo-viride Biourge was cultured at 20°C for 2 weeks in 500 ml Erlenmeyer flasks containing 150 ml of the culture medium listed in the Table. Each result is an average of two flasks.

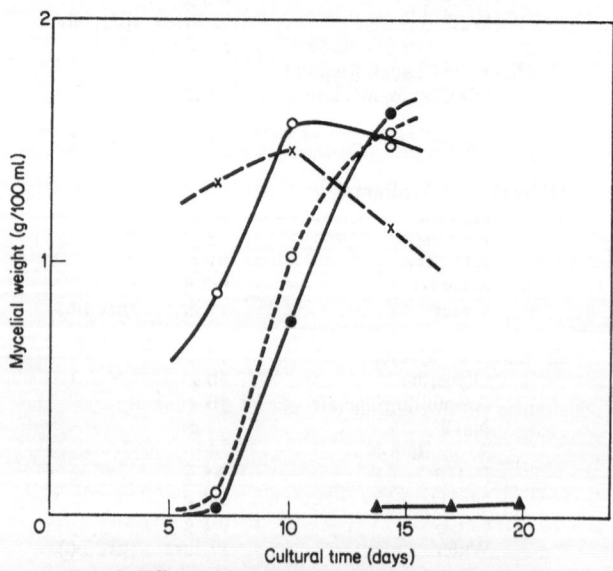

FIG. 8. Effect of temperature on the fungal growth.

▲——▲ 10°C   O——O 27°C
●——● 20°C   ×----× 37°C
O----O 24°C

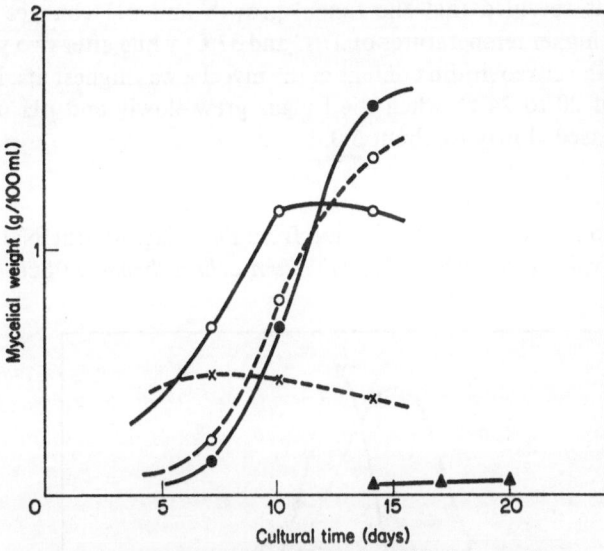

FIG. 9. Production of citreoviridin in Ushinsky's medium at different temperatures.

▲——▲ 10°C   ○——○ 27°C
●——● 20°C   ×----× 37°C
○----○ 24°C

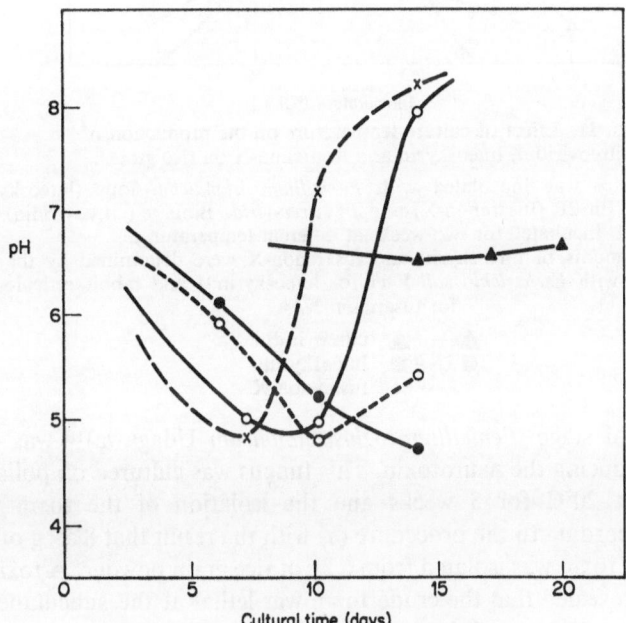

FIG. 10. pH changes in Ushinsky's medium.

▲——▲ 10°C   ○——○ 27°C
●——● 20°C   ×----× 37°C
○----○ 24°C

These results revealed that the fungal growth and pH changes were greatest at the higher temperatures of 27°C and 37°C, while after two weeks of cultivation the citreoviridin content in the mycelia was highest at a lower temperature of 20 to 24°C, when the fungus grew slowly and pH of the medium decreased slowly to about 5·0.

Citreoviridin-producing fungi

According to a private communication from Dr Udagawa (the National Institute of Hygienic Sciences), *Eupenicillium ochrasalmoneum* Scott and

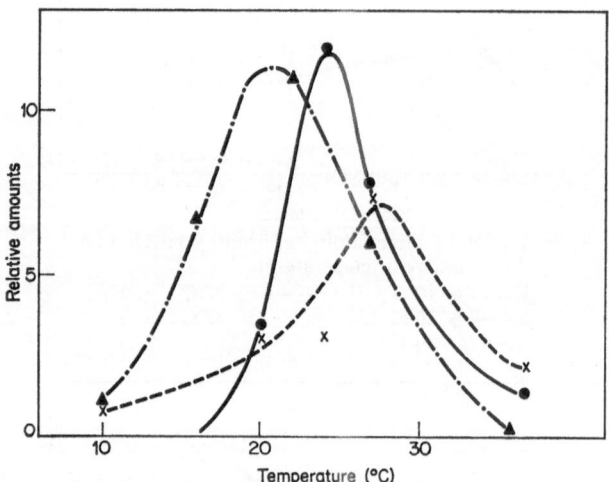

Fɪɢ. 11. Effect of culture temperature on the production of citreoviridin, luteoskyrin and fusarenon-X on rice grains.

The polished rice was inoculated with *Penicillium islandicum* Sopp (luteoskyrin), *Fusarium nivale* Fn 2B (fusarenon-X) and *P. citreo-viride* Biourge (citreoviridin), and incubated for two weeks at different temperatures.

The relative amounts of luteoskyrin and fusarenon-X were determined by the bioassay methods with *Escherichia coli* F-11 for luteoskyrin [11] and rabbit reticulocytes for fusarenon-X.[12]

▲---▲   citreoviridin
●——●   luteoskyrin
×----×   fusarenon-X

Stolk (conidial stage, *Penicillium ochrasalmoneum* Udagawa)[10] was suspected of producing the neurotoxin. This fungus was cultured on polished rice grains at 20°C for 3 weeks and the isolation of the toxin was conducted according to the procedure (*a*) with the result that 8·59 g of the ethanol crude toxin was isolated from 6 kg of rice grain powder. A toxicity test on mice revealed that the crude toxin was lethal at the subcutaneous dose of 2 to 3 mg/10 g, and the acute symptoms were the same as those of the crude and pure toxin of *P. citreo-viride*. Thin-layer chromatography also indicated the presence of citreoviridin and an unknown yellow pigment, and the content of the toxin was calculated as 10 to 15% of the crude extract. These findings strongly suggested that *Eupenicillium ochrasalmoneum* produced citreoviridin on rice, although the relative content of citreoviridin was lower than in the case of *P. citreo-viride*.

DISCUSSION

The neurotoxic mycotoxin in rice polluted by P. citreo-viride

According to Uraguchi,[4] the ethanol soluble fraction of the mouldy rice infested with *P. toxicarium* Miyake was neurotoxic to animals, causing an ascending type of paralysis. Based on this finding, ethanol was used as a solvent and the crude toxin, with a high toxicity, was isolated (Fig. 1 and Table 1). Since the alcohol extract was a yellowish-brown, viscous oil, the yield and the toxicity fluctuated with different batches, and in most cases 2 to 5 g of the ethanol extract with a toxicity of 5 to 10 mg/10 g were obtained from one kilogram of the mouldy rice. The yield and toxicity were similar to those obtained by Uraguchi.[4]

Further purification of the ethanol extract by benzene extraction and *n*-hexane precipitation resulted in the highly toxic powder which contained 25 to 50% toxin. In most cases this powder was not hygroscopic and could be used for toxicity tests.[6]

The effect of temperature on the toxin-producing potency of the fungus was marked. The lethal toxicity of the ethanol extract and the actual content of the neurotoxin was higher when the fungus was cultivated at lower temperature. This relationship also occurred when the fungus was cultured on liquid medium (Fig. 9). In cases of other toxic fungi (Fig. 11) the relative amounts of the mycotoxins produced on rice differ from each other, depending upon the culture temperature. The maximum yield of hepatotoxic luteoskyrin from *P. islandicum* Sopp and cytotoxic fusarenon-X from *Fusarium nivale* Fn 2B occurred at 24°C and 27°C respectively, while that of the neurotoxic citreoviridin of *P. citreo-viride* was at a lower temperature.

This ecological characteristic of *P. citreo-viride* is considered to be very important in the epidemiology of 'Shoshin-kakke'. According to Miyake *et al.*,[1] the growth of *P. toxicarium* Miyake (*P. citreo-viride*) is common when the water content of grains reaches 14·6%, while other fungal species need a water content 1% higher. This indicates that this toxic fungus can grow on rice at an earlier time when the grains become wet. According to Uraguchi,[6] mouldy rice was frequently detected in the district facing the Japan Sea, where the weather is rather cold and less sunny than the districts facing the Pacific Sea. Therefore, the climate favours toxigenicity of *P. citreo-viride*. This ecological investigation of the fungus has given an important key not only to the resolution of the 'Shoshin-kakke' problem but also to studies on the correlation between mycotoxins and human health.

REFERENCES

1. MIYAKE, I., NAITO, H. and TSUNODA, H. (1940). *Beikokuriyo Kenkyujo Hokoku*, **1**, 1. (In Japanese.)
2. MIYAKE, I. (1947). *Nisshin Igaku*, **34**, 161. (In Japanese.)
3. URAGUCHI, K. (1942). *Folia pharmcol. jap.*, **34**, 39. (In Japanese.)
4. URAGUCHI, K. (1947). *Nisshin Igaku*, **34**, 155. (In Japanese.)
5. URAGUCHI, K. (1947). *Nisshin Igaku*, **34**, 224. (In Japanese.)
6. URAGUCHI, K. (1969). *J. stored Prod. Res.*, **5**, 227.
7. URAGUCHI, K. (1969). In: *Encyclopedia of Pharmacology and Therapeutics*. Pergamon Press. In press.
8. URAGUCHI, K. (1970). In: *Microbial Toxins*. Academic Press. In press.
9. SAKABE, N., GOTO, T. and HIRATA, Y. (1964). *Tetrahedron Letters*, **7**, 1825.
10. UDAGAWA, S. (1959). *J. Agr. Sci.* (Tokyo Univ. of Agr.), **5**, 5-21.
11. YAMAKAWA, H. and UENO, Y. (1970). *Chem. Pharm. Bull.*, **18**, 177.
12. UENO, Y., HOSOYA, M. and ISHIKAWA, Y. (1969). *J. Biochem.*, **66**, 419.

STORAGE SURVEYS AND HOW THEY MAY BE USED BOTH TO DETECT AND ESTIMATE FUNGAL CONTAMINATION IN THE DIET

by

G. A. Gilman

Tropical Stored Products Centre (Tropical Products Institute)
London Road, Slough, England

Whether or not proof will eventually be forthcoming regarding the possible association between fungal toxins and liver cancer in man, is still open to question. One thing that is certain, however, is that losses due to fungal deterioration can be considerable and the consumption of damaged food-stuffs is to be discouraged for many reasons. Maximum effort should, therefore, be directed to the prevention of such damage, to which end a thorough knowledge of post-harvest handling and storage methods is essential.

Over the past 2 years a storage survey, designed to assess the extent of fungal contamination in carefully collected food samples, has been carried out in Swaziland and eastern Transvaal. Parallel aflatoxin analyses were also undertaken but this was not considered an important aspect of the survey. The areas investigated, and hence the samples collected, were selected to compare the three tribes encountered, a full range of crops, handling methods, and storage practices, as well as topographical and climatic variations in areas of varying liver cancer incidence.

Swaziland is a landlocked, independent kingdom which adjoins the Republic on three of its sides and Mozambique on its eastern border. It covers an area of 6705 square miles and is conveniently divided into high, middle and low veld areas, which average 3500-4500 feet, 2000-2500 feet and 500-1000 feet respectively, from west to east across the country. In the extreme east, on the Mozambique border, the Lebombo Range occurs as an extension of the middle veld. Rainfall decreases from an average of 50 inches in the high veld to some 26 inches in the low veld while the converse is true of temperature. The low veld has a mean maximum temperature of 29°C which is some 6°C higher than the corresponding high veld figure. The eastern Transvaal covers an area of approximately 15,000 square miles immediately to the north of Swaziland. The areas surveyed were mainly in the low veld between the escarpment in the west and the Kruger National Park in the east. Rainfall, and consequently crop production, decreases from west to east away from the escarpment.

The rural population of Swaziland is almost entirely composed of Swazis and they occur in south-eastern Transvaal in company with the Shangaan tribe. In the northern areas the Sotho and Shangaan groups are established and on the escarpment the former appears to dominate.

Maize is the staple food in all areas, except in the Sotho villages on the eastern Transvaal escarpment where sorghum is preferred. Bulrush millet is a Shangaan crop, although the other tribes may grow it in dry areas, because of its drought resistance. Groundnuts, though preferred by the Shangaans, are grown by all tribes where rainfall permits, especially on the Swaziland middle veld and in south-eastern Transvaal. Other durable food crops produced include jugo beans (*Voandzeia subterranea*), cowpeas (*Vigna sinensis*), sugar beans (*Phaseolus vulgaris*), and various other pulses. Small patches of cassava occur in the low veld although this crop does not appear to be dried.

It was quickly established that storage and crop handling methods varied considerably from district to district. This was influenced more by geographical considerations (especially climate and its effect on crop production), than on tribal preferences. An outline of these methods is now given, in order that the factors influencing food deterioration may be fully understood.

Harvesting and drying

As the rains occur between October and May and groundnuts are harvested between March and May, conditions are usually moist at pulling, and drying is required. When late rains occur, traditional drying methods are not always successful. Small quantities of plants are often bundled and placed on raised platforms, or hut roofs with the pods upwards. Medium amounts are commonly dried in round wind-rows, also with the pods upwards, or in rows with the plants on their sides and some of the pods, inevitably, in contact with the ground. Plants produced in larger quantities are usually stacked with or without prior wind-rowing. These heaps vary from 2 to 4 feet in diameter and are of a similar height. The plants are arranged in a circle on a stone or layer of grass either with the pods outwards or inwards. A light thatch is usually applied. Stacking is relatively uncommon.

Extensive invasion of groundnut kernels by fungi over the harvesting period was not observed, although mould damage to the haulm and surface of the pod was noted in certain stacks and wind-rows, and where the plants had been tightly bundled on platforms. Both stacking and bundling are often carried out without prior wilting when the haulms are still moist. Damage due to subsequent rain is another possibility, especially if the plants are inadequately raised away from the soil.

Picking is done by hand, and final sun drying on a patch of hard ground near the homestead is usually necessary prior to storage. The light weight, immature pods or 'rejects' are separated from the better ones at this time and are eaten first, while the others are stored for sale, seed or later consumption. These rejects are more often damaged by fungi than the mature pods.

Maize and other grain crops are usually cut after the rains when the cobs (or heads) are dry. However, rainfall, both during and after crop maturation considerably influences the moisture content at picking and the amount of fungal damage occurring prior to harvest. This can be considerable in damp weather and further sun drying may be required after picking and before storage. At picking, the small, often immature, maize cobs and those damaged by fungi or cob boring insects are separated from the better ones. The rejects, which may constitute between 5 and 20% of the crop, are usually threshed first; the better quality grain is sorted for consumption, while the remainder (often mouldy) is used in beer making or for feeding to animals.

The knowledge that inferior quality maize and groundnuts are eaten soon after harvesting illustrates one of the important advantages of a survey of this kind. It is normal for such material to be quickly consumed, usually over a period of only two or three weeks, and this important source of fungal contamination in the diet is, therefore, easily overlooked. This season, a special study is being carried out comparing rejected material with the good, as regards fungal deterioration and aflatoxin content.

Storage of threshed grain

The storage of maize on the cob in Swaziland is only temporary. Two or three mounths after harvesting, the cobs are threshed and the grain stored in bulk. In the eastern Transvaal, however, the cobs are stored throughout the rains and are threshed for food as required. Crib storage may be divided into three categories:

   (i) simple platforms built for only small quantities of cobs,
   (ii) cribs constructed inside huts in the better cropping areas, and
   (iii) individual thatched cribs.

Simple platforms, usually unthatched, are more common in the drier, low veld areas. Sometimes a low wall of woven sticks is constructed around the platform to increase its capacity and to give some protection from cattle damage (Fig. 1). Usually these platforms are raised several feet above the ground, sometimes in trees. Thatching is not considered essential as farmers expect to finish their crop before the beginning of the rains or to thresh it before this time. However, if storage is prolonged into the rains, moisture penetrates rapidly and fungal growth soon occurs. This is true even if the cobs are tightly packed and the sheaths are left on.

Cribs built inside huts generally accommodate a larger volume of cobs. These storage huts may be recognised by their open walls, usually of vertical poles, which allow free air circulation. Here the cobs are well protected from rehydration, both above and below, by a good thatched roof and raised platform. They are common in the middle and high veld areas of Swaziland. Individual thatched cribs are popular in the eastern Transvaal. They are raised from 9 to 18 inches above the ground, are usually round in shape, and have an average diameter of 4 to 5 feet with walls of a similar height. Woven sticks, sorghum and millet stalks, tightly bound bundles of grass, or crude planks may be used in their construction according to availability. Roofs are usually of conical thatch but corrugated metal is sometimes used. They vary considerably in sturdiness and thatching is often inadequate to prevent the entry of heavy rain.

Consider now the storage of threshed grain, groundnuts and other legumes. Once again the methods adopted are influenced mainly by the quantities produced, and are either long established methods (traditional) or are a product of our modern community. Corrugated metal grain tanks, jute sacks, and 44 gallon drums fall into the latter category and are being used more and more frequently. However, their unenlightened use can lead to fungal damage. For example, grain may be stored in an enclosed space (e.g. a metal drum) before it has dried sufficiently, or the seams of the metal tanks become damaged thus allowing water to enter. Furthermore, condensation inside a tank can occur if temperature gradients are allowed to develop within the grain as a result of direct exposure to the sun or localised, heavy, insect attack. Jute sacks of grain placed in contact with hard earth (or unproofed concrete) floors for long periods, will absorb moisture at the base with obvious deleterious results. Sacks of groundnuts destined for seed are sometimes hung in trees to reduce rodent attack (Fig. 2), and bundles of maize cobs may be similarly treated. As the surplus seed may be eaten during the rains, after frequent surface wetting, this is another possible source of mycotoxins in the diet.

Three traditional methods of storing grain observed in the areas investigated were, in increasing order of capacity, the clay pot, the 'silulu' (a spherical basket of grass bundles sewn together with leather or tree bark) and the underground pit.

The latter method is of considerable interest here. Firstly, because the high grain moistures which prevail in these pits encourage fungal and bacterial invasion and secondly, although pits were once used throughout the areas investigated they now appear to be confined to certain regions of Swaziland, principally the low veld and Lebombo, where liver cancer is

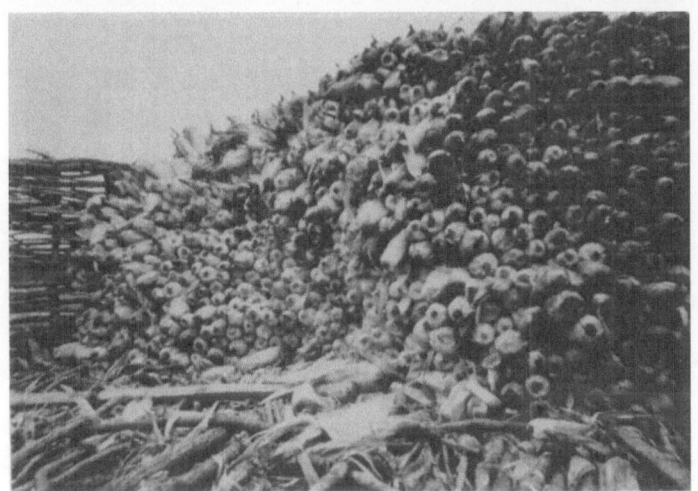

FIG. 1. Maize cobs stored in an open crib, exposed to the weather.

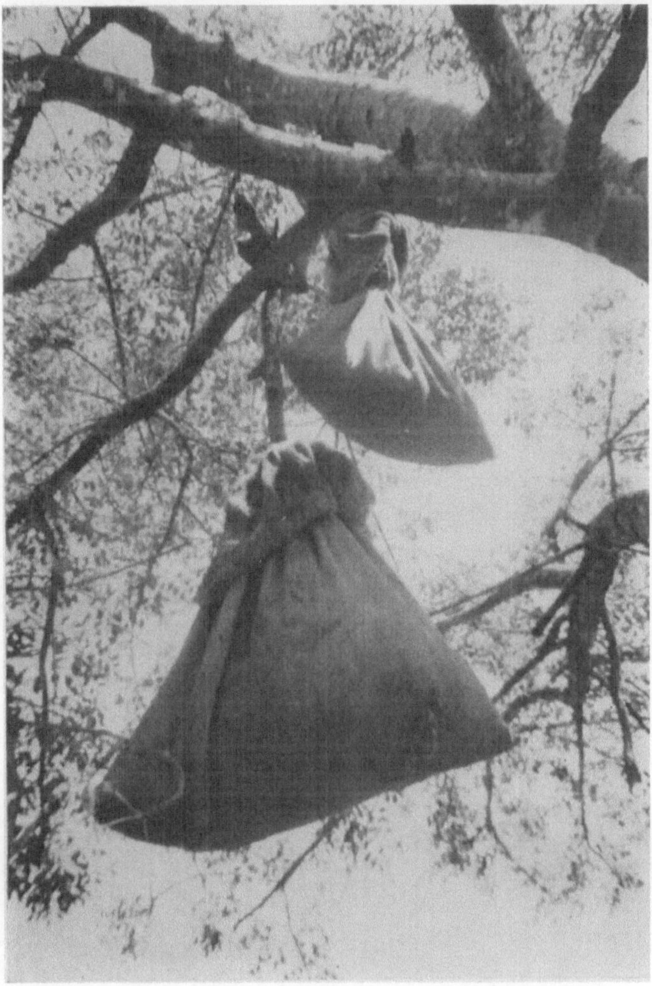

FIG. 2. Sacks of groundnuts hung in a tree to reduce rodent attack.

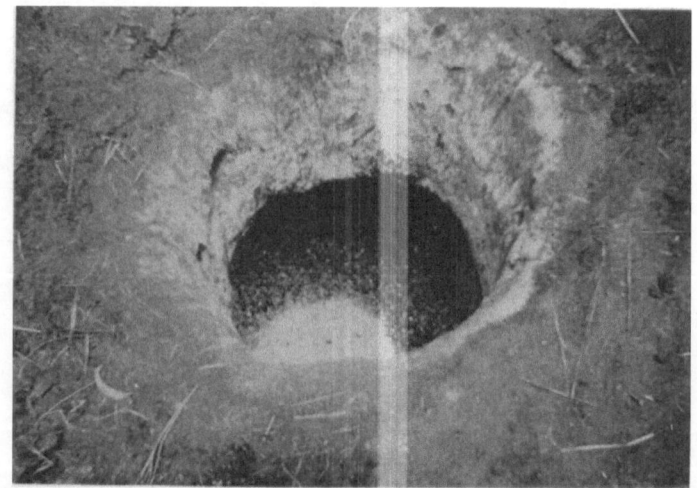

FIG. 3. The entrance to an underground pit showing extensive fungal growth on the walls.

apparently higher than average. Another advantage of the storage approach is thus illustrated. It enables the pattern of food handling and consumption to be traced back many years, which is a useful factor when we are considering liver cancer incidence figures which may have resulted from a situation existing 20 years ago or more.

The underground pit (Fig. 3), which has several advantages over other methods of storage, is used to preserve threshed maize and occasionally sorghum. The grain is safe from fire and is relatively inaccessible, so that wives and others cannot remove food without the knowledge of the farmer. Anaerobic conditions prevail in these pits, especially if they are filled to the top; insect infestation is, therefore, reduced enabling the long-term storage of grain against years of famine. Low grain temperatures also assist here.

In shape, Swazi pits somewhat resemble laboratory conical flasks, although the walls may be more or less rounded. The neck is usually some 20 inches in diameter and from 9 to 24 inches in length. As they are always situated in the cattle kraal, the depth of the neck below ground level depends on the amount of dung present; this is rarely more than 18 inches. Pits vary in depth from 4 to 6 feet and in diameter at the base from 5 to 9 feet. They will accommodate an equivalent of from five to thirty 200 lb bags of grain. A stone or a square of bark cut from the Morula tree is used for covering the pit and before replacing the top soil of decaying manure the edges are sealed with fresh dung. Apart from a thin smear of dung on the walls before the pit is filled, linings are rare, although very occasionally grass mats or bundles of grass may be placed in the bottom. Lining with a grass basket is unusual. New pits are 'fired' before filling, but old ones are only swept out after use.

During a series of good cropping years, it seems probable that one season's produce may be stored for up to 5 years. Recently, however, long-term storage for more than 1 year has become rare. Pits may be opened every 1, 2, 3 or 4 months to remove grain for food or sale. This has to be carefully dried before further storage, because, in spite of the layer of dung on top of the pit, which is supposed to restrict water entry, this is still considerable. Most empty pits examined had damp walls with rotting grain adhering to them, and one pit had 2 inches of water in the bottom. This is especially true of parts of the low veld where the water table can be near the surface. In a full pit, visibly mouldy grain is restricted to the neck, where air is presumably more readily available. Elsewhere, a partial fermentation of the maize occurs varying in colour from pale to dark brown or black, depending on its distance from the walls or the floor; it is strong-smelling and soft as a result of extensive bacterial degradation. *Bacillus megaterium* was the organism most commonly isolated. All the pit maize examined during the rains was above the safe storage moisture content for this grain of about 13·5%. In the vicinity of the walls and floor the moisture content always exceeded 25% while in the centre of the pit it varied between 20 and 23%. This partially fermented grain is considered good to eat by the older Bantu who were observed to consume it either raw, straight from the pit, or as a sour drink or porridge. However, it is not so popular with the younger generation who have been to school and who appreciate better quality maize meal.

Gases present in pits

The Bantu are well aware that it is dangerous to enter a pit until several hours have elapsed from the time of opening. It was decided, therefore, to make a qualitative assessment of the gases which might possibly form during storage using a Drager Multi Gas Detector, Model 23/31. Ammonia and methane, being lighter than air, were measured in the neck before removal of the lid, while the heavier gases, carbon monoxide, hydrogen sulphide and the nitrous gases were measured in the vicinity of the rotting grain after removal of the lid. Carbon dioxide was assessed generally. A total of 13 pits were examined.

Carbon dioxide was present in all pits in concentrations of from 11 to 20% by volume. Traces of carbon monoxide and hydrogen sulphide were each found in two pits. Traces of methane and nitrous gases were each found in four pits. Ammonia and nitrogen dioxide were absent.

The presence of nitrous gases is of some significance as they could be associated with the formation of nitrosamines in the grain; these are substances known to be highly carcinogenic to certain animals. However, when pit-stored maize was examined at the Tropical Products Institute, London, nitrosamines were not detected. However, the dirty nature of the samples made analysis difficult, and existing methods of detection are unreliable.

Aflatoxin has not yet been detected in this pit-stored maize although *Aspergillus flavus* was often present. Anaerobic conditions probably played a part here or this fungus could have contaminated the grain subsequent to its removal from the pit.

General consideration of storage surveys

From this outline of storage and drying methods used by the rural Bantu in the eastern Transvaal and Swaziland, it is clear that fungal-invaded grain is only likely to occur spasmodically and could easily be overlooked. The house to house sampling of grain for microbiological assessment was, therefore, undertaken with two objectives in mind. Firstly, a selective sampling of visibly damaged material in order to estimate the amount of food spoilage together with the fungi involved and secondly, a random sampling of fairly homogeneous grain destined for consumption, thus ensuring that the latter was representative of the family diet. As the housewife is careful to sort grain and other stored crops during food preparation, an analysis of market and pantry samples can be misleading, as the degree of contamination may be overestimated. Throughout this investigation considerable emphasis has been placed on the correct use of recognised sampling techniques. Coning and quartering or the proper application of a sampling spear were two commonly adopted methods. The scooping of grain from the top of a bag is to be discouraged for obvious reasons.

Although the problems associated with a storage approach are many, close contact with the population under study is maintained, enabling specific, complicating factors to be recognised and accounted for. As an example of this, various prepared foodstuffs including maize 'biltong' and a home-made peanut butter are eaten irregularly, rarely as part of the main meal. This first is prepared from 'green' maize by boiling the fresh cobs for a few minutes before hanging them up in a hut to dry. This foodstuff is stored for long periods and frequently goes mouldy if drying is slow. Peanut butter is similarly stored for long periods and is made from roasted, crushed maize and groundnuts. As these and other prepared foodstuffs are often preferred more by one tribe than another, or are restricted to certain areas, the presence or absence of aflatoxin is of considerable significance.

Our aim must be to provide comparative figures for different areas and countries as regards the consumption of foodstuffs invaded by fungi. This is considered to be an important parallel study to that which compares liver cancer incidence with aflatoxin ingestion. The assessment of fungi in foodstuffs, sorted for consumption, is not easy to standardise and hence area comparisons are at present difficult to make. Fungi are ubiquitous, a wide variety contaminate all types of foodstuffs and this is something we cannot prevent. However, surface spores and even small internal infections no more than indicate potential damage should the stored food be re-wetted. In fact, only those species which we find fairly extensively invading grain (either on the surface or internally) can be of major importance from the mycotoxin viewpoint.

The microscopical examination of tissues for hyphae is extremely time consuming, while the rehydration of grain after surface sterilisation is another recognised and more easily applied method for the detection of invading fungi. However, it is felt that this technique leads to an over-estimation, as very small infections will also be detected. These two methods have, therefore, been combined as follows. From each sample, 50 randomly selected maize grains are halved under aseptic conditions, following surface sterilisation and an overnight soaking in sterile water to soften the grain. The first cut is made parallel to the flat surface, and one of these halves is again divided equally, this time cutting in the other plane. Each of the two quarters is then plated on a different agar medium. The remaining half grain is rapidly dried and kept for tissue examination if the corresponding quarters yield fungi. In this way a quantitative assessment is possible at two levels, both as regards the number of grains invaded and the extent of fungal growth within each grain. These techniques are now being adapted for other durable food crops.

CONCLUSIONS

In eastern Transvaal and Swaziland the invasion of foodstuffs by fungi occurs both over the harvesting period and later while in store. Maize is especially prone to damage during the initial drying period.

Storage practices vary considerably with area and certain methods encourage fungal deterioration. The storage of maize in underground pits, and the hanging of sacks of groundnuts in trees, often during rainy weather, are two such methods of local importance.

Stored food is not usually representative of the family diet as cleaning and sorting is invariably carried out prior to cooking. However, in certain areas of Swaziland, maize of very poor quality from underground pits is often consumed.

ACKNOWLEDGEMENTS

I would like to acknowledge the co-operation and assistance given by the Ministry and Department of Agriculture in Swaziland and the Department of Bantu Affairs in South Africa. Financial assistance from the National Cancer Association of South Africa is also gratefully acknowledged.

I am very much indebted to Dr J. S. Harington and staff of the Cancer Research Unit, SAIMR, for their encouragement and to Dr P. Keen for his helpful collaboration in the Swaziland survey.

Finally, I would like to thank the Tropical Stored Products Centre (TPI), Slough, England, for the great assistance received from members of staff. Thanks are also due to Dr D. W. Hall, TPI, London, who, together with the late Dr Oettlé (Cancer Research Unit, SAIMR), was responsible for the initiation of this survey.

THE TOXICOLOGY OF AFLATOXIN

W. H. Butler

Medical Research Council Laboratories, Toxicology Unit
Woodmansterne Road, Carshalton, Surrey, England

That fungi can produce toxic substances has been recognised for centuries. The well-known hazards of the mushrooms, although not strictly relevant to this meeting, are of considerable interest and have been reviewed by Wieland and Wieland.[1] The toxins induce a pathological change in many of the major organs. The mushrooms also produce such pharmacologically interesting compounds as muscarin which has been studied extensively. Accidental ingestion of mycotoxins which are food contaminants have also been recognised for a long time, the best example of which is ergotism. Two basic clinical syndromes are associated with ergot poisoning, the active principals of which are alkaloids of lysergic acid, firstly gangrene and abortion due to effects on smooth muscle and central nervous system effects of convulsions and hallucinations. The action of these compounds on smooth muscle is still used therapeutically in its action upon uterine muscle. However, as a result of improving agricultural methods in those countries where rye is grown, the outbreaks of clinical disease are infrequent and do not really present a problem to public health. To anticipate somewhat any discussion of the problem of other mycotoxins, the decline of ergotism is an example of what can be done with improved agricultural methods.

Although it has been pointed out on many occasions that the study of mycotoxins received a great stimulation following the recognition of aflatoxin, so many mycotoxins have been described that in the time available it would only be possible to list known organisms that produce toxins with their known pathological effects. The work on aflatoxin that has been published since 1960 has resulted in more information being available on aflatoxin than any other mycotoxin. This interest in aflatoxin is justified from the point of view of both its potential hazard to human and animal health and also its interest as an experimental tool. As most of my work has involved aflatoxin, I will concentrate upon this, giving examples of some other mycotoxins in an attempt to justify the view that aflatoxin is of considerable importance.

Most farm animals are susceptible to some mycotoxins although they show varying degrees of susceptibility to aflatoxin. For example, in horses, stachybotryotoxicosis produces changes in the marrow resulting in agranulocytosis, thrombocytopenia and disturbances of clotting mechanisms. Pathological changes have been described in the liver and alimentary tract.[2] This disease has occurred as field cases and has also been produced experimentally. Man is also susceptible to the toxin which produces a dermal toxicity and it has also been shown experimentally to produce leucopenia.[3] I know of no reported incidence of aflatoxicosis in horses. A similar pattern of disease is seen in the syndromes of alimentary toxic aleukia in man. Sheep are susceptible to sporidesmin toxicosis,[4] a condition originally described in New Zealand which causes liver damage and failure of porphyrin metabolism. This results in photosensitisation of the sheep and the resulting name given to the condition of 'facial eczema'. No field cases of aflatoxicosis in sheep have been described although at high dose levels they are susceptible. At Weybridge large doses of aflatoxin killed two rams. These sheep had fatty livers with central lobular necrosis. Recently Armbrecht and his colleagues[5] have described the acute toxicity of aflatoxin B_1 in sheep and have demonstrated a comparatively low LD_{50} in the order of 1 mg/kg. This figure is considerably lower than that found at Weybridge. Pigs are extremely susceptible to some mycotoxins; the best described outbreaks are those of mouldy corn toxicosis in Florida and those attributable to aflatoxin poisoning.[6]

In the latter cases the liver was very severely affected with a centrilobular haemorrhagic necrosis and some fatty change. More chronic exposure results in the lobular pattern of the liver being destroyed by fibrosis, biliary proliferation and nodule formation. There is considerable variation of parenchymal nuclear size.[7, 8] Calves are particularly susceptible to aflatoxin poisoning and field outbreaks have occurred. The liver lesion is again the most striking pathological change and is characterised by massive fibrosis, biliary proliferation and veno-occlusion, similar to that following Ragwort poisoning.[9] Cattle are the only species in which veno-occlusive disease can be induced by aflatoxin.

The original outbreaks of disease attributable to aflatoxin occurred in birds. Turkey poults, ducklings, young pheasants and partridges are all extremely susceptible to aflatoxin and many field cases have been reported.[10] The lesion produced in ducklings is well known and has become the basis for the bio-assay of aflatoxin.[11] This lesion is of some interest from an experimental point of view as it can be produced by nitrosamines but not senecio-alkaloids.[12] Then biliary proliferation, used as the assay system, regresses rapidly so that after 10 days following a single dose, the liver is essentially normal. The mechanism by which this regression is brought about is not understood but would be a useful model for studying the relationship between hepatic parenchymal cells and bile duct cells. As in ducklings the principal lesion occurring in turkey poults and chickens is that of liver cell necrosis and biliary proliferation. It would also seem that in these birds the young bird is more susceptible to the toxin than are older birds.[13]

Most of the work which I have done has been with rats and guinea-pigs. It is of interest that Paget[14] in 1954 described 'exudative hepatitis', a disease of unknown aetiology in guinea-pigs, which was attributed to the diet but for which no causative agent was found. These guinea-pigs were oedematous and had abundant ascites. The liver again was the most severely affected organ with patchy necrosis of the parenchymal cells. The guinea-pig feed contained 15% peanut meal but was changed before it could be investigated for the presence of an aetiologic agent. This disease was experimentally produced by Paterson et al.[15] following the recognition of aflatoxin. The acute LD_{50} in the guinea-pig is 1.4 mg/kg[16]; the lesion most consistently seen is that of centrilobular hepatic necrosis. Ascites and subcutaneous oedema following acute exposure resembled that described by Paget.[14] Another consistent lesion seen in guinea-pigs was haemorrhagic necrosis of the zona reticularis of the adrenal cortex. The animals with ascites and oedema have normal serum sodium levels indicating a sodium retention. At present it is not possible to say whether this is due to an effect of the aflatoxin upon the adrenal or directly upon the kidney. Newberne et al.[17] have demonstrated that dogs are also extremely susceptible to aflatoxin poisoning which induces a centrilobular hepatic cell necrosis followed by a prominent biliary proliferation. The experimental disease is similar to that reported as 'hepatitis X' in 1955 from the south-eastern United States,[18] in dogs fed a commercial feed containing peanut meal.

The acute toxicity and mode of action of aflatoxins have been most extensively studied in the rat. There is considerable sex difference in the LD_{50} values but the lesions induced in males and females are similar[19] and consist of slowly developing periportal hepatic necrosis. The lesion is remarkable in that the usual rapid regenerative response of the liver to injury is not seen. After 1 month following a single LD_{50} dose the liver shows extensive biliary proliferation, fibrosis and occasionally, cholangiofibrosis. The poor regenerative response may be attributable to the inhibition of DNA synthesis which has been reported by De Recondo, and his colleagues[20] after partial hepatectomy subsequent to aflatoxin administration and also by Rogers and Newberne[21] in intact liver. The female rat is less susceptible to the acute effects of aflatoxin (LD_{50} 15 mg/kg) but the lesion is similar and this increased tolerance to aflatoxin is lost in the latter part of pregnancy.[22] When aflatoxin is given on day 16 of pregnancy the foetal weights on day 21 show considerable retardation of growth. We originally considered this was attributable directly to the maternal liver lesion. However, we have since shown that the foetal growth retardation was directly related to the inanition of the animal and not to the liver injury.[23]

The distribution of hepatic lesions induced by aflatoxin B_1 varies from species to species, being periportal in the rat, duckling and cat, centrilobular in the pig, dog, guinea-pig and midzonal in the rabbit.[24] However, aflatoxin G_1 has been studied much less thoroughly than B_1.[25] Similarly in the male rat the LD_{50} value of G_1 is approximately twice that of B_1.[26] Although the lesions induced by G_1 in the duckling are the same as B_1, in the rat they are somewhat different. The zone in the liver lobule that is affected is the same but there is considerable variation between animals and the consistent pattern seen following B_1 is absent. The most consistent lesion following G_1 administration in the rat is that of a necrosis of the straight segment of the proximal tubules in the inner zone of the renal cortex. This is rapidly repaired leaving a residual abnormality of many large tubular nuclei which appear to persist for 2 to 3 months. Another lesion frequently observed is that of an extensive haemorrhagic necrosis of the zona reticularis of the adrenal cortex.[26] This lesion seen in all animals is similar to that following B_1 administration but is much more extensive.

The first metabolite described as originating from aflatoxin was aflatoxin M_1 which is found in cow and rat milk.[27] Subsequently this was shown to occur in urine and was also extracted from blood and liver.[28] The toxicity of this hydroxylated B_1 is similar to that of the parent compound. Since this was described a considerable amount of work has been done in the study of the metabolism of aflatoxin and its mechanism of action in producing liver cell necrosis. Patterson and Allcroft[29] have demonstrated that rat liver microsomes are able to detoxify aflatoxin to a non-fluorescent yellow compound which is, as far as we can tell, completely non-toxic. Following incubation of B_1 with a microsomal system for 1 hr, this metabolite when fed to day-old ducklings fails to induce the typical lesions. The structure of this compound, which has an absorption peak of 400 mμ, is not known. Most species are able to produce this compound but the ability of the liver to do so is not related to the susceptibility of the species.

The ultrastructural lesions seen in the rat liver following administration of aflatoxin B_1 are most striking. The early lesions which are most marked in the periportal zone are similar to those resulting from exposure to other well-known hepatotoxins such as dimethylnitrosamine.[30] The first change seen is that of disaggregation of ribosomes and dilation of the cisternae of the endoplasmic reticulum. Associated with this, but in my experience seen at a later time, is a striking parenchymal cell nucleolar segregation. This nucleolar lesion has been compared with that induced by actinomycin D and has been considered to be the result of binding of the aflatoxin to DNA and subsequent inhibition of DNA-dependent RNA synthesis.

Nucleolar segregation is seen not only in those areas which will eventually undergo necrosis but also in those centrilobular areas which will survive. Six hours after dosing the centrilobular zones exhibit some change in the rough endoplasmic reticulum (RER) but this never becomes as extensive as that in the periportal zone. At 48 hr the periportal parenchymal cells are completely disrupted by large autophagic vacuoles. In the surviving parts of the lobule the most striking change is that of a considerable increase of smooth endoplasmic reticulum (SER). At 18 and 24 hr there is also some increase of SER but this is not as prominent as that observed at 24 hr. This increased abundance of SER is similar to that seen following exposure to phenobarbitone and other compounds.

When the liver is examined 12 hr after the administration of B_1 the cytoplasmic organelles of the hepatocytes in the centrilobular areas are normal. Many nucleoli, however, still show segregation. Betweeen 12th and 24th hr there is a progressive increase of foci of ribosome-like particles within the cytoplasm, not associated with membranes. These particles are characteristically arranged in loose spirals and curved parallel rows. The typical clusters of ribosomes are not seen. At 24 and 48 hr these particles are associated with areas of SER and appear to diminish in abundance with the increase of the SER. In some parts the membrane of the SER appears to be continuous with a row of such particles.[56] Although as yet we do not have any biochemical data as to the character of these particles their appearance resembles reticulosomes described by Pollak and co-workers,[31] who demonstrated that these particles, seen in embryonic chick liver, were RNA-ase resistant and were composed of lipoproteins. They suggested that these particles were precursors of membranes. Although it has been shown that microsomes are able to metabolise aflatoxin[29] we do not know if this increased amount of membrane represents an enhanced capacity of the liver cell to handle and metabolise the compound. Preliminary histochemical investigations indicate that there is an increased activity of both glucose-6-phosphatase and aniline hydroxalase activity when there is considerable proliferation of SER.

Although it is the periportal zone of the liver lobule that becomes necrotic the aflatoxin is distributed throughout the liver lobule. Autoradiographic evidence using tritiated aflatoxin indicates that more of the aflatoxin is bound in the centrilobular cells which do not become necrotic. As mentioned these cells show early changes but this is much less severe than those in the periportal cells. Preliminary results from grain counts indicate that there is about twice as much aflatoxin bound in these centrilobular cells than in the periportal cells. This binding is persistent, enabling a positive autoradiograph to be obtained up to 1 month after dosing. This corresponds to the fractionation studies of Lijinsky who demonstrated a considerable binding of aflatoxin to protein and less to DNA and RNA.[32] Wogan *et al.*[33] using C^{14} labelled aflatoxin B_1 showed that the microsomal fraction was labelled within 4 hr and that the level of labelling remained high in that fraction for 24 hr. In view of these observations it would seem that aflatoxin is able to bind to DNA, RNA and protein and form a persistent bond and, as well as producing cell death it induces the synthesis of SER in surviving cells. The mechanism of this action and that which is at all relevant to its toxic phenomena is not understood.

Interesting as these acute studies on the mechanism of toxicity may be and important as the economic value of livestock killed by the toxin is, the main interest in aflatoxin and some of the other mycotoxins is the demonstration of their carcinogenicity. There is little knowledge of the long-term effects of the other known mycotoxins. Sterigmatocystin has been shown to be carcinogenic.[34] Similary luteoskyrin[35] has been shown to be carcinogenic and will be mentioned later. There is no information concerning the carcinogenicity of most of the other mycotoxins although patulin has been shown to produce subcutaneous sarcomas at the site of injection.[36] Much more is known of the carcinogenicity of the aflatoxins. Lancaster *et al.*[37] were the first to show that the contaminated groundnut meal which was the causative agent in the field cases of aflatoxicosis in poults could induce a high incidence of hepatic carcinoma in rats. Using the same groundnut meal we demonstrated that only low levels of aflatoxin are required to induce hepatic carcinoma in rats and also that short term feeding was sufficient to produce liver neoplasia. Prior to this, however, Schoental[38] found that the toxic meal causing 'exudative hepatitis' in the guinea-pigs described by Paget[14] could induce hepatic carcinomas in rats. Also at this time Salmon and Newberne[39] reported a high incidence of hepatic tumours in rats fed diets containing commercial peanut meal. Le Breton and colleagues[40] also reported a high incidence of hepatic carcinoma in rats fed peanut meal. Since these early reports which conclusively demonstrated the carcinogenic potential of aflatoxin, further experiments have elucidated some of the factors which may influence the induction of hepatic carcinoma in rats.

By feeding aflatoxin-contaminated meal to Carshalton (Porton/Wistar) strain rats we have demonstrated a dose response curve and sex difference. The female rat is less susceptible to the carcinogenic effects of aflatoxin than the male. We have also shown that feeding for as short a period as 3 weeks, followed by a normal diet, induced hepatic carcinomas in rats. Wogan and Newberne[41] using pure aflatoxin B_1 in an inbred strain of Fischer rats have demonstrated that even lower levels of aflatoxin can induce a high incidence of hepatocellular carcinomas. Levels as low as

0·015 mg/kg in the diet resulted in 100% incidence in both males and females. Limited exposure to as little as 0·4 mg to individual rats of 14 days resulted in a significant incidence of hepatic carcinoma in male rats but none in females. It is possible that this difference in response to the contaminated meals of our experiments and the pure B_1 of Wogan and Newberne's experiment reflects a strain difference of the rats. We are at present trying to clarify this difference. Further Carnaghan[42] reported a 50% incidence of hepatic carcinoma after 2 years in female rats which had received a single dose of 7 mg/kg of B_1. I was less successful on the two occasions I repeated this experiment. In the first experiment no rats survived more than 18 months and no hepatic carcinomas were seen. In a second group of rats surviving more than 2 years after receiving an LD_{50} dose of aflatoxin B_1 I saw only 2 hepatic carcinomas. The sub-acute lesions induced by aflatoxin in the rat liver are similar to those seen following other hepatocarcinogens except that the degree of fibrosis is less. The typical lesions comprise considerable variations of parenchymal nuclear size and some oval cell and biliary proliferation.[43] It is only at the very highest dose levels, in the order of 5 mg/kg, that a cirrhotic liver is seen. Nearly all the carcinomas induced by aflatoxin occur in non-cirrhotic livers. Newberne has conclusively demonstrated that the induction of carcinoma is independent of the induction of the cirrhosis.[57]

The response of the rat to aflatoxin can be modified. We have demonstrated that hypophysectomy reduces the incidence of neoplasia.[44] Feeding levels of contaminated meal for 70 weeks, which in intact animals induced 100% incidence of carcinoma, produced no hepatic carcinomas in hypophysectomised animals. More recently Newberne[45] has shown that stilboestrol administration reduces the incidence of hepatic carcinoma. McLean and Marshall[58] have shown that rats receiving phenobarbitone in the drinking water in order to induce microsomal enzyme systems are protected to a certain extent from the carcinogenic action of aflatoxin.

Although most work has been done in rats either mixed aflatoxins or aflatoxin B_1 have been shown to be carcinogenic for trout,[46] ducklings,[47] ferrets (Allcroft, personal communication) and possibly guinea-pigs.[24] Mice appear to be resistant while in sheep only one hepatic carcinoma was seen following a 5 year feeding trial.[48] It is difficult to know whether this tumour is of significance. Of the other purified aflatoxins there is much less extensive information as to the carcinogenicity. Aflatoxin G_1 is a potent hepatocarcinogen in the rat but is somewhat less active than B_1.[49] We have failed to induce any carcinomas with aflatoxin B_2, and G_2 has not been tested. Aflatoxin M_1 which is obviously of considerable public health importance has also been investigated and found to induce subcutaneous sarcomas.[50] More recently it has been shown to induce hepatic tumours in trout. We have tried to demonstrate the carcinogenic action of aflatoxin M_1 in rats. Dr Allcroft of Weybridge prepared large amounts of dried milk from cows fed high levels of contaminated peanut meal. This was fed to rats as 50% of their diet for a 2 year period and we failed to find any hepatic carcinomas. However, the level of M_1 in the diet would have been at the lower level of sensitivity for our strain of rats. As a result of this Newberne and I plan to repeat the experiment using the more susceptible inbred Fischer rats. To date no results have been obtained. Of the other hydroxylated compounds B_{2a}, there is no evidence as to its carcinogenicity although it appears to be considerably less toxic.[51]

Although considerable emphasis is placed upon the hepatocarcinogenicity of the aflatoxins they are able to induce other types of neoplasms. One of the most striking of these is the renal adenocarcinoma induced by aflatoxin G_1.[48] The incidence was low in our initial experiment using G_1 but we have since repeated this and have found a similar number of renal carcinomas. Farber and his group[52] have reported that there is a strain difference in the incidence of renal carcinoma induced by B_1 but they did not test G_1 in the same system. It is interesting that G_1, which is able to induce renal carcinoma, is also a very potent renal toxin in high doses. The other very striking tumour which we induced (although other groups have not confirmed our findings) is carcinoma of the glandular stomach in rats.[53] This tumour is not seen in control animals and is comparatively difficult to induce. We originally reported five such carcinomas but have since seen a further four. It is not possible to say at the moment which of the various aflatoxins is responsible for this action. In all of our experiments using aflatoxin we have seen a variety of other neoplasms. However, most of these did not occur in significant numbers.

We have not mentioned as yet the carcinogenicity of aflatoxin in monkeys. In a 3-year feeding trial undertaken by Glaxo[54] with Cynomologous monkeys no hepatic carcinomas were induced although monkeys are extremely susceptible to relatively high doses of the purified aflatoxin and contaminated meal. In the 3 year survivors receiving 1.8 mg B_1/kg diet, one animal had a coarse nodular cirrhosis of the liver but there was no evidence of carcinoma. In all the remaining test animals the livers were histologically abnormal but no neoplasms were seen. Other experiments are being undertaken at National Cancer Institute, Bethesda, which have been going now for about 5 years and still no carcinomas have been reported.

It is this information concerning the acute and chronic effects of aflatoxins and in particular the demonstration of their carcinogenicity to mammals, birds and fish and the extremely low levels of carcinogen necessary to induce these tumours, which formed the experimental basis for what Oettlé[55] formulated as the 'mycotoxin hypothesis' for the induction of liver cancer in man. At present mycotoxins such as sterigmatocystin, luteoskyrin and aflatoxin and also naturally occurring nitrosamines are seriously considered as presenting hazards to human health.

REFERENCES

1. WIELAND, T. and WIELAND, O. (1959). *Pharmacol. Rev.*, **11**, 87.
2. FORGACS, J. and CARLL, W. T. (1962). *Adv. in vet. Sci.*, **7**, 274.
3. DROBOTKO, V. G. (1945). *Am. Rev. Soviet. Med.*, **2**, 238.
4. DONE, J., MORTIMER, P. H. and TAYLER, A. (1960). *Res. vet. Sci.*, **1**, 76.
5. ARMBRECHT, B. G., SHALKOP, W. G., ROLLINGS, L. E., POHLAND, A. E. and STOLOFF, L. (1970). *Nature* (Lond.), **225**, 1062.
6. SIPPEL, W. L., BURNSIDE, J. E. and ATWOOD, M. B. (1954). *Proc. Am. vet. med. Ass.*, 90th Ann. Meeting, Toronto, 174.
7. HARDING, J. D. J., DONE, J. T., LEWIS, G. and ALLCROFT, R. (1963). *Res. vet. Sci.*, **4**, 217.
8. LOOSMORE, R. M. and HARDING, J. D. J. (1961). *Vet. Rec.*, **73**, 1362.
9. HILL, L. R. (1963). *Vet. Rec.*, **75**, 493.
10. ALLCROFT, R. (1969). In: *Aflatoxin* (Ed. Goldblatt, L. A.), pp. 237-274. Academic Press.
11. SARGEANT, K., O'KELLY, J., CARNAGHAN, R. B. A. and ALLCROFT, R. (1961). *Vet. Rec.*, **73**, 1219.
12. BUTLER, W. H. (1964). *J. Path. Bact.*, **88**, 189.
13. MAGWOOD, S. E., ANNAU, E. and CORNER, A. H. (1966). *Can. J. comp. Med.*, **30**, 17.
14. PAGET, G. E. (1954). *J. Path. Bact.*, **47**, 393.
15. PATERSON, J. S., CROOK, J. C., SHAND, A., LEWIS, G. and ALLCROFT, R. (1962). *Vet. Rec.*, **74**, 639.
16. BUTLER, W. H. (1966). *J. Path. Bact.*, **91**, 277.
17. NEWBERNE, P. M., RUSSO, R. and WOGAN, G. N. (1966). *Path. Vet.*, **3**, 331.
18. NEWBERNE, J. W., BAILEY, W. S. and SEIBOLD, H. R. (1955). *J. Am. vet. med. Ass.*, **127**, 59.
19. BUTLER, W. H. (1964). *Br. J. Cancer*, **18**, 756.
20. DE RECONDO, A. M., FRAYSSINET, C., LEFRAGE, C. and LE BRETON, E. (1965). *C.R. Acad. Sci.*, (D) (Paris), **261**, 1409.
21. ROGERS, A. E. and NEWBERNE, P. M. (1967). *Cancer Res.*, **27**, 855.
22. BUTLER, W. H. and WIGGLESWORTH, J. S. (1966). *Br. J. exp. Path.*, **47**, 242.
23. BUTLER, W. H. (1970). *Fd. Cosmet Toxicol.*, **9**, 57.

24. NEWBERNE, P. M. and BUTLER, W. H. (1969). *Cancer Res.*, **29**, 236.
25. CARNAGHAN, R. B. A., HARTLEY, R. D. and O'KELLY, J. (1963). *Nature* (Lond.), **200**, 1101.
26. BUTLER, W. H. (1970). *J. Path.*, **102**, 209.
27. DE IONGH, H., VLES, R. O. and VAN PELT, J. G. (1964). *Nature* (Lond.), **202**, 466.
28. BUTLER, W. H. and CLIFFORD, J. L. (1965). *Nature* (Lond.), **206**, 1045.
29. PATTERSON, D. S. P. and ALLCROFT, R. (1970). *Fd. Cosmet. Toxicol.*, **8**, 43.
30. BUTLER, E. H. (1966). *Am. J. Path.*, **49**, 113.
31. POLLAK, J. K., WARD, K. and SHOREY, C. D. (1960). *J. mol. Biol.*, **16**, 564.
32. LIJINSKY, W. (1968). *N.Z. med. J.*, **67**, 100.
33. WOGAN, G. N., EDWARDS, G. S. and SHANK, R. C. (1967). *Cancer Res.*, **27**, 1729.
34. PURCHASE, I. F. H. and VAN DER WATT, J. J. (1970). *Fd. Cosmet. Toxicol.*, **8**, 289.
35. URUGUCIII, J. *et al.* (1961). *Jap. J. exp. Med.*, **31**, 135.
36. DICKENS, F. and JONES, H. B. H. (1961). *Br. J. Cancer*, **51**, 85.
37. LANCASTER, M. C., JENKINS, F. P. and PHILP, McL. (1961). *Nature* (Lond.), **192**, 1095.
38. SCHOENTAL, R. (1961). *Br. J. Cancer*, **15**, 812.
39. SALMON, W. D. and NEWBERNE, P. M. (1963). *Cancer Res.*, **23**, 571.
40. LE BRETON, E., FRAYSSINET, C. and BOY, J. (1962). *C.R. Acad. Sci.* (Paris), **255**, 784.
41. WOGAN, G. N. and NEWBERNE, P. M. (1967). *Cancer Res.*, **27**, 2370.
42. CARNAGHAN, R. B. A. (1967). *Br. J. Cancer*, **21**, 811.
43. BUTLER, W. H. and BARNES, J. M. (1963). *Br. J. Cancer*, **17**, 699.
44. GOODALL, C. M. and BUTLER, W. H. (1969). *Int. J. Cancer*, **4**, 422.
45. NEWBERNE, P. M. and WILLIAMS, G. (1969). *Arch. Envir. Hlth*, **19**, 489.
46. HALVER, J. E. (1965). In: *Mycotoxins in Foodstuffs* (Ed. Wogan, G. N.). MIT Press.
47. CARNAGHAN, R. B. A. (1965). *Nature* (Lond.), **208**, 308.
48. LEWIS, G., MARKSON, L. M. and ALLCROFT, R. (1967). *Vet. Rec.*, **80**, 312.
49. BUTLER, W. H., GREENBLATT, M. and LIJINSKY, W. (1969). *Cancer Res.*, **29**, 2206.
50. PURCHASE, I. F. H. and VORSTER, L. J. (1968). *S. Afr. med. J.*, **42**, 219.
51. DUTTON, M. F. and HEATHCOTE, J. G. (1968). *Chem. Ind.*, p. 418.
52. EPSTEIN, S. M., BARTUS, B. and FARBER, E. (1969). *Cancer Res.*, **29**, 1045.

53. BUTLER, W. H. and BARNES, J. M. (1966). *Nature* (Lond.), **209**, 90.
54. CUTHBERTSON, W. F. J., LAURSEN, A. C. and PRATT, D. A. H. (1967). *Br. J. Nutr.*, **21**, 893.
55. OETTLÉ, A. G. (1965). *S. Afr. med. J.*, **39**, 817.
56. BUTLER, W. H. (1971). *Chemico. Biol. Inter.* In press.
57. NEWBERNE, P. M., HARRINGTON, D. H. and WOGAN, G. N. (1966). *Lab. Invest.*, **15**, 962.
58. MCLEAN, A. E. M. and MARSHALL, A. (1971). *Br. J. exp. Path.*, **52**, 322.

HEPATIC AND RENAL PATHOLOGY INDUCED IN MICE BY FEEDING FUNGAL CULTURES

by

S. J. van Rensburg, I. F. H. Purchase and J. J. van der Watt

National Institute for Nutritional Diseases
South African Medical Research Council

Our search for toxic fungi originated from the concept that mycotoxins may be responsible for liver cancer in certain tribes in Africa. In order to provide a practical screening technique for the toxicity of fungal cultures, ducklings have frequently been used because of their known susceptibility to aflatoxin and because they will eat foods which are unpalatable to mammals. The drawback of these acute toxicity tests is that death (or weight loss) is the only criterion on which to judge toxicity and that acute toxicity is used as an index for carcinogenicity. The economic implications of using very long-term screening tests for carcinogens and the fact that the vast majority of carcinogens are also acutely toxic have so far prevented large-scale chronic toxicity studies. The only practical way of overcoming the objection to using death as the only end point is to examine animals fed fungal cultures for pathological lesions. We have found that the histopathological examination of organs from ducklings consuming fungal cultures is unrewarding except in a few cases such as *Aspergillus flavus* toxicity.

This study reports the histopathological changes occurring in mice fed fungal cultures so that a comparison can be made of the pathology produced by fungal cultures and so that an assessment can be made of the criteria for selecting toxic fungi.

METHODS

The 22 fungal strains tested (Table 1) were isolated from domestic cereal and legume products.[1] They were grown on sterilised maize meal as described by Scott[1] and dried, milled and incorporated as 50% by weight in the balanced laboratory animal diet.

Groups of ten young adult male mice were housed three or four mice per cage in an air-conditioned room in which the temperature and humidity were controlled to $26°C \pm 1°C$ and $50\% \pm 5\%$ respectively and which was illuminated for 12 hours per day. The test material was fed *ad lib.* for up to 36 days if the available quantity permitted. Three control groups were fed a similarly constituted, but unmoulded, ration.

Liver and kidney specimens were removed at post-mortem examination

Table 1

The Incidence of Mortality, Duration of the Experiment and the Body Weight of Test Mice

Group	Fungus	Number died/survived	Average mortality time (days)	Duration of experiment (days)	Mean initial body weight	Mean weight of survivors when killed
1	*Aspergillus clavatus*	1-9	6	22	20·9	19·3
2	*Aspergillus flavipes*	0-10	—	19	20·5	22·0
3	*Aspergillus flavus*	0-10	—	19	21·2	17·3
4	*Aspergillus fumigatus*	0-10	—	22	21·8	23·4
5	*Aspergillus mangini*	0-10	—	20	21·5	22·3
6	*Aspergillus mangini*	0-10	—	7	21·6	21·9
7	*Aspergillus nidulans*	0-10	—	20	21·6	17·4
8	*Aspergillus versicolor*	0-10	—	14	21·1	23·3
9	*Cunninghamella elegans*	2-8	3	7	21·4	18·1
10	*Fusarium moniliforme*	1-9	3	20	20·9	15·7
11	*Fusarium roseum*	10-0	15	—	20·5	—
12	*Fusarium roseum*	10-0	10	—	20·0	—
13	*Fusarium species*	1-9	4	14	22·1	21·7
14	*Helminthosporium species*	0-10	—	36	15·9	17·8
15	*Mycelia sterilia*	10-0	5	—	15·3	—
16	*Paecilomyces varioti*	0-10	—	20	21·9	22·3
17	*Penicillium cyclopium*	10-0	14	—	22·0	—
18	*Penicillium oxalicum*	10-0	4	—	16·0	—
19	*Penicillium oxalicum*	10-0	12	—	22·5	—
20	*Penicillium variabile*	0-10	—	14	22·8	22·7
21	*Rhizopus arrhizus*	10-0	3	—	16·4	—
22	*Sphaeropsidales species*	1-9	3	20	21·1	19·8
23	Control	0-10	—	36	16·7	20·4
24	Control	0-10	—	34	20·5	—
25	Control	0-10	—	30	22·7	25·7

from mice which had died and were fixed in 10% buffered formalin. Mice which survived until the conclusion of the test were killed with ether and similar specimens were taken. Haematoxylin and erythrosin stained sections (0·5 μ) were prepared from paraffin-wax embedded liver and kidney tissue from each of the 250 mice in the experiment. Histopathological alterations were recorded in tabular form for each group and description of a lesion implies that it was found in the majority, if not all, test animals in the group.

RESULTS

The occurrence of mortality, duration of each test and the initial and final body weight of survivors are recorded in Table 1.

Significant mortality was encountered with only five species of fungi, which killed all ten test mice in 3 to 15 days. They were *Fusarium roseum*, *Mycelia sterilia*, *P. cyclopium*, *P. oxalicum* and *Rhizopus arrhizus*. One or two of the ten test mice died in trials with four other fungal species and the survivors in each of these groups lost weight during the test. In the remaining nine groups no mortality was encountered, as in the three control groups, and significant weight loss was only encountered in the *A. flavus* and *A. nidulans* groups. The latter two species are known to be capable of producing aflatoxins and sterigmatocystin respectively.

The histopathological findings of each group, in alphabetical order as in Table 1, are described below.

1. Aspergillus clavatus. This fungus has been incriminated in chicken mycotoxicosis and as a cause of bovine hyperkeratosis. During the test one mouse died on the 6th day and the remainder showed slight weight loss.

Kidney glomerular cell nuclei were somewhat pycnotic and slight degenerative changes were evident in the epithelial cells of the proximal convoluted tubules. The outstanding changes, however, were proliferation of tubular epithelial cells and, interstitially, fibroblasts and macrophages. In the liver, mild periportal vacuolar degeneration and many large hepatocyte nuclei with pachychromatic chromatin were noted. The bile ducts were prominent, and in some livers the vascular and biliary elements of the portal triads were surrounded by a cellular infiltrate.

2. Aspergillus flavipes. Apparently non-toxic, this isolate nevertheless induced histologically distinct degenerative changes in the kidney tubules. Sporadic pycnosis of medullary tubule cell nuclei was invariably present and occasionally cortical cells were also affected. The liver appeared relatively normal except for unusual prominence of Kupffer cells, many of which had pycnotic nuclei.

3. Aspergillus flavus. Strains of this species have been demonstrated to produce a variety of toxic substances in addition to aflatoxins, yet in this mouse test the culture only induced weight loss without mortality. The kidney glomeruli were hyperaemic, with pycnotic nuclei. Obliteration of Bowman's space was apparent in the majority of instances. Hyaline degeneration of the proximal tubules near the cortico-medullary junction was sometimes evident and numerous tubular cell nuclei at and immediately below the junction were pycnotic.

Mild hepatic hydropic degeneration, particularly central, was present and there was much variation in the size of the hepatocytes. Large nuclei frequently had condensed chromatin creating a 'cartwheel' appearance and moderate single cell necrosis was apparent. Mild proliferative changes of the bile duct cells were usually present.

4. *Aspergillus fumigatus*. Potent nephrotoxic fungal metabolites have been associated with this species.[2] In this trial only mild hydropic degeneration of the proximal tubules and occasional pycnosis of epithelial cells at the cortico-medullary junction were noted. A diffuse vacuolar change of the hepatic parenchyma was also present, yet the mice grew well and suffered no obvious clinical ill-effects.

5, 6. *Aspergillus mangini*. The two isolates tested both failed to cause mortality but permitted only slight growth. Renal lesions in both groups were similar and consisted of congestion of the cortex, glomeruli and medulla and degeneration of the proximal tubular epithelium, particularly near the cortico-medullary junction. In both groups moderate numbers of medullary tubular cells were necrotic, and in the 20-day test group many tubule cell nuclei had peripheral chromatin with frequent signet-cell formation.

Hepatic changes observed in both groups were congestion of all vasculature including the parenchymal sinusoids, large numbers of hepatocytes with small nuclei in the periportal areas and occasional midzonal single cell necrosis. Consistent dilation or distention of the smaller bile ducts and prominent cellularity of the smaller bile ductules was clear in the shorter test and in the 20-day test very early bile duct proliferative changes were noted in a few mice.

7. *Aspergillus nidulans*. The hepatotoxic and carcinogenic mycotoxin sterigmatocystin and an unusual metabolite, nidulol, are known to be produced by this species.[3] In this test, lasting 20 days, serious weight loss was encountered without any mortality.

The renal glomeruli were hyperaemic and there was considerable distention of Bowman's space. The convoluted tubules consistently exhibited hydropic and hyaline droplet degeneration, particularly in the vicinity of the cortico-medullary junction. Lysis of isolated proximal tubular cells was invariably accompanied by some pycnosis and necrosis of the medullary tubular epithelial cells.

Generalised hydropic-like degeneration was present in the liver parenchyma; in some animals the vacuolation was more pronounced in the centrilobular area and in others the midzonal or periportal regions were most affected. Hepatocytes with unusually large nuclei were particularly noticeable in the midzonal region. Early proliferation of bile ducts was clear in all the mice.

8. *Aspergillus versicolor.* Sterigmatocystin is also produced by this species, and the lesions have some resemblance to those induced by *A. nidulans*. Degenerative changes were present in the renal glomeruli and necrosis of individual tubular cells appeared to be present throughout the nephron but was particularly prevalent in the medulla. Vacuolar degeneration of the liver cells varied inconsistently between mice; but Kupffer cell prominence was constant. Many hepatocyte nuclei in the vicinity of the portal triads were unusually small.

9. *Cunninghamella elegans.* Two of the ten test mice died during the short 7-day test with this culture, and the remainder exhibited severe weight loss.

Mild renal glomerular congestion and moderate pycnosis of its cellular elements were constantly present. Within the renal cortex sporadic single cell or, in some mice, focal proximal tubular necrosis was evident. Endothelial cells of the interstitial vascular system were pycnotic and were possibly the cause of small scattered cortical haemorrhages. The majority of medullary tubules exhibited severe degenerative and necrotic changes.

The portal and sinusoidal hepatic vascular system was severely congested in the majority of specimens. Endothelial cells of particularly the portal veins appeared to have a disrupted arrangement and the nuclei were pycnotic; areas of focal haemorrhagic necrosis in some mice appeared to be associated with these degenerative vascular changes. The hepatocyte cytoplasm was reduced and small nuclei were frequent in the periportal areas, whereas in the midzonal area large pachychromatic nuclei and single cell necrosis were frequent. Bile duct proliferation varied from a slight to a moderate degree.

10. *Fusarium moniliforme.* Although only one mouse died during the 20-day test period, the survivors exhibited a severe loss of weight. The renal glomeruli were slightly hyperaemic and vacuolar degenerative changes were present in the proximal tubules. Occasional cells of the convoluted tubules were necrotic and in the medullary rays moderate numbers of nuclei were pycnotic.

Hepatocyte nuclei exhibited considerable variation in size and many were binucleate. Cytoplasmic vacuolar change was irregularly present but occasional single cell necrosis was noted in all mice. The outstanding hepatic alteration was, however, a pronounced bile duct proliferation.

11, 12. *Fusarium roseum.* Lesions induced by these lethal cultures were similar with both strains tested. Focal to massive necrosis of the proximal convoluted tubules was the salient renal alteration; moderate pycnosis of the medullary tubule cells was less severe than the hyaline degeneration and coagulative necrosis of the proximal tubules. Glomerular congestion and pycnosis as well as congestion of the medulla were also constant findings.

There was congestion of the entire hepatic vascular bed and marked atrophy of the hepatocytes, including the nucleus, particularly in the periportal zones. In this area cellular degeneration and at times marked necrosis, in addition to the frequent scattered single cell necrosis, was most evident. The bile ducts of some mice appeared to be proliferating.

13. Fusarium species. The histological lesions of this group were similar to those caused by *F. moniliforme* (group 10), although to a somewhat milder degree.

14. Helminthosporium species. Considering the long period of this 36-day test, the mice grew only very slightly, but pathological alterations were exceedingly mild. The proximal tubules exhibited nephrosis and occasional cells throughout the nephron, particularly in the portion constituting the medullary rays, were necrotic. Occasional distended proximal tubules and an increase in the size of Bowman's space emphasised the chronic nature of the tubular degeneration. Some of the liver sections had mild vacuolar changes.

15. Mycelia sterilia. This culture of mycelia which failed to sporulate proved to be acutely toxic within a short period. The renal glomeruli were congested and there was necrosis of individual tubular epithelial cells, particularly in the medulla. Bowman's space was increased and sporadic nephrons were distended.

The loss of hepatocyte cytoplasm resulted in densely packed nuclei and atrophic livers in all mice. The portal and central veins were also congested.

16. Paecilomyces varioti. Although consumption of this culture had no obvious clinical ill-effects on mice, mild pathological changes were present in both the kidney and liver. Degenerative changes in the renal tubular epithelium appeared to culminate in occasional necrosis of individual cells, particularly in the medulla. There was some oedema of Bowman's space and portions of the capsule appeared thickened.

Considerable variation in the size of the hepatocyte nuclei was present and many large nuclei had condensed chromatin imparting a 'cartwheel' effect. Necrosis of individual hepatocytes was rare but the nuclei of the bile duct epithelium tended to have peripherally arranged chromatin resulting in a vacuolated appearance.

17. Penicillium cyclopium. The mycotoxin cyclopiazonic acid has been described as the major toxic metabolite.[4] Wilson, Wilson and Hays[5] described a tremorogenic toxin but their three strains of *P. cyclopium* apparently failed to produce cyclopiazonic acid. The fungus does, however, appear to be highly toxic under all circumstances, apparently even causing mortality in sheep and horses. The lesions found in our mouse test bear an exceedingly close resemblance to those produced by pure cyclopiazonic acid.[6]

The renal glomeruli were congested and the nuclei tended to be pycnotic. Mild sporadic necrosis of the epithelial lining cells of all tubules was present and the medulla was usually congested. The amount of hepatocyte cytoplasm was severely reduced and many Kupffer cells, the majority with pycnotic nuclei, were present. Much variation in the size of hepatocyte nuclei was apparent and the cytoplasm exhibited moderate degenerative changes. Bile duct cells were pycnotic and the tubules themselves were frequently distended. Oedema and some proliferative changes were present in the walls of both the portal and central veins.

18, 19. *Penicillium oxalicum.* The cultures of the two strains tested proved to be even more toxic to mice than those tested by Carlton, Tuite and Mislivec.[7]

Renal changes of those mice dying as early as the 3rd day consisted mainly of severe congestion of the cortex and glomeruli with focal haemorrhages which usually appeared to be situated immediately adjacent to a glomerulus. The proximal convoluted tubule cells were degenerated and the chromatin of the nuclei was marginally arranged. In those mice dying a day or two later, focal proximal tubular necrosis and pycnosis was severe. The majority of medullary and distal convoluted tubule cell nuclei had marginal chromatin imparting a vacuolated appearance. Mice dying on about the 12th day as in group 19 had pycnotic glomerular tuft cells and mild glomerular congestion, moderate sporadic necrosis of tubular cells and occasional cast formation and distention of nephrons.

Acute hepatic alterations were dominated by severe generalised congestion characterised in particular by dilation of portal vessels and the sinusoidal spaces. Degenerative changes in the endothelial cells and at times slightly thickened blood vessel walls were clear to those animals in which the hepatocyte single cell necrosis had progressed in focal necrosis. Slight ductule cell proliferation was seen in acute deaths, but those dying later had marked pycnosis of all bile duct epithelial cells. Kupffer cells were not prominent but their nuclei were pycnotic.

20. *Penicillium variabile.* In agreement with the result of Carlton *et al.*[7] this culture was found to inhibit the growth of mice without causing mortality.

The renal cortices and glomeruli were mildly hyperaemic and occasional cells within the glomerular tufts had pycnotic nuclei. Slight hyaline degeneration and lytic necrosis of the tubules at the cortico-medullary junction was present but, deeper within the medulla, scattered tubular necrosis characterised by pycnosis was frequent.

G

Vacuolar changes within the liver usually affected all hepatocytes but were more pronounced in the centrilobular areas. Occasional hepatocytes in the interzonal areas were necrotic and slight proliferative changes of bile ductule cells were constantly present.

21. *Rhizopus arrhizus.* This previously untested culture proved to be the most toxic species tested and virtually all mice died on the 3rd day. On post-mortem examination all had mosaic-patterned livers.

Histologically, all renal tubular epithelium had undergone hyaline or vacuolar degeneration; many proximal tubules were necrotic and the distal tubules frequently had enlarged vesicular nuclei with marginal chromatin. Intratubular casts, distended nephrons and haemorrhages in the upper portion of the medulla were common.

Hepatic periportal coagulative necrosis, frequently accompanied by haemorrhage and congestion, was severe in all mice. There was considerable macrophage activity within and around the necrotic areas and the remaining hepatic parenchyma was severely degenerated. Slight bile duct proliferative changes were seen in a few specimens.

22. *Sphaeropsidales* species. The one mouse that died in this group had pathological changes which suggested that death was not directly related to treatment. Weight loss was, however, exhibited by the remainder and all had mild degenerative changes in the renal tubular epithelium with a moderate amount of scattered necrosis in the medulla. There was marked centrilobular hydropic-like vacuolar degeneration and occasional single cell necrosis. Margination of nuclear chromatin of the bile duct cells was constant.

23, 24, 25. *Controls.* Slight sporadic pycnosis of medullary renal tubule cells was seen in about half of the control animals. Microscopically, the hepatic lobules regularly exhibited slight centrilobular changes. Similar changes, when described in the test groups above, were all of greater severity.

DISCUSSION

None of the groups of mice fed moulded maize grew quite as well as the controls, and some pathological changes were found to be induced by every fungus studied. Cytotoxic effects on the renal nephron were invariably present and normal livers were rarely found. The degree to which the liver or kidney was altered within a group appeared to depend largely on the duration of exposure and it was therefore usually not possible to classify a culture as primarily 'nephrotoxic' or 'hepatotoxic'. The presence of only moderately advanced degenerative changes in the kidneys usually had little effect on the mice but when hepatic pathology of any consequence was present, mortality occurred or the mice lost weight.

The value of pathological examinations was illustrated with our *A. flavus*, *A. nidulans* and *A. versicolor* cultures. These fungi are known to produce potent hepatotoxins, yet with the test material used no mortality was encountered. All three groups of mice did, however, have considerable variation in the size of the hepatocyte nuclei in addition to various parenchymal degenerative changes and proliferation of bile ductule cells. Eight other fungal species (groups 1, 5, 6, 9, 10, 11, 20, 21 and 22) whose toxic metabolites have not been characterised, induced at least similar or more advanced hepatotoxic alterations and thus warrant further investigation by chemical means. The pathology induced appeared to be quite independent of the genus of the fungus.

ACKNOWLEDGEMENTS

Mrs W. Bourquin and Mr D. M. T. Tagg provided excellent technical assistance.

REFERENCES

1. SCOTT, DE B. (1965). *Mycopathol. et Mycol. Appl.*, **25**, 213.
2. KROGH, P. and HASSELAGER, E. (1968). *Studies on fungal nephrotoxicity.* Royal Veterinary and Agricultural College, Copenhagen, Denmark. Yearbook, pp. 198-214.
3. AUCAMP, P. J. and HOLZAPFEL, C. W. (1968). *J. S.A. Chem. Inst.*, **21**, 26.
4. HOLZAPFEL, C. W. (1968). *Tetrahedron*, **24**, 2101.
5. WILSON, B. J., WILSON, CHRISTINA H. and HAYS, A. W. (1968). *Nature* (Lond.), **220**, 77.
6. PURCHASE, I. F. H. (1971). *Toxicol. App. Pharmacol.*, **18**, 114.
7. CARLTON, W. W., TUITE, J. and MISLIVEC, P. (1968). *Toxicol. Appl. Pharmacol.*, **13**, 372.

TOXICOLOGICAL AND BIOLOGICAL PROPERTIES OF FUSARENON-X, A CYTOTOXIC MYCOTOXIN OF *FUSARIUM NIVALE* Fn-2B

by

Yoshio Ueno

Microbial Chemistry, Faculty of Pharmaceutical Sciences
Science University of Tokyo, Ichigaya, Tokyo, Japan

With the aim of finding out the factors responsible for intoxication caused by mouldy foodstuffs, extensive research was carried out, with the co-operation of mycologists, toxicologists and chemists, into the 'rice-fungus-toxin'. The hepatotoxic luteoskyrin and chlorine-containing peptide of *Penicillium islandicum* Sopp,[1] the nephrotoxic citrinin of *Penicillium citrinum* Thom,[2] and the neurotoxic citreoviridin of *Penicillium citreo-viride* Biourge[3, 4] were isolated.

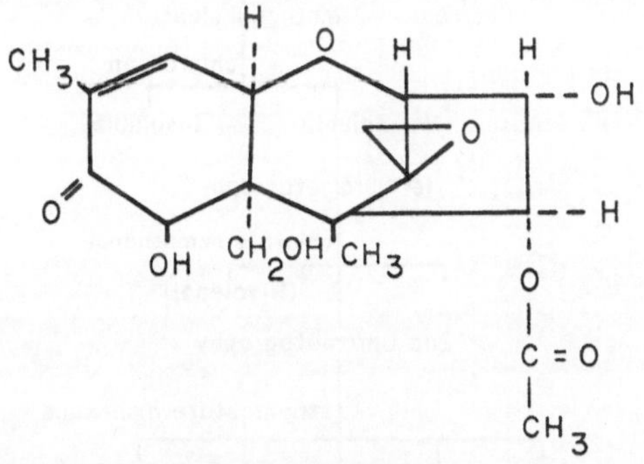

FIG. 1. Fusarenon-X.

Recently further work was conducted on the 'wheat-fungus-toxin'. As a result of extensive screening, several toxic *Fusaria* were isolated from damaged wheat. The new scirpene mycotoxin, named nivalenol (3,4,7,15-tetrahydroxyscirp-9en-8one),[5, 6] was isolated from rice grains artificially inoculated with *Fusarium nivale* Fn-2B. Recently the author isolated fusarenon-X (3,7,15-trihydroxyscirp-4-acetoxy-9en-8one) as a main toxic metabolite of the same fungus[7, 8, 9] (Fig. 1) when grown on peptone supplemented Czapek medium.

In the present paper, the acute toxicity and biological properties of fusarenon-X are reported.

MATERIALS

Fusarenon-X

Fusarenon-X was isolated from the culture filtrate of *F. nivale* Fn-2B according to the method previously reported.[7, 8] *F. nivale* Fn-2B was cultured stationally at 25-27°C for 10-14 days on Czapek medium supplemented with 10 g/l of peptone. The culture filtrate (20 l) was mixed with 200 g of activated charcoal. After standing overnight at 4°C, the charcoal was filtered, and the active principle was eluted with 3 litres of methanol. The methanol-eluate dissolved in a small amount of methanol was mixed with

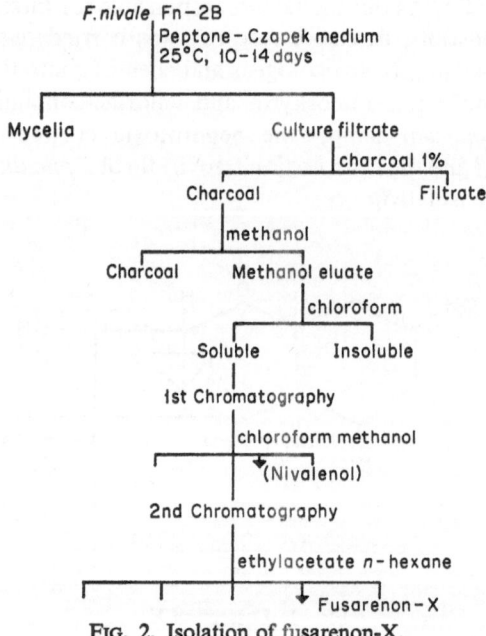

FIG. 2. Isolation of fusarenon-X.

five volumes of chloroform, and the chloroform-methanol soluble fraction was chromatographed on a silicagel column with chloroform-methanol (9:1) as solvent. Rechromatography of fusarenon-X fraction with ethyl-acetate-*n*-hexane (3 : 1) gave a white powder, from which fusarenon-X was crystallised with dichloromethane-*n*-pentane, as shown in Figure 2.

Other scirpene mycotoxins

Diacetoxyscirpenol and T-2 toxin were kindly provided by Dr Taeshler (Sandoz Ltd) and Dr Strong (University of Wisconsin, U.S.A.), respectively. Trichothecolon, verrucarin-A, trichothecin and nivalenol were a generous gift from Dr Tatsuno (Institute of Physical and Chemical Research, Saitama-ken).

Crude toxin of mouldy rice

A 500-ml flask containing 200 g of polished rice grains, which were previously immersed in tap water for 30 minutes, was inoculated with *Fusaria* and incubated for 2 weeks at 27°C. The mouldy rice was powdered, extracted with *n*-hexane, and then with methanol. The chloroform-soluble material of the charcoal-adsorbable fraction in the methanol extract was referred to as the crude toxin.[9]

RESULTS

Detection of fusarenon-X

(*a*) Chemical method: Thin-layer chromatography is the most useful way for detecting the mycotoxin. Fusarenon-X and other scirpene toxins exhibit no fluorescence under UV-light and no absorption in the UV-region. Therefore, the chemical detection of these mycotoxins on chromatoplates was carried out with H_2SO_4-spraying. Rf values of fusarenon-X and the

Table 1

Rf Values of Scirpene Toxins

Developers	Fusarenon-X	Nivalenol	Diacetoxy-scirpenol	T-2 toxin
Chloroform-Methanol (5:1)	0·89	0·44	0·95	0·95
Chloroform-Methanol (97:3)	0·19	0·05	0·55	—
Ethylacetate-Toluene (3:1)	0·36	0·09	0·50	0·56
Ethylacetate-*n*-Hexane (3:1)	0·37	0·17	0·63	0·69

Thin-layer chromatography was carried out at 25°C with Kieselgel G and developers listed in the Table.

others in different sorts of developer are listed in Table 1. Of the four mobile phases, chloroform:methanol (5:1) and ethylacetate-*n*-hexane (3:1) generally gave the best results. Spot testing with H_2SO_4 showed a time-dependent change of colour as follows: fusarenon-X, purple to brown; nivalenol, pink to brown; diacetoxyscirpenol and T-2 toxin, brown. In cases of the last two toxins, even a small amount of the toxins fluoresced sky-blue under a UV-lamp after spraying with H_2SO_4.

(*b*) Biological method: As previously reported,[10, 11] the uptake of C^{14}-amino acid by rabbit reticulocytes was highly sensitive to the scirpene toxins. In order to confirm this, the inhibitory effect of fusarenon-X was compared with the other newly isolated toxins. As shown in Figure 3, all seven scirpenes inhibited the uptake of C^{14}-leucine, and the activity was almost proportional to the logarithmic concentration of the toxins, indicating that the amount of toxin could be determined biochemically. In addition protein synthesis in the reticulocyte was inhibited only by the scirpene

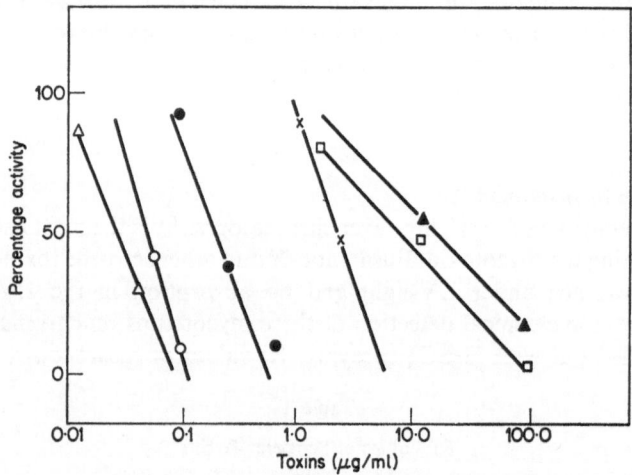

FIG. 3. Inhibition of protein synthesis in rabbit reticulocytes by the scirpene mycotoxins.

Reticulocytes 0·1 ml, Locke-Ringer's solution 0·7 ml, and the toxin 0·1 ml were pre-incubated at 37°C for 15 min, and C^{11}-leucine 0·1 ml (0·05 μC) was added to continue the incubation for 40 min. Radioactivity in acid-insoluble material was counted.

○ —— ○	Diacetoxyscirpenol	▲ —— ▲	T-2 toxin
● —— ●	Fusarenon-X	× —— ×	Nivalenol
△ —— △	Trichothecolon	□ —— □	Verrucarin-A

toxins (Table 2), although the inhibitory potency differed depending on the chemical structure.

Toxic Fusaria: Several strains of *Fusaria* and *Gibberella* were subjected to the biological assay as well as the chemical test. As indicated in Table 3, the crude toxin from all of the strains of *F. nivale* were positive in the lethal toxicity to mice, the reticulocyte bioassay, the skin test with rabbit; and TLC-analysis, with the exception of NRRL-A-B-318 which was negative in the latter two assay methods. Further, *G. zeae* (*F. roseum*), was also lethal to mice and inhibitory to protein synthesis in rabbit reticulocytes.

Acute toxicity of fusarenon-X

(a) Mice: Male and female mice (6-8 weeks old) were administered fusarenon-X dissolved in saline. The 7-day LD_{50} of fusarenon-X was 3·3

Table 2

Specificity of Reticulocyte Bioassay

Specificity	Mycotoxins	50% Inhibition (μg/ml)
Marked	T-2 toxin	0·02
	diacetoxyscirpenol	0·05
	fusarenon-X	0·25
	trichothecin	0·5*
	nivalenol	2·5
Moderate	verrucarin A	
	trichothecolon	10–15
	patulin	
	zearalenone	
Slightly	luteoskyrin	
	rugolosin	50–
	penicillic acid	
None	rubratoxin B	
	aflatoxin B	
	ascradiol	
	citrinin	
	sporidesmin	—
	butenolide	
	Cl-peptide	

* 80% inhibition.

and 3·4 mg/kg intraperitoneally (male and female, respectively), 4·5 and 4·0 mg/kg subcutaneously (male and female, respectively), and 4·5 mg/kg orally (female). New-born mice were highly sensitive to the toxin and the subcutaneous LD$_{50}$ was estimated as 0·1 mg/kg.

Mortality occurred in 24 to 72 hours irrespective of doses and route of administration. As to the acute symptoms, the mice became inactive with ruffled hair and stopped eating and drinking. Respiration seemed to be slowing down and the next day they lay down. No convulsions or unusual behaviour were observed even when external stimuli were applied to the mice.

In the fatal cases, dilatation and haemorrhage of the intestine, atrophy and ecchymosis of the thymus, hyperaemia in the periphery of the liver lobules, and sometimes diarrhoea were observed.

Table 3

Screening of Toxic *Fusaria*

The fungi were cultured on polished rice grains at 27°C for 2 weeks and the crude toxin was isolated as described in the Methods

Fungi	Strain	Lethal toxicity* (dead/used)	Reticulocyte† bioassay (per-cent activity, %)	Skin‡ test	F-X	N
			Biological activity of crude toxin		TLC§	
F. nivale	Fn-2B	3/3	43·2	+	+	+
	Fn-2-L-A	3/3	8·7	+	+	+
	Fn-2-L-B	3/3	8·4	+	+	+
	NRRL A-13-318	3/3	10·5	±	−	
	Fn-M	3/3	15·9	+	+	+
	Fn-M-L	3/3	35·8		+	+
F. sp.	MR-39-1	0/3	75·0		−	−
G. zeae	Ohoita-2	3/3	16·8	+ +		
	Ishii	3/3	46·1	+		
	NRRL-2830	1/3	45·7	+		

* 20 mg/10 g mice, i.p.; † 100 μg/ml; ‡ 1 mg to rabbit skin;
§ F-X, fusarenon-X; N, nivalenol.

(*b*) Rats: Male Wistar rats (9 weeks old) were administered orally five doses of 2·4-5·0 mg/kg of fusarenon-X, and the death rate on the 7th day gave LD_{50} of 4·4 mg/kg. When 4·0 mg of fusarenon-X per kg body weight was administered intraperitoneally, after 1 to 2 hours the respiration was increased and the capillaries in the ear were dilated, and after 5 to 10 hours the rats became inactive and drowsy.

In the fatal cases, yellow intestine with expanded capillaries, hyperaemia in the liver lobules and spleen, ecchymosis of the thymus and dilated capillaries around the body wall were noted. Diarrhoea was marked in all cases.

(*c*) Guinea-pigs: A male guinea-pig weighing 860 g died 11 hours after the intraperitoneal administration of fusarenon-X (0·5 mg/kg) and a pregnant female weighing 950 g died 8 hours after the intraperitoneal injection of 5 mg/kg. In both cases, the heart rate was temporarily increased and the respiration was markedly disturbed.

The toxin is highly toxic to new-born guinea-pigs. When three guinea-pigs were injected subcutaneously, within 24 hours of birth, with the mycotoxin, a male weighing 94 g (dose 1 mg/kg) died after 18 hours, a female weighing

77 g (dose 0·1 mg/kg) died after 18 hours, and a female weighing 77 g (dose 0·01 mg/kg) survived. From the preliminary data described above, the subcutaneous LD_{50} of fusarenon-X to the new-born guinea-pig is assumed to be less than 0·1 mg/kg.

(d) Cats: A male cat, weighing 1·58 kg, received 5 mg/kg subcutaneously and vomited 30 minutes after the administration and died overnight. No convulsions or tremors were observed, but the cat became inactive with ruffled hair. Subcutaneous administration of 1 mg/kg of fusarenon-X was fatal to a 1-week-old cat.

(e) Ducklings: When Pekin ducklings (10 days old) weighing 80-100 g, were administered the toxin, the mortality was 100% at 5 mg/kg subcutaneously and orally, and around 50% at 2 mg/kg subcutaneously. No fatal cases were observed at 1 mg/kg. In all cases, marked vomiting was evoked. For example, the duckling receiving subcutaneously 2·0 mg/kg vomited 7 minutes after administration, and then took drinking water. This vomiting-drinking was repeated for the following 20 minutes with an interval of 2 minutes. This symptom appeared even with a smaller dose of 0·5 mg/kg irrespective of the route of administration.

Table 4

Skin-irritant Toxicity of Scirpene Mycotoxins

0·01 ml of the acetone solution containing varied amounts of the toxin was applied on the shaved skin of the back, and the degree of skin lesion was indicated: − seemingly normal, + slight, + + medium and + + + heavy and scabby

	Dose (µg)	Animals		
		Rabbit	Guinea-pig	Mouse
Diacetoxyscirpenol	0·2	−	+	−
	1·0	+	+	±
	10·0	+ +	+ + +	+
	100·0	+ + +	+ + +	+ +
Fusarenon-X	0·2	−	+	±
	1·0	−	+	±
	10·0	+	+ +	+
	100·0	+ + +	+ + +	+ +
Nivalenol	1·0	−	−	−
	10·0	+	−	−
	100·0	+	+ +	+

Ueno et al. (1970).[12]

(*f*) Fish: *Oryzias latipes* Temmink et Schlegel (Himedaka in Japanese), 15-20 mm in length, were reared in open 500-ml petri dishes. Each dish contained 400 ml of charcoal-treated water and seven fishes. With 5 μg/ml of the toxin, the death rates were 1/7 and 4/7 at the 51st and 70th hour respectively, and with 10 μg/ml the death rates were 2/7, 5/7 and 7/7 at 45, 51 and 70 hours of incubation, respectively. These data indicated that the LD$_{50}$ of the toxin on the 3rd day was around 5 μg/ml.

(*g*) Chicken embryo: With the co-operation of Drs Kurata and Ichinoe (the National Institute of Hygienic Sciences, Tokyo), the lethal toxicity of fusarenon-X to chicken embryo was examined. When the aqueous solution containing varied amounts of the toxin was injected into the yolk of 96 hour fertile White Leghorn eggs, 10 μg of fusarenon-X per egg caused 90% mortality at 24 hours incubation, and the calculated LD$_{50}$ at 48 hours incubation was 6 μg/egg.

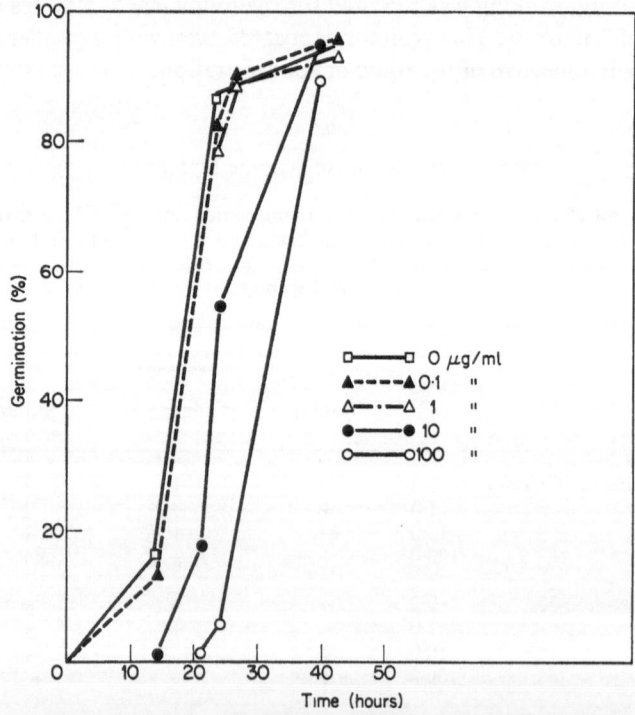

FIG. 4. Inhibitory effect of fusarenon-X on the germination of
Brassia oleracea L.

One hundred seeds of *Brassia oleracea* L. were plated on a petri dish containing 1·5% agar, and incubated at 20-22°C for a few days. Each point in the Figure represents an average of four petri dishes.

(*h*) Skin tissue: As previously reported,[12] fusarenon-X was highly irritant to skin tissue of mouse, rabbit and guinea-pig, causing haemorrhage and necrosis of the epidermis, degeneration and necrosis of hair follicles and dermis. The comparative studies on fusarenon-X and the other scirpene toxins revealed (Table 4) that the skin-irritant toxicity of fusarenon-X was slightly less than that of diacetoxyscirpenol.

Biological activity

(*a*) Phytotoxic effect: The phytotoxic action of fusarenon-X was examined with the seed of the cauliflower, *Brassia oleracea* L. When 100 seeds were inoculated on an agar plate at room temperature (20-22°C) they started to germinate 15 hours later and the germination reached 95% after 40 hours. When fusarenon-X was added to the plate, germination was retarded in the presence of 10 μg to 100 μg of the toxin per ml (Fig. 4).

(*b*) Antimicrobial effect: The antibacterial effect of fusarenon-X was investigated using the cup method. 5 to 25 μg/ml of the toxin did not inhibit the growth of *Bacillus subtilis*, *Alcaligenes faecalis*, *Pseudomonas aeruginosa*, *Escherichia coli*, *Mycobacterium tuberculosis* or *Serracia marcescence*.

Heat treatment of the protozoon *Tetrahymena pyriformis* GL induces synchronous cell division. When the mycotoxin was added to the culture medium just after the end of heat treatment, 5 μg/ml inhibited multiplication completely and even 1·0 μg/ml of the toxin was inhibitory to the synchronous cell division, giving an estimated LD_{50} of 2 μg/ml (Fig. 5).

(*c*) Mutagenicity to yeast cells: It is well established that chemical agents, including carcinogens, induce a respiratory-deficient mutant (RD-mutant) in yeast cells, *Saccharomyces cerevisiae*.

When the cells were cultured at 27°C for a week in the presence of fusarenon-X 250 μg/ml (7×10^{-4} M) the increase of cellular turbidity did not differ from the control, indicating no cytostatic effect. However, when a drop of the treated cell suspension was plated on colour plates which contained tryphan blue and eosin, white colonies formed about 4% of the total. TTC-overlay method also afforded about 3·8% of RD-mutant with the same concentration of fusarenon-X.

Further experiments carried out with a differential spectrophotometer revealed that the mutant cells lacked absorption peaks at 565 mμ (cytochrome b) and 605 mμ (cytochrome a). These results confirmed that the toxin actually induced RD-mutants in yeast cells.

(*d*) Induction of prophage in *Escherichia coli* K-12: According to a private communication of Dr Iwahara (the National Institute of Hygienic Sciences, Tokyo), fusarenon-X neither induced the prophage nor inhibited the growth of *Escherichia coli* K-12 at a concentration of 10-100 μg/ml.

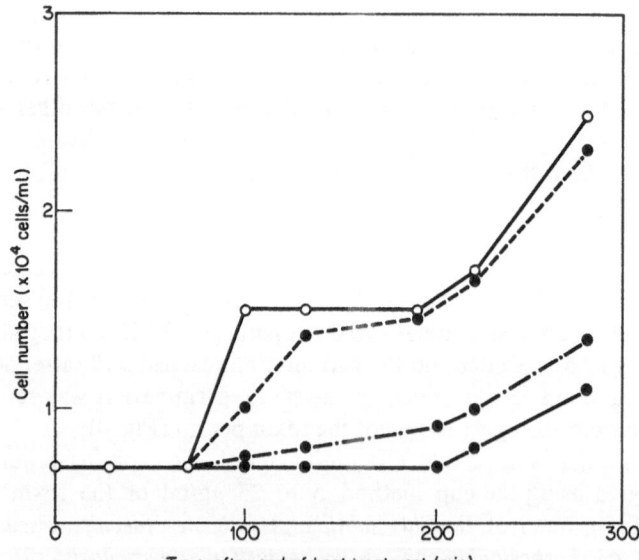

FIG. 5. Inhibitory effect of fusarenon-X on the synchronously
dividing cells of *Tetrahymena pyriformis* GL.

The cells were cultured in 2% proteose-peptone No. 3 (Difco) supplemented with
1% yeast extract and 0·6% glucose, and the synchronous cell division was induced
by seven applications of alternative heat treatment at 34°C and 28°C with 30 min
intervals.

Biochemical mode of action

The pathological effect of the toxin is cellular damage to actively-dividing
cells such as thymus, small intestine, bone marrow, testis, and ovary. In
this respect, the author examined an inhibitory effect of fusarenon-X and
the other scirpenes on macromolecule synthesis in Ehrlich ascites tumour,
rabbit reticulocyte and rat liver.

Ehrlich ascites tumour cells (4N strain) maintained in ddS male mice
were suspended in Lock-Ringer's solution, and after pre-incubation of the
cells with the toxin for 15 minutes at 37°C, the incorporation of C^{14}-labelled
thymidine and leucine into DNA and protein was estimated. As shown in
Figure 6, diacetoxyscirpenol, fusarenon-X and nivalenol inhibited protein
and DNA synthesis, and the percentage inhibition in both cases was clearly
parallel to a logarithmic concentration of the toxin. The 50% inhibitory
concentration (ED_{50}) for protein synthesis was 0·035 $\mu g/ml$, 0·35 $\mu g/ml$ and
6 $\mu g/ml$ for diacetoxyscirpenol, fusarenon-X and nivalenol, respectively.

In the case of rabbit reticulocytes and rat liver, the protein synthesis was
examined with the cell-free system. As illustrated in Figures 7 and 8 and
Table 5, the poly U-dependent synthesis of polyphenylalanine in the

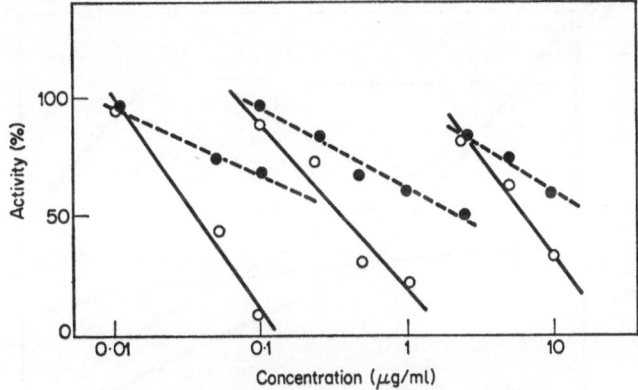

FIG. 6. Inhibition of protein and DNA synthesis in
Ehrlich tumour cells.

The tumour cells suspended in Locke-Ringer's solution were preincubated with the
toxin at 37°C, and after 15 min C14-labelled compound (0·01 μC) was added to continue
the incubation for 40 min. Total volume was 1·0 ml.

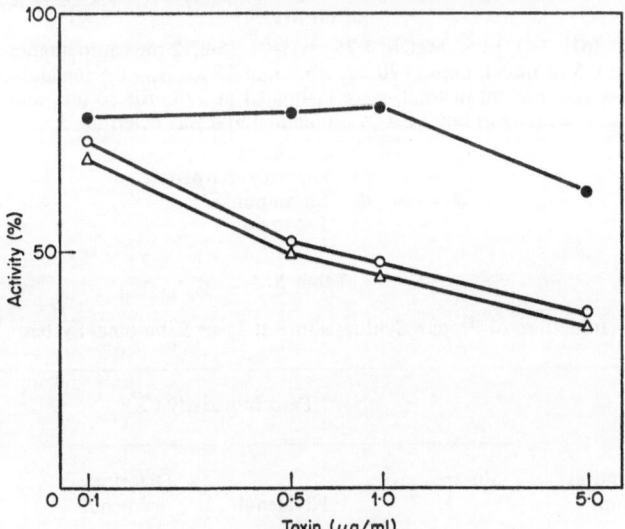

FIG. 7. Inhibition of protein synthesis in ribosomal system
of rabbit reticulocytes.

Tris buffer (pH 7·8) 10, Mg-Acetate 2, KCl 24, 2-mercaptoethanol 1·2, ATP 0·24,
GTP 0·012 (μ mole), poly U 20 μg, ribosome 50 μg, pH 5, enzyme 0·2 mg and C14-
phenylalanine 0·05 μC, 0·4 ml in total, were incubated at 37°C for 30 min and the
radio-activity in hot TCA-insoluble material was determined.

●———● Diacetoxyscirpenol
○———○ Nivalenol
△———△ Fusarenon-X

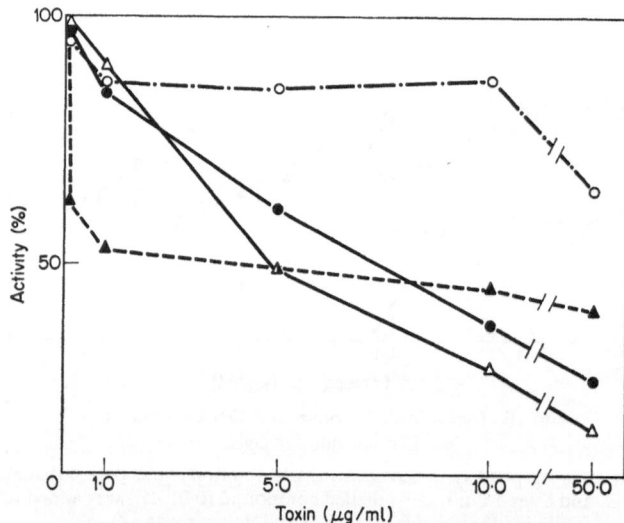

FIG. 8. Inhibition of protein synthesis in ribosomal systems
of rat liver.

Tris buffer (pH 7·4) 12·5, MgCl$_2$ 1·75, NH$_4$Cl 15·0, 2-mercaptoethanol 2·5, GTP
0·025, ATP 0·5 (μ mole), poly U 20 μg, ribosome 45 μg, S$_{100}$ 0·5 mg and C^{14}-phenyl-
alanine 0·05 μC, 0·25 ml in total, were incubated at 37°C for 30 min and the radio-
activity in hot TCA-insoluble material was determined.

           O —— —— O   Nivalenol
           O ——·—— O   Diacetoxyscirpenol
           ● ———— ●   Fusarenon-X
           △ ----- △   T-2 toxin

Table 5

Inhibition of Protein Synthesis in Rat Liver Ribosomal System

Concentration (μg/ml)	Percent activity (%)			
	Fusarenon-X	Nivalenol	Diacetoxy-scirpenol	T-2 toxin
0·1	102	103	100	61
1·0	88	94	89	51
5·0	61	47	88	—
10·0	46	36	91	43
50·0	22	12	67	38

ribosomal system was inhibited by 0·1-10 μg/ml of fusarenon-X, nivalenol and T-2 toxin, and this inhibition was not demonstrated with diacetoxyscirpenol up to 50 μg/ml.

These findings strongly indicate that fusarenon-X as well as nivalenol and T-2 toxin are potent inhibitors of protein synthesis in animal cells.

DISCUSSION

Historical background of Fusaria mycotoxicosis in Japan

Mycotoxicosis caused by so-called 'scabby grains' is widely distributed in the world, especially in countries where barley and wheat are consumed as foodstuffs.

In Japan, 'Akakabi-byo', a disease of wheat and barley, develops after an interval, and heavy outbreaks occur after a rather cold spring and heavy rain. Miyake[13] and Hara[14] isolated Gibberella saubinetti from rice plants and scabby wheat, and Urakura[15] observed that the scabby grains induced vomiting and diarrhoea in men. Takahashi[16] reported mortality in mice dosed with an ether extract of scabby grains. Hirayama et al.[17] demonstrated that the culture filtrate of Fusarium sp. isolated from rationed rice caused mortality in mice, and Nakamura et al.,[18, 19] when food poisoning occurred in Hokkaido, a northern part of Japan, noted a toxicity of F. graminearum Schw.-moulded wheat.

In 1953, heavy rain continued during the harvest time of barley and wheat, causing a prevalence of scab disease. According to Nishikado[20] in Okayama, where 50-100% of the total yield was damaged by this disease, a young bull (10 months old) fed with the scabby wheat for several days lost his appetite, and the decrease of body weight and diarrhoea was marked. This syndrome was more severe in the young bull than in an adult cow. Microbiological examination on the scabby grains indicated the presence of Gibberella zeae, Alternaria sp., and Penicillium sp., the commonest of which was G. zeae.

In the summer of 1956, 25 young men from Tokyo consumed Fusarium sp. contaminated rice and suffered from nausea, vomiting and drowsiness; 5% of the total fungi isolated from the damaged grains were Fusarium sp. F2 (later identified as F. roseum) and F. nivale.[21] Uraguchi[22, 23] conducted a toxicological investigation on the former fungus, revealing that the culture filtrate and its charcoal-adsorbable materials caused a fall in body weight, haemorrhage around the testis and infiltration of the lung and liver in mice. Matsunami et al.[24] carried out a toxicity test on F. nivale and reported a high toxicity when it was cultured on unpolished rice grains.

Recently, Tsunoda et al.[25] re-examined toxic Fusaria, and F. nivale Fn-2B, isolated from actually damaged wheat at the Agricultural Station of Kumamoto, a southern district of Japan, was proved to be toxic to mice and rats. As a result of extensive research, nivalenol[5, 6] and fusarenon-X[7, 8] were isolated from the mouldy rice and the culture filtrate of this fungus respectively. The author's microbiological study[9] suggested that fusarenon-X is the main toxic metabolite of the fungus and nivalenol was assumed to be derived, chemically or enzymatically, from fusarenon-X. Therefore, the toxicological properties of this mycotoxin were investigated in relation to the *Fusaria* mycotoxicosis described above.

Detection of fusarenon-X

Fusarenon-X can be detected chemically by thin-layer chromatography. Further, fusarenon-X is skin-irritant, and the bioassay method using rabbit reticulocyte is highly specific for scirpenes among the 19 mycotoxins examined. Therefore, the screening of toxic *Fusaria* was carried out with the multisystem as follows:

Biological screening—(1) reticulocyte bioassay, (2) skin test, and (3) toxicity test with mice.
Chemical screening—thin-layer chromatography.

The results indicated that beside *F. nivale* Fn-2B and Fn-2L, *F. nivale* Fn-M, *G. zeae* Ohoita-II, *G. zeae* Ishii are positive in the biological screening test and from the culture filtrate of *F. nivale* Fn-M (later identified as *Caronectoria graminicola* by Dr Tsunoda), fusarenon-X was isolated (unpublished). An interesting finding was that the crude toxin of *G. zeae* (*F. roseum*)-mouldy rice was toxic to mice and inhibitory to protein synthesis. Judging from the specificity of reticulocyte bioassay it is highly possible that *G. zeae* produces scirpene metabolite(s) on rice. In fact, the author's preliminary experiment with chromatographic analysis revealed the presence of toxic metabolite(s) which caused radiomimetic injury to mice.

Fusarenon-X as a suspected causal factor of Fusaria *mycotoxicosis*

Fusarenon-X is toxic to mice, rats, guinea-pigs, cats and ducklings, and among these laboratory animals guinea-pigs proved to be most sensitive to lethal toxicity and skin toxicity. In the case of mice, no marked difference in the value of LD_{50} was observed with male and female or with the route of administration. The narrow range between the maximum and minimum lethal dose and similarity in LD_{50} values with different administration routes indicates that the toxin was absorbed quickly and reached the target organ without degradation. New-born mice and guinea-pigs are more sensitive to the toxin than adults which is in agreement with the observation of Nishikado[21] that the immature animal was more sensitive than the adult.

This high sensitivity of the new-born animal to the toxin is presumed to be caused by the interference of the cellular proliferation and the macro-molecule synthesis in the tissue.

The symptoms of *Fusaria* mycotoxicosis in Japan are vomiting, nausea, drowsiness, diarrhoea and haemorrhage. The toxicity tests conducted with several species of animals revealed that diarrhoea occurred in all cases and marked vomiting and nausea-like symptoms were noted in cats and ducklings. In this respect, Dr Ohkubo[8, 25] reported that the crude toxin of *F. nivale* Fn-2B and the isolated fusarenon-X caused haemorrhage in the brain of mice and rabbit. These toxicological and pathological findings strongly suggest that fusarenon-X is one of the causal factors of *Fusaria* mycotoxicosis, causing a disturbance of the central nervous system of the animals. A noticeable finding was that the administration of only 10 micro-grams of the toxin caused vomiting in ducklings within a few minutes of the injection. This toxicological behaviour of ducklings provides a simple tool for screening of toxic cereal grains or foodstuffs, although the pharmaco-logical reason for this symptom remains to be investigated.

Biological activity

Fusarenon-X interferes with the multiplication of a protozoon *Tetra-hymena pyriformis* at a low concentration. However, the other microbes such as bacteria, yeast and fungi are resistant, although the toxin induced RD-mutants in yeast. Further, the germination of plant seeds was retarded only in the presence of higher doses of the toxin. From these findings, it seems likely that fusarenon-X has a high affinity to animal cells only. In this respect, fusarenon-X is definitely a cytotoxic zootoxin.

The biochemical studies conducted with Ehrlich tumour cells, rabbit reticulocytes and rat liver has proved that the toxin is inhibitory to DNA and protein synthesis. This biochemical feature of the toxin is assumed to be one of the reasons for the cellular damage characterised by karyorrhexis and degeneration in the proliferating tissues. The different LD_{50} of the toxins to protein synthesis observed with the whole cells (reticulocytes and Ehrlich tumour cells) is presumed to be due to differences in cellular permeability as suggested in the previous paper.[11]

REFERENCES

1. URAGUCHI, K., TATSUNO, T., SAKAI, F., TSUKIOKA, M., YONEMITSU, O., ITO, H., MIYAKE, M., SAITO, M., ENOMOTO, M., SHIKATA, T. and ISHIKO, T. (1961). *Jap. J. exp. Med.*, **31**, 19.
2. SAKAI, F. (1955). *Folio pharmacol. japon.*, **51**, 431. (In Japanese.)
3. URAGUCHI, K. (1969). *J. stored Prod. Res.*, **5**, 227.

4. UENO, Y. (1970). Production of citreoviridin, a neurotoxic mycotoxin of *Penicillium citreo-viride* Biourge. This symposium.
5. TATSUNO, T., SAITO, M., ENOMOTO, M. and TSUNODA, H. (1968). *Chem. Pharm. Bull.* (Tokyo), 16, 2519.
6. TATSUNO, T., FUJIMOTO, Y. and MORITA, Y. (1969). *Tetrahedron Letters*, 33, 2823.
7. UENO, Y., SAITO, K. and TSUNODA, H. (1969). *Hawaiian Conference on Toxic micro-organisms*. In press.
8. UENO, Y., UENO, I., TATSUNO, T., OHKUBO, K. and TSUNODA, H. (1969). *Experientia*, 25, 1062.
9. UENO, Y., ISHIKAWA, Y., SAITO-AMAKAI, K. and TSUNODA, H. (1970). *Chem. Pharm. Bull.* (Tokyo), 18, 304.
10. UENO, Y., HOSOYA, M., MORITA, Y., UENO, I. and TATSUNO, T. (1968). *J. Biochem.* (Tokyo), 64, 479.
11. UENO, Y., HOSOYA, M. and ISHIKAWA, Y. (1969). *J. Biochem.* (Tokyo), 66, 419.
12. UENO, Y., ISHIKAWA, Y., AMAKAI, K., NAKAJIMA, M., SAITO, M., ENOMOTO, M. and OHTSUBO, K. (1970). *Jap. J. Exp. Med.*, 40, 33.
13. MIYAKE, I. (1969). *The Botanical Magazine*, 8, 89. (In Japanese.)
14. HARA, Y. (1910). *Nogyokoku*, 4, 34. (In Japanese.)
15. URAKURA, U. (1933). *Byochugai Zashi*, 20, 390. (In Japanese.)
16. TAKAHASHI, E. and SHIRAHAMA, K. (1934). *J. Sapporo Soc. Agr. Forest*, 25, 375. (In Japanese.)
17. HIRAYAMA, S. and YAMAMOTO, M. (1950). *Bull. Nat. Hyg. Lab.*, 66, 85. (In Japanese.)
18. NAKAMURA, Y., TAKEDA, S., OGASAWARA, K., KARASHIMADA, T. and ANDO, K. (1951). *Hokkaido Eisei Kenkyujoho*, 2, 35. (In Japanese.)
19. NAKAMURA, Y., TAKEDA, S. and OGASAWARA, K. (1951). *Hokkaido Eisei Kenkyujoho*, 2, 47. (In Japanese.)
20. NISHIKADO, G. (1958). *Nogyo-Kairyo-gijutsu-shiryo*, 97, 107. (In Japanese.)
21. TSUNODA, H., TSURUTA, U., MATSUNAMI, S. and ISHII, S. (1957). *Proc. Food Res. Inst.*, 12, 27. (In Japanese.)
22. URAGUCHI, K. (1958). *Shokuhin Eisei Kenkyu*, 8, 25. (In Japanese.)
23. URAGUCHI, K., SAKAI, Y., TATSUNO, T., TSUNODA, H. and WAKAMATSU, H. (1958). *Folia pharmacol. japon.*, 54, 127.
24. MATSUNAMI, Y. and IKEBUCHI, J. (1961). *The 70th Memorial Bull. of Tokyo Univ. Agr.*, pp. 41-49.
25. TSUNODA, H., TOYAZAKI, N., MOROOKA, S., NAKANO, N., YOSHIYAMA, H., OHKUBO, K. and ISOKA, M. (1968). *Proc. Food Res. Inst.*, 23, 89.

FIELD SURVEY OF MYCOTOXIN-PRODUCING FUNGI CONTAMINATING HUMAN FOODSTUFFS IN JAPAN, WITH EPIDEMIOLOGICAL BACKGROUND

(II) Biological effects of the mycotoxins produced by the
fungi isolated from foodstuffs

by

Mamoru Saito, Makoto Enomoto, Makoto Umeda,
Kohichiro Ohtsubo*, Toshitaka Ishiko†,
Shunichi Yamamoto and Hiroyuki Toyokawa‡

Approximately 250 strains selected from 2940 strains of fungi isolated as food contaminants were assayed for their toxic effects on cultured cells and animals.

Tissue culture experiment

The modified method of Toplin's plastic panel technique using HeLa S_3 cells was employed for bioassay of the culture filtrates or chloroform extracts of the fungi. The filtrates were diluted in the culture medium at concentrations of 10, 3·2, 1·0 and 0·32%. The mycelial extracts were dissolved in dimethyl sulphoxide and diluted with the medium at final concentration of 100, 32, 10 and 3·2 $\mu g/ml$. Each cup (Disposo-tray FB-54) with a round cover glass received 0·5 ml of the diluted samples and 0·5 ml of a cell suspension containing 1×10^5 cells. After 3 days of incubation in a CO_2-incubator at 37°C, the cells in cups were stained for estimation of the degree of toxicity and cytological examination.

Animal experiment

The test animals, male mice of DDD strain, weighing approximately 20-25 g each, were housed individually. The mice were each given intraperitoneally 0·8 ml of the culture filtrate daily for 3 or 5 days and sacrificed on the day after the last injection. One to 3 mg of the mycelial extracts were suspended in olive oil, injected subcutaneously and the mice sacrificed 3 days after injection. Observation of symptoms and measurement of the body weight of each mouse was done daily after administration of the sample. Complete necropsies as well as histological examinations were performed on the dead or sacrificed mice.

* Institute of Medical Science, University of Tokyo.
† Kanto Communication Hospital.
‡ Medical School, University of Tokyo.

The degree of toxicity was graded, depending on lethal or growth-inhibitory effects and histological damage. The biological properties of the mycotoxins were characterised by their target tissues.

Results of biological assay

The names of the fungi found to be exhibiting toxicity by any of the above tests are shown in Table 1. Twenty fungi producing known mycotoxins are

Table 1

Names of Toxic Fungi Isolated from Foodstuffs
(Examination of Filtrate and Mycelium Extract)—1968-1969

Arthrinium sacchari   *Ascochyta* sp.

A. aculeatus	*A. chevalieri*	*A. clavatus*	*A. flavus*
A. foetidus	*A. fumigatus*	*A. heteromorphus*	*A. niger*
A. ochraceus	*A. oryzae*	*A. ostianus*	*A. petrakii*
A. phoenicis	*A. putterillii*	*A. sclerotiorum*	*A. sulphureus*
A. tamarii	*A. terreus* var. *africanus*		*A. tubingensis*
A. umbrosus	*A. versicolor*		

Chaetomium cochlioides	*Chaetomium globosum*	*Diaporthe phaseolorum*
Epicoccum nigrum	*Eupenicillium* sp.	*Gliocladium* sp.
Helminthosporium oryzae	*Hemispora stellata*	*Nigrospora oryzae*

P. charlesii	*P. chrysogenum*	*P. citreo-viride*
P. citrinum	*P. cyaneofulvum*	*P. cyclopium*
P. implicatum	*P. islandicum*	*P. italicum*
P. lanosum	*P. lilacinum*	*P. notatum*
P. oxalicum	*P. puberulum*	*P. purpurogenum*
P. roqueforti	*P. rugulosum*	*P. steckii*
P. telikowskii	*P. urticae*	*P. variabile*
P. viridicatum		

Phyllospicta spp.	*Phoma* spp.	*Pithomyces chartarum*
Trichothecium roseum		

included (Table 2). Usually, histological examination of the mice after acute death revealed no remarkable findings other than acute visceral congestion. Products of many fungi showed specific target effects on the actively dividing cells of the animals, such as the crypt cells of the intestinal mucosa, germ centre of the lymph follicles in the spleen, lymph nodes and other lymph apparatus, thymus and bone marrow. Sometimes the deep gland cells of the stomach and the cellular components of spermatogenesis in the testis were also involved in the cytotoxic damage. The findings in these regions of active cellular proliferation are hydration and swelling of the cytoplasm, hyperchromatosis of the nuclear membrane, pycnosis, fragmentation of the nuclei, atypical mitosis and subsequent cell necrosis. The mitotic injury

Table 2

Mycotoxin-producing Fungi isolated from Foodstuffs . . . And their
Target Effects

(Examination of Filtrate and Mycelium Extract)—1968–1969

Fungus	Known mycotoxins	No. of strains toxic/ examined	Target effect in culture cell and organs of mouse
A. aculeatus	—	3/3	Mitosis Injury, Kidney (F)
A. chevalieri	Xanthocillin X Gliotoxin	7/7	Mitosis Injury (F)
A. clavatus	Patulin, Ascladiol	3/3	Mitosis Injury (F, M)
A. flavus	Aflatoxin	2/2, 18/50	Liver
A. fumigatus	Fumigatin	2/2	Lethal, Mitosis Injury (M)
A. ochraceus	Ochratoxin Penicillic Acid	2/2, 29/33	Liver, Mitosis Injury
A. oryzae	(Aflatoxin)	1/1	Liver
A. tamarii	Kojic Acid	3/3	Lethal (M)
A. terreus var. africanus	—	1/1	Mitosis Injury (M), Lethal (F)
A. versicolor	Sterigmatocystin	1/1	—
Chaetomium globosum	Chaetomin	8/8	Mitosis Injury (F, M), Liver (M)
Hemispora stellata	Sporidesmolides	2/2	Mitosis Injury (F)
P. chrysogenum	—	1/1	Mitosis Injury (M), Kidney, Brain (F)
P. citreo-viride	Citreoviridin	1/1	Brain
P. citrinum	Citrinin	1/1	Kidney, Lethal
P. cyclopium	Cyclopiazonic Acid	3/3	Mitosis injury (F, M), Liver
P. implicatum	Citrinin	2/3	Lethal (F), Kidney (M)
P. islandicum	Luteoskyrin Cyclochlorotine	1/1, 10/10	Liver (M) Liver (F)
P. notatum	Xanthocillin X	2/2	Mitosis Injury, Liver
P. oxalicum	Oxalic Acid	3/3	Mitosis Injury, Liver (M)
P. puberulum	Cyclopiazonic Acid	3/3	Liver, Kidney (F)
P. purpurogenum	Rubratoxins	2/3	Mitosis Injury, Liver, Kidney
P. roqueforti	—	2/2	Mitosis Injury (F)
P. rugulosum	Rugulosin	1/1	Liver, Mitosis Injury (M)
P. steckii	—	1/2	Lethal (M)
P. urticae	Patulin, Griseofulvin	1/1	Lethal (F)
P. viridicatum	—	6/6	Mitosis Injury, Liver, Kidney (F)
Phoma spp.	—	4/6	Lethal (F)
Pithomyces chartarum	Sporidesmolides	1/1	—
Trichothecium roseum	Trichothecin	2/2	—

(F) Filtrate   (M) Mycelium extract.

and appearance of the abnormal chromosomes was more definitely demonstrated in the culture cells than the animal tissues. The metabolites of *Chaetomium globosum* showed a very interesting toxic effect causing multipolar mitosis with multinuclear cell formation.

Other than the effect on actively dividing cells described above, the patterns of toxicity can be classified into the following categories according to the particular organ affected: hepatotoxic, nephrotoxic and neurotoxic patterns (Table 2). Several mycotoxins revealed polyfunctional effects which can be summarised as combinations of two or more toxic patterns. Both culture filtrate and mycelial extracts of *Penicillium cyclopium* showed hepatotoxicity with fatty degeneration of the liver cells and damage of the actively dividing cells. The filtrate of *Penicillium purpurogenum* gave toxic effects on liver and kidneys and also disorders of mitosis. Further investigation on the metabolites of *Penicillium purpurogenum* resulted in successful isolation and identification of rubratoxin B as the causal agent of these biological properties.[1]

The interesting finding concerning the difference in mycotoxin-producing activity among the strains belonging to the same species of fungus, was that all the tested strains of *Penicillium islandicum* showed hepatotoxic effects (Table 2). As for *Aspergillus ochraceus*, 29 out of 33 strains were toxic on HeLa cells probably as a result of penicillic acid-production, which was shown in 28 strains of this fungus. However, ochratoxin production was proved in only two strains.[2]

DISCUSSION

Since we found in 1958[3] that the metabolites of *Penicillium islandicum* produced liver cirrhosis and liver tumours in experimental animals, the role of fungi in human as well as animal health, especially through contamination of foods, has been our great concern. As for diseases of man and animals attributed to mycotoxins in Japan, there are several reported cases of acute intoxication in man and animals probably caused by food infected with *Penicillium*, *Aspergillus* and *Fusarium*.[4] However, the relation of mycotoxins to human disease, especially cancer and other chronic diseases, is not well defined.

In the present study, 30 kinds of toxic fungi, 20 of which are capable of producing the known mycotoxins including aflatoxin, ochratoxin and rubratoxin, were isolated from the foodstuffs. This fact indicates the importance of the mycotoxin problem in the field of food hygiene in Japan. It is especially interesting that many of the toxic fungi produce metabolites showing target effects on rapidly dividing cells, which might reflect the carcinogenic, teratogenic or mutagenic properties of the products. Further study on their chronic effects when ingested by the animals should be carried out.

In addition to the difficulties of obtaining accurate statistics of cause of death in the selected districts, lack of quantitative data on distribution and contents of the mycotoxins in the foodstuffs in the present study, makes it difficult to evaluate the connection of mycotoxin-contamination with human disease. Food habit survey (food consumption and attitude analysis) revealed, however, some difference in the kind of foodstuffs and the food intake between the districts. This result suggests the possibility of the spatial clustering of the diseases induced by mycotoxins.

The methods of accumulating evidence, which supersede mere speculation on this problem, require further exploration. In particular methods of chemical and biological assay for detection of mycotoxins, in parallel with the efforts in obtaining the further epidemiological backing, is required.

REFERENCES

1. NATORI, S., SAKAKI, S., KURATA, H., UDAGAWA, S., SAITO, M., UMEDA, M. and OHTSUBO, K. (1970). *Appl. Microbiol.*, **19**, 613.
2. NATORI, S., SAKAKI, S., KURATA, H., UDAGAWA, S., ICHINOE, M., SAITO, M. and UMEDA, M.   In preparation.
3. KOBAYASHI, Y., URAGUCHI, K., SAKAI, F., TATSUNO, T., TSUKIOKA, M., SHIKATA, T. and ISHIKO, T. (1958 and 1959).
4. TSUNODA, H. (1968). In press.

EXPERIMENTAL EVIDENCE THAT LUPINOSIS OF SHEEP IS A MYCOTOXICOSIS CAUSED BY THE FUNGUS *PHOMOPSIS LEPTOSTROMIFORMIS* (KÜHN) BUBÁK

by

K. T. van Warmelo*, W. F. O. Marasas*, T. F. Adelaar†, T. S. Kellerman†, I. B. J. van Rensburg† and J. A. Minne†

Lupines (*Lupinus* spp.) are known to cause two distinct forms of poisoning in animals, *viz.* lupine or alkaloidal poisoning and lupinosis. The first of these is a nervous disorder caused by the alkaloids present in bitter lupines. The second is an icteric disease caused by a hepatotoxin (ictrogen) of unknown structure and origin.[1]

Lupinosis is a problem of long-standing importance with sporadic occurrence in Europe,[1, 2] Australia,[1, 3, 4, 5, 6, 7] New Zealand[8] and South Africa.[9, 10] A detailed historical review of lupinosis has been given by Gardiner.[1] Lupinosis has been induced in sheep by means of aqueous extracts of toxic lupine material.[11] The toxin appeared to be phenolic in character.[11]

Kühn[12] in 1880 first suggested that toxic metabolites of saprophytic fungi growing on the lupines may be the cause of lupinosis. In an attempt to determine the causal fungus, Kühn compared the mycoflora of toxic and non-toxic lupines. A fungus which he described as a new species, *Cryptosporium leptostromiforme* Kühn,[12] was found on the stems of toxic as well as non-toxic lupine plants. The toxicity of individual fungal species was not determined and the aetiologic role of fungi in lupinosis was thus not proved.

Gardiner[13] in 1966 proved that non-toxic lupine material could be rendered toxic by inoculating and incubating it with a mixed fungal suspension from toxic lupines. The fungi responsible for toxin formation were not definitely established, although either *Cytospora* sp. or *Pleospora* sp. appeared to be a probable cause. Gardiner[1] concluded that one or more fungi were definitely involved in the development of lupinosis, but that the species of fungus responsible was unknown.

This paper reports on the occurrence of a field outbreak of lupinosis of sheep in South Africa, on the induction of lupinosis in sheep fed lupine material from this field, and on the experimental reproduction of lupinosis in sheep fed a pure culture of *Phomopsis leptostromiformis* (Kühn) Bubák.

* Plant Protection Research Institute, Pretoria.
† Veterinary Research Institute, Onderstepoort.

isolated from this toxic material and cultured on autoclaved lupine seeds. A detailed report of this work has been submitted for publication.[14]

DESCRIPTION OF THE FIELD OUTBREAK OF LUPINOSIS IN SHEEP

During October, 1969 approximately 850 breeding ewes on the farm Burgersdrif, Hermon district, Cape Province, were grazed on a field of sweet white lupines (*Lupinus albus* L. cult. Pflugs Gela), many of which were bearing pods in various stages of development. The lupine plants were approximately 9 in. tall and growing amongst a variety of grasses. Rain fell over this field on approximately the 12th and 5th day before the first mortalities occurred on October 19.

The ewes were immediately removed from this field after the first mortalities occurred and were fed lucerne hay. Mortalities increased on October 20 and 21 and then decreased. By October 25 a total of 530 ewes had died.

Examination of this field on October 25 revealed that the sheep had selectively grazed on the lupine pods containing seeds while the rest of the plant had been avoided. The external surface of the dry pods appeared black. Dark brown, water-soaked lesions were evident on some green pods. The discoloured pods were infected internally with a conspicuous, white fungal mycelium. Many of the seeds were also infected internally and were discoloured brown. The white mycelium was found only under areas showing an external discolouration.

ISOLATION OF THE CAUSAL FUNGUS

The fungus was readily isolated in pure culture from pieces of infected pods and seeds placed directly on $1\frac{1}{2}\%$ malt extract agar containing 100 mg/l of sodium novobiocin. The same white fungus grew without the development of any contaminants from a total of 57 such platings. The complete dominance of this fungus on lupine pods from this field provided strong circumstantial evidence that it was responsible for the toxicosis.

CULTURAL CHARACTERISTICS OF THE CAUSAL FUNGUS

A dense white surface mycelium is formed on $1\frac{1}{2}\%$ malt extract agar. Irregular stromatic masses develop in the mycelial layer. These masses gradually develop into black, stromatic pycnidia. Conidia are borne on conidiophores in locules within the stromatic pycnidia. Mature conidia are exuded through an ostiole in a round, pink to orange spore mass. Sporulation can be induced within 21 days on sterilised lupine stems, $1\frac{1}{2}\%$ malt extract agar, $\frac{3}{4}\%$ malt extract agar and corn meal agar, provided that cultures are incubated at 16-18°C and are exposed to light.

IDENTITY OF THE CAUSAL FUNGUS

Cultures of the fungus isolated from the toxic *L. albus* material were submitted to Dr B. C. Sutton, Commonwealth Mycological Institute, Kew, England and to Dr J. A. von Arx, Centraalbureau voor Schimmelcultures, Baarn, Netherlands, for identification. We also compared the fungus with authentic material of *Cryptosporium leptostromiforme* Kühn from Germany. The fungus was finally identified as *Phomopsis leptostromiformis* (Kühn) Bubák[15] (= *Cryptosporium leptostromiforme* Kühn).[12]

P. leptostromiformis is pathogenic to lupines and causes a disease characterised by grey to light tan, bleached out, sunken, linear stem lesions containing black stromatic masses.[12, 16, 17, 18] The fungus is known to occur in Denmark,[15] England,[19] Germany,[12, 16] Poland,[17] Portugal[20] and the United States.[18] *P. leptostromiformis* survives on pieces of lupine stem for at least 3 years[16, 17] and in *L. luteus* seed for at least 2 years.[18]

In nature *P. leptostromiformis* is known to be pathogenic to *L. luteus*[16,17,18] and *L. angustifolius* var. *leucospermus*.[16] Artificial inoculations have shown that only *L. luteus*[17, 18] and *L. albus*[18] are infected by *P. leptostromiformis*.

PREPARATION OF PURE CULTURES OF *P. LEPTOSTROMIFORMIS* ON AUTOCLAVED LUPINE SEEDS FOR USE IN FEEDING TRIALS

L. albus seeds were autoclaved for 3 hours at 15 psi in 1-quart jars (200 g seed in 150 ml distilled water/jar) and inoculated with 10 ml of a *P. leptostromiformis* spore suspension containing 1×10^6 spores/ml. The jars were shaken to distribute the spores evenly and incubated in the dark at 25°C for 21 days. The contents of the jars were then minced in a meat mincer, care being taken that the material was not heated, and stored at 4°C in a refrigerator. Uninoculated seeds from the same batch that were treated in the same manner but not incubated, were used as controls.

In all the experiments reported here, wet, minced lupine seeds were dosed to sheep per stomach tube. In subsequent experiments it was found that the minced, inoculated seeds retained their toxicity after air-drying at room temperature for 24 hours or more.

TOXICITY TRIALS WITH FIELD MATERIAL

Material from the field where the outbreak had occurred was milled and dosed per stomach tube to sheep. Shelled pods appeared to be more toxic than either the seeds or stalks when dosed at levels varying between 2·5 g/kg and 10 g/kg body weight, but all induced typical lupinosis.

The sheep were clinically examined every day and chemical pathological determinations were periodically done on the blood.

Increased levels of serum glutamic oxaloacetic transaminase (SGOT) and total bilirubin (T.Br.) were the most significant chemical pathological changes observed. Clinically a progressive inappetence, lethargy and severe terminal icterus were seen.

Necropsy findings

Generalised icterus and atrophy, fatty degeneration and cirrhosis of the liver were the most important and constant features of the examination. Impaction of the large intestine, splenomegaly, ascites, hydrothorax and hydropericardium were often present whilst enterorrhagia was present in two cases and in one sheep the kidneys were pigmented brown.

Histopathological findings

The histopathological lesions comprised severe inter- and intralobular cirrhosis, leading to disturbance of the gross architecture of the livers. In haematoxylin and eosin stained sections a granular brown pigment was present in the cytoplasm of many cells. By special staining techniques this pigment proved to consist of lipoproteins (Sudan Black positive), lipo-fuchsins (Schmorl's positive), mucopolysaccharides (Periodic Acid Schiff positive) and haemosiderin (Berlin Blue positive). Furthermore the reticulo-endothelial cells were prominent and proliferation of bile ducts and bile duct epithelial cells was conspicuous. Megalocytosis, multinucleation, vesiculation of nuclei, karyopyknosis and karyorrhexis were noticed in a number of hepatocytes. Eosinophilic globules—often larger than the nucleus, occurred in the cytoplasm of some hepatocytes and fat meta-morphosis was fairly obvious.

Haemosiderosis of the spleen and periportal lymph node was a common finding while the kidney of one case contained brown pigment granules in the epithelial cells of the convoluted tubules.

TOXICITY TRIALS WITH PURE CULTURES OF *P. LEPTOSTROMIFORMIS*

Pilot trial

A pilot trial was performed by the daily dosing of pure culture material to two sheep at the levels of 5·0 g/kg and 2·5 g/kg respectively. Both these sheep died within 14 days after showing typical clinical symptoms of lupinosis. One of these was too decomposed for examination whilst the other exhibited a severe generalised icterus, venous congestion, petechiae and ecchymoses in the subcutaneous tissue and intermuscular fascia, as well as on the gut wall and epicardium. It also had a severe fatty degeneration and slight cirrhosis of the liver as well as impaction of the caecum and colon, splenomegaly, nephrosis and congestion of the lungs. The urinary bladder was distended with dark reddish-brown urine.

Histopathologically the gross architecture of the liver was indistinct and the intralobular architecture was greatly disturbed. There was severe midzonal fat metamorphosis in the lobules, early centrilobular fibrosis and proliferation of bile ducts in the portal tracts.

Kupffer cells were prominent while several of these as well as some of the hepatocytes contained coarse yellowish-brown granules. The staining characteristic of the pigment was similar to that already described.

Eosinophilic globules varying in size but often larger than the nuclei were present in the cytoplasm of a minority of the hepatocytes. Megalocytosis and vesiculation of nuclei occurred fairly commonly.

The myocardium showed large areas of necrosis, with proliferation of fibroblasts in these areas.

Two sheep used as controls remained normal.

Main trial

Five sheep were dosed with pure culture material at the levels of 10 g/kg, 7·5 g/kg, 5·0 g/kg and 2·5 g/kg body weight respectively per day while five sheep receiving uninoculated seed from the same batch served as controls.

The sheep were clinically examined every day and chemical pathological determinations were done periodically on the blood.

Results

The sheep in the control group remained normal and survived the experiment.

Clinical signs

All the treated sheep became depressed and developed an anorexia after about 36 hours. Seventy-two hours after the onset of treatment all the sheep had pronounced icterus and after day 6, one of the sheep showed rumenal stasis.

Chemical pathology

The most significant changes were sudden increases in the levels of SGOT and T.Br. in the blood (see Table 1).

Table 1

Effect of Dosing Pure Cultures of *P. leptostromiformis* on Blood SGOT and T.BR. Levels of Merino Sheep

Day	SHEEP No.									
	1		2		3		4		5	
	SGOT*	T.BR†	SGOT	T.BR	SGOT	T.BR	SGOT	T.BR.	SGOT	T.BR
1	139	0·0	173	0·0	125	0·0	166	0·0	152	0·0
2	200	0·0	132	0·0	112	0·0	159	0·0	206	0·0
4	187	0·8	212	1·6	152	3·2	247	4·8	226	2·8
8	274	7·6	—	—	—	—	—	—	—	—
9	296	9·4	—	—	—	—	—	—	—	—
10	342	5·1	—	—	—	—	—	—	—	—

* SGOT in King units
† T.BR. in mg%

Necropsy findings

The lesions observed at necropsy resembled those described above. Icterus, severe fatty degeneration of the liver (but no fibrosis) impaction, of the caecum and colon, haemorrhages in the subcutaneous tissue and oedema of the lungs were the most constant features.

Histopathological findings

The gross architecture of the liver was preserved but the intralobular architecture was disturbed by a massive fat metamorphosis that distended the hepatocytes and frequently distorted the nuclei. The central vein, moreover, was compressed and difficult to distinguish in many lobules.

Few of the reticulo-endothelial cells and hepatocytes in the central areas of the liver lobules contained pigment.

A small percentage of hepatocytes contained eosinophilic globules or had vesicular nuclei.

The myocardium of the sheep that received 2·5 g/kg of the toxic material revealed distinct areas of fibrosis.

The lesions in the other organs resembled those already described (i.e. nephrosis and haemosiderosis of spleen and lymph nodes).

DISCUSSION

Lupinosis of sheep has been studied since the latter part of the previous century. Since 1880 the fungus *P. leptostromiformis* has also been known to cause a serious disease of lupines. Although this fungus was actually described as a new species in one of the first papers dealing with lupinosis,[12] the relationship between the fungal disease of lupines and the icteric disease of sheep has remained obscure until now.

The histopathological lesions seen in the livers of sheep that died in the field outbreak were similar to those of the trials described in this paper, and by Gardiner.[21] We therefore believe that the same toxic principle was present in both the field and pure culture material, and that the aetiology of the disease known as lupinosis has now been elucidated. Differences in the disease produced in these experiments are due to the relative acuteness or chronicity of the intoxication. The field material produced chronic intoxication whilst that of the pilot and main trials was either sub-acute or acute. It appeared that the pods were more toxic than the seeds or stalks.

Preliminary chemical work in our laboratories confirmed that the toxic principle of lupinosis is not aflatoxin.[11] The macro- and microscopic lesions of the disease, however, do resemble those of aflatoxicosis in sheep. Although very little has been published on this subject,[22, 23, 24] J. D. Smit (Veterinary Research Institute, Onderstepoort, personal communication,

H

1970) described the most significant macroscopic lesions of experimental aflatoxicosis in sheep, as generalised icterus, and fatty degeneration of the liver. Microscopically fatty degeneration, pigmentation and bile duct proliferation are present in the liver. Difficulty may also be experienced in differentiating between the histopathological lesions of chronic lupinosis and those of chronic enzootic icterus and seneciosis.

Three possible approaches to the practical control of lupinosis are currently being investigated.

1. Detoxification of toxic lupine material by steaming under pressure, as was first suggested by Kühn.[12]
2. Forecasting of epiphytotics of the fungal disease of lupines by studying weather conditions which favour infection.
3. Breeding of lupine varieties resistant to *P. leptostromiformis*.

ACKNOWLEDGEMENT

We are grateful to Dr N. P. J. Kriek and Dr J. de Wet, Regional Veterinary Investigation Centre, Stellenbosch, for their assistance with the field investigation and for establishing the toxicity of the material by a preliminary feeding trial.

REFERENCES

1. GARDINER, M. R. (1967). *Adv. vet. Sci.*, **11**, 85.
2. HACKBARTH, J. (1961). *J. Aust. Inst. agric. Sci.*, **27**, 61.
3. GARDINER, M. R. (1961). *Aust. vet. J.*, **37**, 135.
4. GARDINER, M. R. (1964). *J. Agric. West Aust.*, **5**, 890.
5. BENNETTS, H. W. (1957). *Aust. vet. J.*, **33**, 277.
6. BENNETTS, H. W. (1960). *J. Agric. West. Aust.*, **1**, 47.
7. NEIL, H. G., TOMS, W. J. and RALPH, C. M. (1960). *J. Agric. West. Aust.*, **1**, 565.
8. BRASH, A. G. (1943). *N.Z. Journ. Agric.*, **67**, 83.
9. FLIGHT, L. H. (1956). *Fmg S. Afr.*, **32**, 37.
10. GROENEWALD, J. W., SMIT, J. D. and ADELAAR, T. F. (1954). *Je S. Afr. vet. med. Ass.*, **25**, 29.
11. PETTERSON, D. S. and PARR, W. H. (1970). *Res. vet. Sci.*, **11**, 282.
12. KÜHN, J. (1880). *Ber. landw. Inst. Univ. Halle*, **2**, 115.
13. GARDINER, M. R. (1966). *Br. vet. J.*, **122**, 508.
14. VAN WARMELO, K. T., MARASAS, W. F. O., ADELAAR, T. F., KELLERMAN, T. S., VAN RENSBURG, I. B. J. and MINNE, J. A. (1970). *Je S. Afr. vet. med. Ass.*, **41**, 234.
15. LIND, J. (1913). In: *Danish Fungi as Represented in the Herbarium of E. Rostrup*, p. 648. Copenhagen.

16. FISCHER, M. (1893). *Bot. Zbl.*, **54**, 289.

17. KOCHMAN, J. (1957). *Acta agrobot*, **6**, 117. (In Polish.)

18. OSTAZESKI, S. A. and WELLS, H. D. (1960). *Pl. Dis. Reptr.*, **44**, 66.

19. GROVE, W. B. (1935). In: *British Stem and Leaf Fungi*, Vol. 1, p. 488. Cambridge Univ. Press.

20. LUCAS, MARIA T. and DA CAMARA, E. DE S. (1954). *Agronomia lusit*, **16**, 81.

21. GARDINER, M. R. (1965). *Path. vet.*, **2**, 417.

22. NEWBERNE, P. M. and BUTLER, W. H. (1969). *Cancer Res.*, **29**, 236.

23. ABRAMS, L. (1965). *Je S. Afr. vet. med. Ass.*, **36**, 5.

24. ARMBRECHT, B. H., SHALKOP, W. T., ROLLINS, L. D., POHLAND, A. E. and STOLLOFF, L. (1970). *Nature* (Lond.), **225**, 1062.

AFLATOXIN CARCINOGENESIS IN RATS: DIETARY EFFECTS*

by

Paul M. Newberne and Adrianne E. Rogers

Laboratory of Nutritional Pathology
Department of Nutrition and Food Science
Massachusetts Institute of Technology, Cambridge, Massachusetts

Malnutrition and aflatoxins co-exist in many areas of the world where there is a high incidence of cirrhosis and primary hepatic carcinoma in native population groups.[1-6] Despite the often referred to association between malnutrition, cirrhosis and liver carcinoma in man, relatively few reports have appeared in the literature describing experimental studies in animals. The early reports of Salmon et al.[7] described the induction of nutritional cirrhosis in rats in which a significant number developed liver cell carcinoma. Later work[8] indicated that cirrhosis was neither a necessary prerequisite nor concomitant to the development of liver cancer in rats exposed to aflatoxin although nutritional cirrhosis may modify the response under some conditions.[9] Further work using chemically defined, purified amino acid diets[10] has shown that nutritional cirrhosis alone is not sufficient to induce liver cell cancer in rats. In retrospect, it seems reasonable to assume that the diet of Salmon et al. was contaminated with aflatoxin and that cirrhosis was an additional complicating factor induced by the choline deficient diet possibly interacting with the carcinogen.

Whether malnutrition is a factor contributing to the induction of cirrhosis and liver carcinoma is an open question. However, general considerations of geographical distribution of hepatocarcinoma and its association with liver disease and cirrhosis led us to an examination of interactions between nutritionally induced liver disease and experimental aflatoxin carcinogenesis. Although aflatoxin is not associated with cirrhosis in animals, the interaction of diet and carcinogen under precise conditions may well suggest an explanation to the enigmatic distribution of liver cancer and cirrhosis in human populations about the world. The remarkable differences in response to aflatoxin of rats fed diets severely deficient, marginally deficient or adequate, relative to lipotropes, indicate that the degree and perhaps the time of nutritionally-induced liver injury is highly significant in determining the final outcome of the interaction between dietary treatment and carcinogen. Furthermore, dietary lipotropes, especially methionine

* Contribution No. 1699. This work was supported in part by NIH grants CAO8870, AM11158 and a grant from William S. Merrell Company.

and Vitamin B_{12}, may be critically low in some areas where liver disease and mycotoxins co-exist, providing additional reasons to investigate this interesting but little studied area of carcinogenesis.

MATERIALS AND METHODS

The general design of the various experiments reported here was the same although certain minor modifications were used; these are referred to

Table 1

Dietary Composition

Component	Control		Lipotrope deficient	
	(Diet 1)	(Diet 2)	(Diet 3) severe	(Diet 4) marginal
Casein*	6·0	22·0	6·0	3·0
Peanut Meal *	25·0	0·0	25·0	12·0
Gelatin	0·0	0·0	0·0	6·0
Fibrin	0·0	0·0	0·0	1·0
Sucrose	41·7	18·3	42·0	12·1
Dextrose	0·0	19·7	0·0	12·1
Dextrin	0·0	19·7	0·0	12·1
Corn Oil	0·0	15·0	0·0	2·0
Beef Fat or Lard	20·0	0·0	20·0	30·0
Celluflour	0·0	0·0	0·0	2·0
Vitamin Mix†	2·0	1·0	2·0	2·0
Salts Mix‡	5·0	4·0	5·0	5·0
Cystine	0·0	0·0	0·0	0·5
Choline	0·3	0·3	0·0	0·2
Methionine	0·0	0·0	0·0	0·2
Vitamin B_{12}§	+	+	−	+

* Alcohol extracted.
† Complete for rat except for choline and B_{12}.
‡ Rogers and Harper.
§ Choline and B_{12} added where indicated in solution at time diet was mixed at levels of 0·3 and 50 micrograms respectively.

in the text or in the tables where appropriate. Male weanling rats of either the Charles River, Sprague-Dawley strain (Charles River Breeding Laboratories, Wilmington) or the Fischer strain (A. R. Schmidt Co., Madison, Wisconsin) were housed in individual screen-bottomed cages in temperature-controlled animal facilities with feed and water supplied *ad libitum*. The composition of the diets is shown in Table 1. Two types of control diets were used in order to compare results with reports in the literature; in some experiments, casein was the only protein source while in others, a mixture of casein and peanut meal was used. Severe or marginal lipotrope deficiency was achieved by altering the dietary content of choline, methionine, cystine and Vitamin B_{12}: the dietary peanut meal was solvent extracted with N-hexane, then with methanol and assayed for aflatoxin (Food and Drug Research Laboratories, Maspeth, New York). Aflatoxin B_1 (AFB$_1$), provided by Professor G. N. Wogan or purchased from Makor Chemicals, Jerusalem, Israel, was administered in dimethylsulfoxide (DMSO, Metheson, Coleman and Bell, East Rutherford, N.J.) by gastric intubation or in a few instances by intraperitoneal injection. The standard dosing schedule was 25 micrograms AFB$_1$ daily for 15 days although in a few instances, in acute studies, different doses were given.[11] Penicillin, used in one experiment, was added to the diet at a level of 0·1% and fed continuously.

Rats were sacrificed by decapitation after an overnight fast and tissues preserved in 10% neutral buffered formalin; when autoradiographs were made, thymidine-methyl-^{3}H (Schwarz Bioresearch, Orangeburg, N.Y.) was injected intraperitoneally, 1 microcurie/g body weight 2 hours before sacrifice. Tissues for histologic evaluation and autoradiography were processed according to techniques described previously.[12] Biochemical determinations of aminopyrine demethylase,[13] p-nitroanisole demethylase,[14] benzpyrene hydroxylase,[13] glucose-6-phosphatase,[15] and acid phosphatase[16] were done on liver tissue of rats from the various groups. In the case of acid phosphatase, 'bound' and 'free' fractions were assayed. Total liver lipid was measured by standard extraction and gravimetric techniques.[17]

RESULTS

Effects of cirrhosis, induced by severe lipotrope deficiency, on aflatoxin tumour induction is shown in Table 2. Severe lipotrope deficiency-induced cirrhosis appeared to decrease slightly rather than increase the incidence of liver carcinoma after 12 months (64% vs. 41%).

The addition of penicillin to the diet of severely deficient rats treated with aflatoxin significantly decreased liver tumours (41% vs. 6%) although the usual inhibition of cirrhosis[17, 18] was not observed. These results are characteristic of other experiments in which there has been no definite effect of nutritional cirrhosis on development of AFB$_1$-induced liver tumours although low lipotropes do influence tumour induction.[9, 12, 19, 20]

The less severe lipotrope deficiency (diet 4) has consistently resulted in a higher incidence of liver tumours in a shorter period of time[12] compared to controls or to severely deficient animals (Table 3). Furthermore, livers of

Table 2

Effect of Severe Lipotrope Deficiency and Penicillin on
Aflatoxin Carcinogenicity—12 Months*

Group no.	Dietary treatment	Average body weight (gm)	Number with:			
			Cirrhosis		Carcinoma	
			No.	%	No.	%
B# 1	Control #1 + aflatoxin	504	0/14	0·0	9/14	64·0
2	Control #1 + aflatoxin + penicillin	530	0/20	0·0	14/20	70·0
3	Lipotrope deficiency #3 + aflatoxin	392	15/17	88·0	7/17	41·0
4	Lipotrope deficiency #3 + penicillin	465	4/15	27·0	0/15	0·0
5	Lipotrope deficiency #3 + aflatoxin + penicillin	478	11/18	61·0	3/18	6·0

* Charles River, Sprague-Dawley strain, sacrificed 12 months after total dose of 375 micrograms AFB_1.

Table 3

Effect of Lipotropes on Parenchymal Hyperplasia and AFB_1 Tumour
Incidence*

Dietary treatment	Appearance of hyperplastic cell clusters	Tumour incidence (%) Months after AFB_1 exposure		
		6	9	12
Control #2	6 months	0	30	71
Severe deficiency #3	none	0	50	60
Marginal deficiency #4	3 weeks	40	95	95

* Rats dosed with 15 daily doses, 25 micrograms each of AFB_1.

marginally deficient rats have an associated focal hyperplasia of paren-chymal cells immediately after a carcinogenic dose of AFB_1; these are not observed in severely deficient rats and only in the late stages of tumour induction in rats fed control diets. We feel that this phenomenon is highly significant and represents a morphologic manifestation of a period during which there is transformation from normal to neoplastic liver cells. The remainder of the paper will be devoted to illustration and discussion of the

Table 4

Effect of Diet on Acute Toxicity of Single Dose Aflatoxin B_1

Dosage AFB_1*	Rat strain Route admin.	Diet	Two-weeks mortality No. rats	%
	Sprague-Dawley rats			
7 mg/kg	Intragastric	control #2	3/5	60
		marginal lipotrope #4	0/5	0
9 mg/kg	Intragastric	control #2	4/5	80
		marginal lipotrope #4	0/10	0
7 mg/kg	Intraperitoneal	control #2	5/5	100
		marginal lipotrope #4	0/5	0
	Fischer rats			
7 mg/kg	Intragastric	control #2	10/10	100
		marginal lipotrope #4	0/10	0

* AFB_1 dissolved in 0·1 ml DMSO.

acute and chronic response of rats fed the marginal lipotrope diet No. 4 and dosed or fed AFB_1.

Because of earlier, long-term experiments in which the marginal lipotrope diet enhanced AFB_1 carcinogenesis, we have examined the acute toxicity of AFB_1 in rats fed the control or the marginal lipotrope diet. Results are shown in Table 4 and are characteristic of several trials.

The marginal lipotrope diet (number 4, Table 1) protected rats against doses of AFB_1 which were lethal to 60-100% of rats fed the control diet (Table 4). That this effect was not mediated through differences in gastro-intestinal absorption or alteration within the tract of AFB_1 is shown by the fact that rats were protected against an intraperitoneal dose.

Table 5

Dietary Effects on Hyperplasia and Neoplasia by AFB_1

Treatments	Interval treatment to sacrifice	No. rats	3H-labelled hepatic nuclei %—SE	Percent rats with:		
				Focal hyperplasia	Bile duct adenomas	Hepato-carcinomas
Control Diet 2						
DMSO	3 days	4	0·049±0·021	0	0	0
AFB_1	3 days	5	0·816±0·422	0	0	0
AFB_1	3 weeks	5	0·300±0·080	60	0	0
DMSO	6-12 months	5	0·033±0·013	0	0	0
AFB_1	6 months	10	0·102±0·027	50	0	0
AFB_1	9 months	10	0·040±0·015	30	0	0
AFB_1	12 months	7	0·074±0·026	71	0	0
Marginal lipotrope Diet 4						
DMSO	3 days	4	0·403±0·170	0	0	0
AFB_1	3 days	5	2·497±1·320	60	0	0
AFB_1	3 weeks	5	1·386±0·193	40	0	0
DMSO	6-12 months	9	0·138±0·052	0	0	0
AFB_1	6 months	10	0·307±0·128	60	10	10
AFB_1	9 months	10	0·203±0·059	60	30	10
AFB_1	12 months	10	0·157±0·066	30	40	20

The rats that succumbed to acute AFB_1 toxicity had haemorrhagic necrosis of the liver with variable degrees of bile duct hyperplasia. Surviving rats had increased size of periportal hepatocytes, some focal necrosis and bile duct proliferation. About 20 % of the rats fed diet #4 marginal lipotrope, and administered AFB_1 had focal areas of abnormal hepatocytes which were hyperplastic as measured by increased uptake of ^3H-thymidine. We have described these areas in rats given repeated doses of AFB_1 sufficient to induce hepatocellular carcinomas and suggest that they represent a preneoplastic change in the liver cell.[12] The appearance in animals fed marginal lipotrope diets of these microscopic hyperplastic foci correlate well with short-term tumour induction time in these animals. They appear late in tumourigenesis in animals fed control diets.

A large group of Fischer strain rats was used to further examine chronic toxicity and carcinogenicity of AFB_1 under conditions of normal and marginal lipotrope dietary treatments. Male weanling rats were fed control diet 2 for 1 week, then fed marginal lipotrope diet 4 for 2 additional weeks. All were then dosed with ten doses, each 25 micrograms of AFB_1, rested for a week and then given another four doses of 25 micrograms each for a total of 350 micrograms, a known carcinogenic dose. Representative numbers from each group were sacrificed at intervals and gross observations and histopathologic examination plus autoradiography were done on liver tissue. Results are shown in Table 5. The marginal lipotrope diet alone increased uptake of ^3H-thymidine by liver parenchymal cells. Aflatoxin B_1 induced a generalised hyperplasia in both groups which persisted for at least 3 weeks. Focal hyperplasia in areas which may be preneoplastic was seen 3 days after the full dose of AFB_1 was given to the marginal lipotrope group but did not appear in the group fed the control diet until 3 weeks later; and here they were frequent only after 9-12 months. Liver carcinomas appeared in the marginal lipotrope group after 6 months and the control group after 18 months.

To determine the effect of diet alone on liver drug metabolising enzymes, another group of male weanling Fischer rats were fed control diet 2 for 1 week then divided and half given the marginal lipotrope diet for 2 additional weeks. Both groups were then sacrificed and enzyme assays done on whole liver homogenate or the post-mitochondrial 9000 × g supernatant fraction. Results are listed in Table 6. In each case, the marginal lipotrope diet alone resulted in a significant decrease in enzyme activity.

In further experiments on effects of diet and repeated dosing of AFB_1 on liver microsomal and lysosomal enzymes, 40 Fischer rats were fed control diet 2 for 1 week, then 25 were fed the marginal lipotrope diet 4 an additional 2 weeks. Both groups were then dosed with either DMSO only or AFB_1 dissolved in DMSO for either 5 or 14 doses. After the 1st week and at the

Table 6

Dietary Effects on Hepatic Drug-metabolising Enzymes

Diet	No. rats*	Aminopyrine homogenate	Demethylase† PMS‡	P-nitroanisole homogenate	Demethylase† PMS‡	Benzpyrene homogenate	Hydroxylase† PMS‡
Control (2)	4	481±55	450±55	1132±74	824±64§	184±16	162±13
Marginal lipotrope (4)	4	305±23	234±28	536±116	480±68	99±11	97±11
P Value‖		<0·05	<0·02	<0·01	0·01	<0·01	<0·01

* Four rats each enzyme assay, total of 12 animals per diet.
† All enzyme values expressed per g dry, fat-free liver±SE.
  Units: aminopyrine demethylase, μg aminoantipyrine/hour, p-nitroanisole demethylase, μg p-nitrophenol/hour; quinine units.
‡ Postmitochondrial supernatant.
§ Only case where PMS differed significantly from homogenate, P 0·02.
‖ Students 't' test using two-sided probability for control vs. marginal lipotrope diets.

Table 7

Effect of Aflatoxin B$_1$ and Lipotropes on Liver Microsomal and Lysosomal Enzymes

Diet and treatment*	Aminopyrine demethylase†	P-nitroanisole demethylase†	Benzpyrene hydroxylase†	Acid p'tase† Total	% free	Glucose-6-p'tase†
Control+DMSO	284±6	1423±58	147±15	2109±240	24·3±2·0	40±8
Control+AFB$_1$ 125 µg	460±22	1684±34§	60±5¶	3504±982	29·2±6·0	16±2‡
Marginal lipotrope+DMSO	220±13	1147±77	36±9	3165±146	18·6±1·6	37±4
Marginal lipotrope+AFB$_1$ 125 µg	217±37	1274±79	35±4	2788±296	17·1±1·4§	16±2¶
Control+DMSO	228±8	1148±11	201±15	2190±166	25·1±1·5	63±2
Control+AFB$_1$ 350 µg	650±109§	1535±51¶	100±18§	2415±123	42·7±1·8¶	59±1
Marginal lipotrope+DMSO	156±47	863±108	69±10	2523±91	25·6±2·3	85±2
Marginal lipotrope† AFB$_1$ 350 µg	154±	944±	47±	2646±	42·0±	56±

* 25 mg AFB$_1$ in 0·1 ml DMSO or DMSO only was given by gastric tube, 5 or 14 doses; rats sacrificed 24 hours after last dose and amino-pyrine demethylase+p-nitroanisole demethylase determined. The other three enzymes determined 48 hours after last dose.

† Enzymes expressed per g dry, fat-free liver±S.E.; units respectively, µg aminoantipyrine/hour, µg p-nitrophenol/hour, quinine units, µM p-nitrophenol/hour and µM phosphate/minute.

‡ Difference from DMSO-treated controls significant P<0·05.

§ Difference from controls significant P<0·02.

¶ Difference from controls significant P<0·0.

end of dosing, rats from each group were sacrificed 24 or 48 hours after the 5th or after the final dose of AFB_1 or DMSO and liver enzymes assayed. Total lipid was extracted and measured gravimetrically, histopathologic assessment made, and results statistically analysed for significance by Students 't' test. Results are listed in Table 7.

The marginal lipotrope diet alone resulted in a significant decrease in the three drug-metabolising enzymes when measured in either the whole liver homogenate or the postmitochondrial fraction (Table 6). A similar difference between dietary responses was observed again in groups used to examine effect on response to repeated small doses of AFB_1 (Table 7). Rats fed the control diet had an increase in the two demethylating enzymes and a decrease in hydroxylase. This was in contrast to rats fed the marginal

Table 8

Effect of Diet and AFB_1 on Liver Lipids

Diet and treatment	Total liver lipid % wet weight
Control #2	$7·5 \pm 0·2$
Control #2 + AFB_1	$12·0 \pm 0·6$
Marginal lipotrope #4	$11·3 \pm 1·1$
Marginal lipotrope #4 + AFB_1	$17·8 \pm 1·4$

lipotrope diet in which there was no significant change in any of the three enzyme systems following 5 or 14 doses of AFB_1. Total acid phosphatase was not affected by diet but the percentage of free enzyme was elevated after 5 or 14 doses of AFB_1. Glucose-6-phosphatase generally was depressed in the marginal lipotrope group dosed with AFB_1.

Lipid levels were increased in the liver of both groups of rats as a result of AFB_1 exposure; on a wet weight basis, lipid increased from $7·5 \pm 0·2$ to $12·0 \pm 0·6\%$ in rats fed control 2 diet and from $11·3 \pm 1·1$ to $17·8 \pm 1·4$ in rats fed marginal lipotrope diet 4 (Table 8).

After five doses of AFB_1 histological changes, consisting of moderate bile duct proliferation and increased size of periportal hepatocytes, were about the same in both dietary groups. After 14 doses, however, the marginal lipotrope group had more extensive bile duct hyperplasia accompanied by small foci of abnormal hyperplastic parenchymal cells with increased mitoses.

DISCUSSION

Geographic patterns of neoplastic diseases emphasise the importance of investigating the interactions between nutritional status and exposure to environmental toxins and carcinogens. Furthermore, some of the conflicting reports of effects of environmental toxins from different laboratories are surely related to variations in diet. From those studies on the influence of diet on liver carcinogenesis[21] the most significant and consistent observation has been that reduced calorie or protein intake tends to decrease or postpone the development of neoplasms. Although little, if any, substantive evidence has been derived from the experiments as to mechanism of action, it has been postulated that the action results from direct effects on cell division and/or by altered metabolism of the carcinogen in the liver.

The metabolism of AFB_1 has been only partially elucidated and the nature of its active metabolites, if indeed any exist, is unknown. Two metabolic changes most often referred to are O-demethylation and hydroxylation[22, 23] reactions probably carried out by two of the enzyme systems examined in this study (p-nitroanisole demethylase and benzpyrene hydroxylase). The hydroxylated metabolite is toxic but probably not carcinogenic, and the properties of other metabolites have not been reported.

Cirrhosis induced in rats before, during or after exposure to aflatoxin has shown a variable but indefinite effect on liver tumour induction.[9, 11, 12] In general, the severe nature of the diets used to induce cirrhosis appears to decrease incidence of tumours, conceivably by decreasing the general clinical condition of the animal to a point below which a standard response to the carcinogen is precluded. Lack of cell division was not a significant factor since parenchymal cell hyperplasia proceeds at a higher than normal rate in lipotrope deficiency.[12]

It is difficult to interpret the tumour inhibition by dietary penicillin, although it has been observed that penicillin largely prevents cirrhosis induced by choline deficiency[17, 18] as shown in Table 2. Whatever the mechanism in these experiments, the cirrhosis-inhibiting effect of penicillin was overridden by addition of aflatoxin but liver tumour incidence was significantly decreased. The effects may be mediated through the intestinal microflora but not through Vitamin B_{12} contamination of the penicillin since microbiological assay revealed none was present in the antibiotic.

In contrast to reports of other dietary carcinogen interactions, we have found that diets marginal in lipotropes consistently enhanced the carcinogenic activity of AFB_1[12, 19, 20] and affect the acute toxicity, the latter depending on whether the dose is single or multiple. Rats fed the marginal lipotrope diet were resistant to the effects of a single dose of 7 or 9 mg/kg of AFB_1 but exhibited increased sensitivity to the toxicity of repeated doses, measured both by acute mortality and by long-term induction of liver cell carcinoma. In our earlier study using the marginal lipotrope diet[12] the rats were fed for a longer period of time (14 weeks versus 2 weeks before exposure to AFB_1). They were, therefore, more deficient and they developed tumours in an even shorter period of time; 40% of rats sacrificed at 6 months and 100% of the rats sacrificed at 9 months had hepatocarcinomas compared to 10% at each of those times in the present study. This suggests that age does not afford protection and may actually increase sensitivity to aflatoxin when the diet is inadequate.

We have also found that the resting levels of the microsomal drug-metabolising enzymes were low in livers of rats fed the marginal lipotrope diet and that they were not raised (demethylases) or lowered (hydroxylase) in response to AFB_1 administration as were the enzymes in rats fed a complete diet. If the diet is exerting its effect through decreased synthesis or activity of these enzymes, then the evidence suggests the following:

1. AFB_1 is not itself toxic but must be metabolised to a toxic product. The adequately-fed rats are capable of metabolising a sufficient amount of a single dose to be toxic but lipotrope-deficient rats cannot make the conversion. When confronted with small, repeated doses, the normal liver develops enzyme systems capable of further metabolising a portion of the toxic compound to a non-toxic product while the deficient liver produces sufficient amounts of one or another toxic product to induce severe liver damage after a cumulative dose of about $250~\mu g$ or approximately $1 \cdot 5$ mg/kg body weight. It does not develop enzyme systems to metabolise the product further. The observed changes in the enzymes may indicate also that hydroxylation is important in production of the toxic product and that the normal but not the deficient liver is able to reduce its hydroxylase level while elevating the levels of detoxifying enzymes.
2. The same changes in relative as well as absolute enzyme levels enhance production of the carcinogenic metabolite(s).

There are, of course, other equally valid hypotheses suggested by the results of current experiments. The inherent sensitivity of the hepatocyte to the toxic and carcinogenic action of AFB_1 may be altered by the deficient diet. In that case, however, one would expect a similar rather than an opposite effect on sensitivity to one exposure or to repeated doses.

The level of cell division in the liver may affect the manner in which it responds to AFB_1. Numerous studies have shown that AFB_1 has profound effects on nucleic acid metabolism and on cell division in both acute and chronic studies.[12, 23, 24] In a single dose it depresses DNA and RNA synthesis but in repeated doses it induces generalised and focal hyperplasia under certain dietary conditions. In examining the effects of hyperplasia induced by partial hepatectomy on AFB_1 carcinogenesis, we have found no consistent enhancement or depression or tumour development related to the level of cell division during or after AFB_1 administration.[25] Therefore, the level of cell division, alone, in the lipotrope-deficient livers is probably not an important factor in determining their response to AFB_1 although rate of cell turnover remains high under such dietary conditions.

The significance of one or more episodes of generalised hyperplasia of hepatocytes during chemical liver carcinogenesis has been referred to in several studies[24, 26-28] and transient or generalised hyperplasia has been shown to occur with exposure to some of them. The matter is of clinical as well as theoretical interest; liver regeneration consequent to injury, whether induced by malnutrition, viruses, toxins or parasites, may be a significant promotional force in the genesis of liver carcinoma in geographic areas where it commonly occurs.[29] In other studies[25] we have found severe effects on DNA synthesis and hepatic mitosis accompanying AFB_1 and partial hepatectomy but no change in latent period or in incidence of liver carcinomas. Thus, it appears that with AFB_1, liver regeneration induced by partial hepatectomy has no influence and, in this case, generalised hyperplasia of hepatocytes is unrelated or unimportant to tumour development. This then appears to parallel the case with nutritional cirrhosis[12, 20] in which generalised hepatocyte hyperplasia occurs and provides two systems in which this is obtained.

The early appearance of hyperplastic foci in the livers of AFB_1 treated rats and the correlation of their presence with carcinogenicity supports our earlier study[11, 12] and emphasises the need for ultrastructural and biochemical examination of those areas. It is interesting that we have markedly enhanced AFB_1 carcinogenesis by feeding a diet that both lowers liver drug metabolising enzymes, and induces liver cell hyperplasia. Conversely, viewed in a positive light, good nutrition protects against the carcinogenic effects of AFB_1. It now seems likely that the use of dietary treatments to predispose the liver of animals to the action of aflatoxin may be the most direct approach to learning more about the real or potential hazards of this class of compounds to man. This concept is even more credible when one considers that in areas where aflatoxin, liver disease, and neoplasia co-exist, diet is usually less than adequate. If we are to learn more about the human situation then we must strive to duplicate environmental conditions, including diet, as closely as possible.

REFERENCES

1. ALPERT, M. E., HUTT, M. S. R. and DAVIDSON, C. S. (1968). *Lancet*, **1**, 1265.
2. ROSENBERG, H. (1969). *Naturwissenschaften*, **56**, 350 2.
3. KOROBKIN, M. and WILLIAMS, E. H. (1968). *Yale J. Biol. med.*, **41**, 69.
4. WOGAN, G. N. (1968). *Fed. Proc.*, **27**, 932.

5. DAVIDSON, C. S. (1970). *Am. J. Clin. Nutr.*, **23**, 427.

6. ALPERT, M. E. and DAVIDSON, C. S. (1969). *Am. J. Med.*, **117**, 325.

7. SALMON, W. D., COPELAND, D. H. and BURNS, M. J. (1955). *J. Nat'l. Cancer Inst.*, **15**, 1549.

8. SALMON, W. D. and NEWBERNE, P. M. (1963). *Cancer Res.*, **23**, 571.

9. NEWBERNE, P. M., HARINGTON, D. H. and WOGAN, G. N. (1966). *Lab. Investigation*, **15**, 662.

10. NEWBERNE, P. M., ROGERS, A. E., BAILEY, C. and YOUNG, V. R. (1969). *Cancer Res.*, **29**, 230.

11. ROGERS, A. E. and NEWBERNE, P. M.   In press.

12. ROGERS, A. E. and NEWBERNE, O. M. (1969).   *Cancer Res.*, **29**, 1965.

13. MCLEAN, A. E. M. and MCLEAN, E. K. (1966).   *Biochem. J.*, **100**, 564.

14. KINOSHITA, F. K., FRAWLEY, J. P. and DUBOIS, K. P. (1966).   *Tox. and Appl. Pharmacol.*, **9**, 505.

15. HARPER, A. E. (1963).   In: *Methods of Enzyme Analysis* (Ed. Bergmeyer, H. V.).   Acad. Press.

16. SIGMA (1963).   *Technical Bulletin*, **104**.

17. SALMON, W. D. and NEWBERNE, P. M. (1962).   *J. Nutr.*, **76**, 483.

18. RUTENBERG, A. M., SONNENBLICK, E., KOREN, I., APRAHANUASH, H., REINER, L. and FINE, J. (1957).   *J. Exp. Med.*, **106**, 1.

19. NEWBERNE, P. M., ROGERS, A. E. and WOGAN, G. N. (1968).   *J. Nutr.*, **94**, 331-343.

20. NEWBERNE, P. M. and ROGERS, A. E. (1970).   Symposium on naturally occurring Carcinogens. The Czek Oncological Society, Prague, April 14-15.

21. TANNENBAUM, A. (1959).   Nutrition and Cancer.   In: *Physiopathology of Cancer* (Ed. Homberger, F.), 2nd Edition, pp. 517-562. Hoeber-Harper Company, New York, N.Y.

22. EDWARDS, G. (1970).   In: *Aflatoxin-structure Activity Studies and a Site of Action in the Hepatocyte Nucleus*. Ph.D. Thesis, M.I.T.

23. WOGAN, G. N. (1968).   *Bacteriol. Revs.*, **30**, 460.

24. ROGERS, A. E. and NEWBERNE, P. M. (1967).   *Cancer Res.*, **27**, 855.

25. ROGERS, A. E. and NEWBERNE, P. M. (1971).   In press.

26. DAOUST, R. and MOLNAR, F. (1964).   *Cancer Res.*, **24**, 1898.

27. DAOUST, R. and SIMRAD, A. (1968).   *Cancer Res.*, **28**, 874.

28. MCDONALD, R. A. (1957).   *Arch. Internal. Med.*, **99**, 266.

29. STEINER, P. E., CAMAIN, R. and NETIK, J. (1959).   *Cancer Res.*, **19**, 567.

THE ACUTE AND CHRONIC
TOXICITY OF STERIGMATOCYSTIN

by

I. F. H. Purchase

and

J. J. van der Watt

Division of Toxicology, National Institute for Nutritional Diseases
South African Medical Research Council

The widespread occurrence of toxigenic fungi in foods and the potent carcinogenic action of aflatoxin to various laboratory animals have caused much speculation on the possible relationships between mycotoxin ingestion and the high incidence of malignant hepatoma in man in Africa. The possibility that mycotoxins other than aflatoxin may be responsible has been stressed and sterigmatocystin, a metabolite of the moulds *Aspergillus nidulans*, *Aspergillus versicolor* and a *Bipolaris* sp., chemically related to aflatoxin, was therefore studied.

The 10-day LD_{50} values of sterigmatocystin in Wistar rats and Vervet monkeys were first determined and thereafter the subacute toxicity was studied in Wistar rats. Chronic feeding experiments using Wistar rats and male Vervet monkeys formed the final phase of this study.

MATERIALS AND METHODS

Test material

Sterigmatocystin used in these experiments was extracted from maize meal contaminated with a species of *Bipolaris* and purified by column chromatography on formamide-impregnated cellulose. The sterigmatocystin was recrystallised and determined to be 95% pure.

Animals and dosage

Wistar derived MRC strain rats from our own colony were used for the acute, subacute and chronic rat toxicity studies and male Vervet monkeys (*Cercopithecus aethiops*) weighing between 0·5 and 5·5 kg were used for the LD_{50} determinations and long-term primate toxicity studies.

The methods employed during the course of the experiments on rats and the acute toxicity studies on monkeys have been published.[1-4]

The long-term studies on monkeys entailed the intragastric administration of sterigmatocystin at a rate of 20 mg/kg body weight fortnightly.

Control animals received only solvent solutions. Wedge biopsies of the livers of the experimental and the control animals were performed under anaesthesia at 9-week intervals for a period of 12 months.

RESULTS

LD$_{50}$ values

The 10-day LD$_{50}$ values were determined using either groups of rats with four animals per group or groups of monkeys with two animals per group. The results, with 95% confidence limits, are given in Table 1.

Table 1

10-Day LD$_{50}$ Values (with 95% confidence limits) of Sterigmatocystin as determined in Rats and Monkeys by Different Routes

Animal	Sex	Solvent	Route	LD$_{50}$ (mg/kg with 95% confidence limits)
Rat	Male	Dimethylformamide	Oral	166 (113-224)
Rat	Male	Dimethylformamide	Intraperitoneal	60 (46-77)
Rat	Female	Wheat-germ oil	Oral	120 (92-155)
Rat	Male	Wheat-germ oil	Intraperitoneal	65 (37-109)
Monkey	Male	DMSO	Intraperitoneal	32 (15-70)

Pathology

Animals that received the highest doses of toxin in the acute experiments showed signs of liver and kidney damage on post-mortem examination. Liver damage in the monkeys was severe and icterus was prominent. Petechia could be observed on all the serosal surfaces and in all the parenchymal organs. In the lower dose groups, all monkeys showed some macroscopic signs of liver and kidney damage.

The most prominent lesions observed microscopically in rats from the acute experiments were hepatic and renal necrosis. Liver lesions varied according to the route of administration of the toxin, being periportal after intraperitoneal injection and central after *per os* administration.

The hepatic changes varied from cloudy swelling at the lowest doses to haemorrhagic necrosis with increasing amounts of toxin. Nuclear pleomorphism of the hepatocytes was prominent.

In contrast to the situation in the liver, the route of administration had no influence on the type of kidney lesions. Lesions varied according to dose, from cortical haemorrhages and degeneration of the cortico-medullary tubular cells to degeneration and necrosis of the glomeruli. Hyalinisation

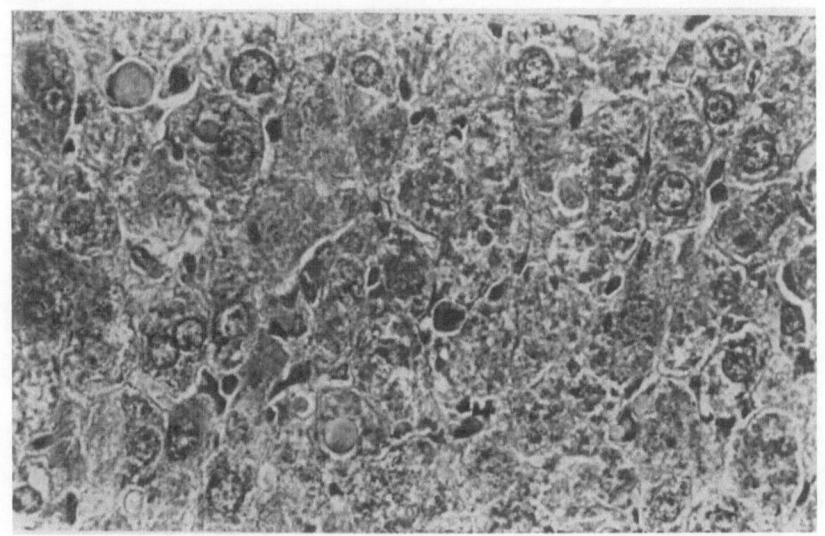

FIG. 1. Rat liver after 14 days on a diet containing sterigmatocystin. (H. & E. ×400)

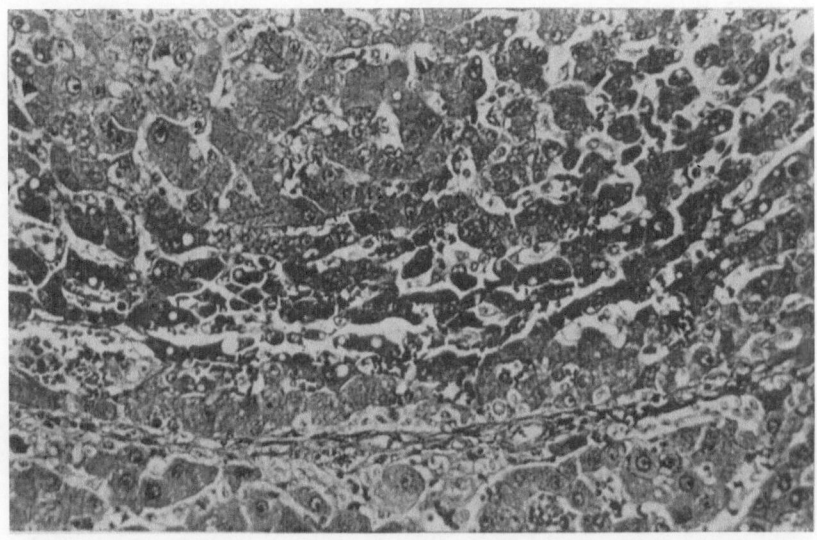

FIG. 2. Rat liver after 12 weeks on a diet containing sterigmatocystin showing edge of a macroscopically visible hyperplastic nodule. (H. & E. ×400)

of Bowman's capsule and massive haemorrhages throughout the entire kidney were induced by the highest dose of toxin.

After rats were fed a diet containing 100 mg/kg of sterigmatocystin *ad libitum* for 21 to 14 days, alterations in the liver consisted of diffuse single-cell and focal necrosis. The necrosis seen at this stage was relatively mild and a round-cell response was not elicited. Many degenerated hepatocytes contained round, eosinophilic hyaline bodies within the cytoplasm and certain liver cells had a swollen reticulated cytoplasm (Fig. 1). These pathological changes progressed in severity over the next 4 weeks resulting in distinct periportal necrosis and round cell infiltration. After 8 weeks, necrosis affecting the entire lobule could be observed. Small hyperplastic or regenerating foci could be seen at this stage. These foci enlarged and were macroscopically visible after 12 weeks exposure to the toxin (Fig. 2).

With continued feeding of sterigmatocystin-contaminated food the sequence of hepatocellular necrosis and hyperplasia in the rat liver continued and at 40 weeks after the first exposure, the first hepatic neoplasm was observed. All animals surviving 50 weeks developed malignant hepatomas with the females tending to be affected at a later stage than males. From the evidence obtained from the experiments in rats, it was concluded that sterigmatocystin is a hepatocarcinogen and not carcinogenic due to its cirrhogenic properties.

Vervet monkeys are also susceptible to the toxic effects of this mycotoxin and even at the lowest doses employed in the LD_{50} determinations, macroscopic evidence of hepatic and renal damage was observed. Microscopic examination of kidney sections revealed degeneration of the glomeruli with oedema in Bowman's space. Hyaline droplet degeneration was also present in the proximal and distal convoluted tubules. In the medullary rays fatty changes and necrosis of the tubular epithelium was prominent.

Microscopically, the liver sections from animals in the lowest dose groups showed predominantly centrilobular changes consisting of small foci of necrosis, fatty vacuolation of hepatocytes and ballooning degeneration. Macrophages, plasma cells and round cells infiltrated the necrotic areas.

Both the liver and kidney lesions increased in severity with an increase in the dose of toxin and at the highest doses employed, the livers of the monkeys were enlarged, yellow and friable; petechia and haemorrhages were present in the kidneys, gastrointestinal tract, epicardium and on all the serosal surfaces.

Histological examination revealed that there were diffuse haemorrhages throughout the renal parenchyma with hyalinisation of the glomeruli or fragmentation of the capillary loops. The epithelial cells of the nephrons showed hyaline degeneration, fatty changes and necrosis. The livers showed diffuse fatty changes, extensive single cell and central haemorrhage necrosis. Intracellular bile stasis was present in most of the surviving parenchymal cells. Zenker's hyaline degeneration was present in the myocardium.

Oral dosing of monkeys with sterigmatocystin at a rate of 20 mg/kg every 14 days for a period of 4 to 6 months resulted in chronic hepatitis. This condition was characterised by portal fibrosis with fibrous elements extending a short way into the parenchyma from the enlarged portal tracts (Fig. 3). The lobular structure at this stage remained intact but the portal tracts were infiltrated with round cells and plasma cells. With continued exposure to the toxin this preceding phase was followed by chronic aggressive hepatitis. Single-cell necrosis of the hepatocytes and progressive growth of the fibrous septa led to disruption of the lobular architecture. Bands of reticulum fibres, commencing in the enlarged portal tracts, extended between the foci of hepatocytes (Fig. 4). Kupffer cell prominence and bile duct epithelial proliferation could also be observed.

Simultaneously focal reactive hyperplasia of the liver cells commenced, and after 12 months' exposure large hyperplastic nodules, up to 8 mm in diameter, were observed throughout the entire organ (Figs. 5 and 6). These hyperplastic foci and the grossly disturbed inter-hyperplastic parenchyma contained hepatocytes of varying dimensions with pleomorphic nuclei. The cytoplasm of these cells was hypochromatic and the chromatin could be seen as basophilic masses situated mainly at the periphery of the nucleus.

Animals dying at this stage had essentially the same histological alterations in the liver, but the entire organ was in addition affected by marked fatty changes of the hepatocytes within hyperplastic nodules and the surrounding parenchyma.

CONCLUSIONS

Sterigmatocystin, in contrast to the aflatoxins, has enjoyed very little attention as a potential carcinogen. The above studies in rats have emphasised the possible importance of mycotoxins other than aflatoxin as carcinogenic agents. The studies conducted in primates indicated that this toxin is cirrhogenic to the primate liver. Since hepatoma in man is invariably accompanied by cirrhosis this is an important consideration in the search for a possible cause of liver cancer in man. This toxin must now also be considered as a possible aetiological agent responsible for the high incidence of cirrhosis in human populations in Africa where liver cancer is most prevalent. Similarities between the hepatic lesions seen in the Bantu in Mozambique suffering from liver damage of unknown aetiology and rats exposed to sterigmatocystin have been described. These similarities, when it is considered that they occur in the primate liver also, are even more striking.

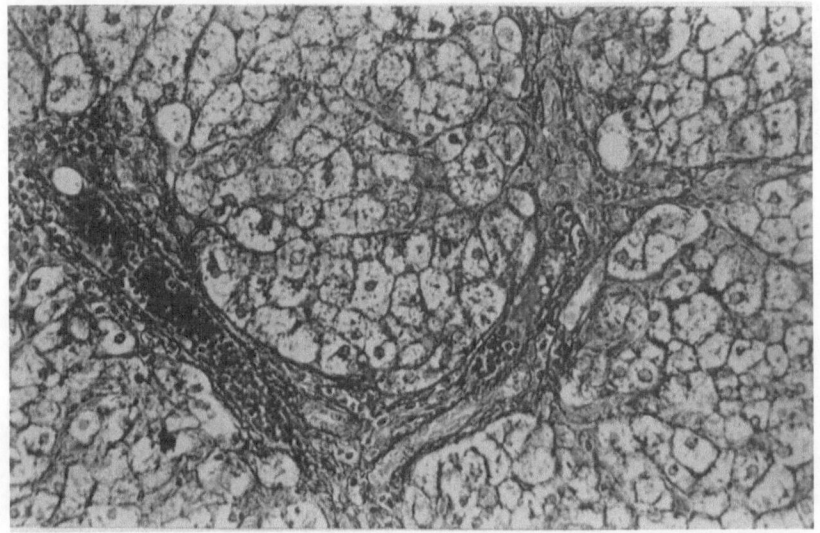

FIG. 3. Biopsy specimen of a monkey liver after 6 months of sterigmatocystin dosage. Portal fibrosis and early parenchymal infiltration of fibrous elements can be observed. (Reticulin stain × 160)

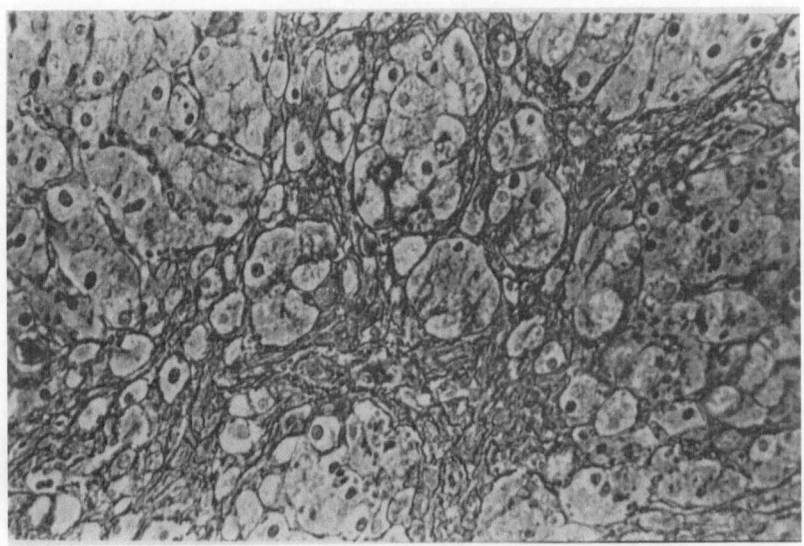

FIG. 4. Monkey liver after 10 months of sterigmatocystin dosage showing bands of reticulin fibres extending between and surrounding foci of parenchymal cells. (Reticulin stain × 160)

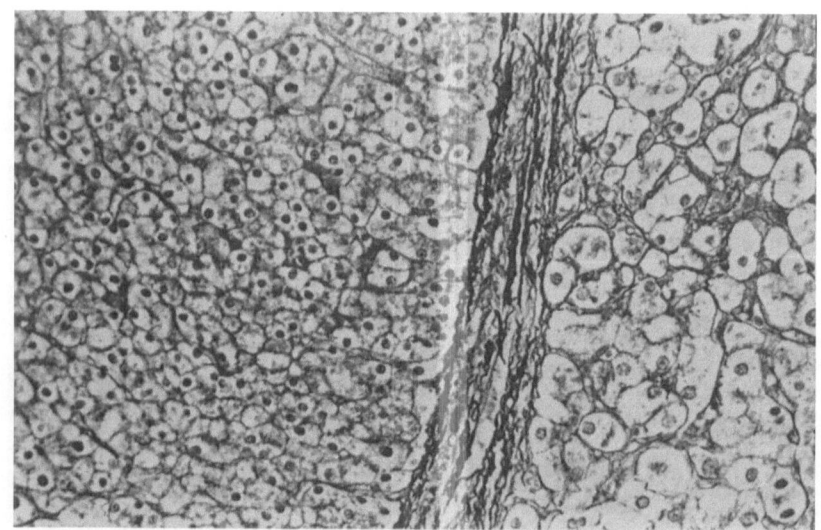

FIG. 5. Monkey liver showing edge of hyperplastic nodule seen 12 months after sterigmatocystin dosage. (Reticulin stain × 160)

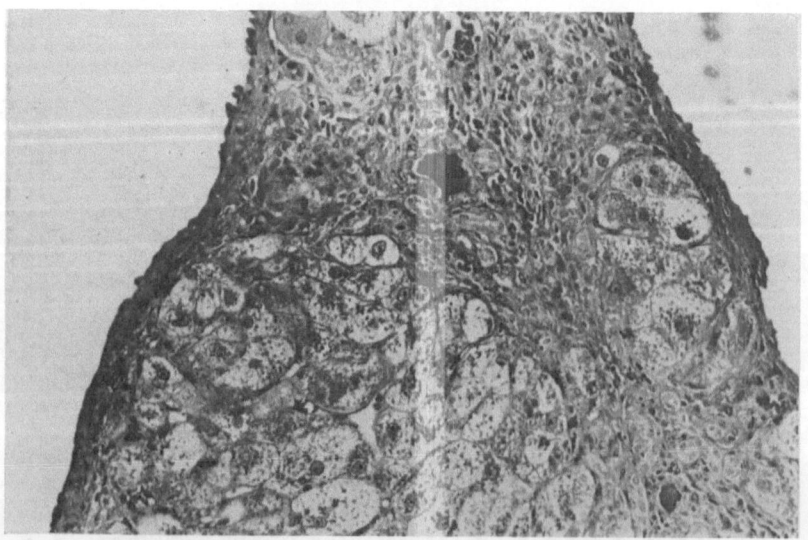

FIG. 6. Hyperplastic nodules in a cirrhotic monkey liver as seen 14 months after sterigmatocystin dosage. (H. & E. × 160)

Epidemiological studies at present being conducted in Mozambique should shed more light on the hypothesis that mycotoxins and especially sterigmatocystin may be implicated in the aetiology of chronic liver disease in man in Africa.

ACKNOWLEDGEMENTS

We wish to thank Mrs W. Bourquin and Mr D. M. T. Tagg for technical assistance with these experiments.

REFERENCES

1. PURCHASE, I. F. H. and VAN DER WATT, J. J. (1968).   *Fd. Cosmet. Toxicol.*, **6**, 555-556.
2. PURCHASE, I. F. H. and VAN DER WATT, J. J. (1969).   *Fd. Cosmet. Toxicol.*, **7**, 135-139.
3. VAN DER WATT, J. J. and PURCHASE, I. F. H. (1970).   *S.A. med. J.*, **44**, 159-160.
4. VAN DER WATT, J. J. and PURCHASE, I. F. H. (1970).   *Br. J. exp. Path.*, **51**, 183-190.
5. TORRES, F. O., PURCHASE, I. F. H. and VAN DER WATT, J. J. (1970).   *J. Path.*, **102**, 163-169.

THE EFFECTS OF AFLATOXIN B₁ AND STERIGMATOCYSTIN ON TWO DIFFERENT TYPES OF CELL CULTURES

by

Johanna C. Engelbrecht

Division of Toxicology
National Institute for Nutritional Diseases
South African Medical Research Council

Sterigmatocystin was isolated in 1954 from *Aspergillus versicolor* and structurally identified in 1962.[1] This mycotoxin is chemically closely related to the aflatoxins. Dickens *et al.*[2] have shown it to be carcinogenic on subcutaneous injection in rats and Purchase and Van der Watt[3] found it to be hepatocarcinogenic on oral administration. Sterigmatocystin is, however, 200 times less carcinogenic than aflatoxin B₁, on subcutaneous injection in Wistar rats and 10 times less on oral administration. Holzapfel *et al.*[4] isolated sterigmatocystin from two additional moulds: *Aspergillus nidulans* and *Bipolaris* sp. It is produced in much larger quantities than aflatoxins and although less toxic in experimental animals, it may be as hazardous to human health as aflatoxin B₁.

There are several reports on the effects of aflatoxin B₁ on the morphology of various cell cultures.[5, 6, 7, 8] These effects include nucleolar fragmentation, segregation of nucleolar components, giant cell formation and vacuolation of the cytoplasm.

The effects of sterigmatocystin on cell cultures have not been studied previously. A comparative morphological study of the effects of aflatoxin B₁ and sterigmatocystin on the same batch and type of cell culture was of interest. In the first series of experiments monolayers of primary monkey epithelial cells were exposed to aflatoxin B₁ and sterigmatocystin, respectively. In a subsequent series of experiments, monolayers of a continuous line of mouse liver fibroblasts were exposed to the mycotoxins.

METHODS

The monolayers of primary kidney epithelial cells of *Cercopithecus aethiops pygerythrus* were exposed to 1·0 μg aflatoxin B₁/ml medium and 1·0 μg sterigmatocystin/ml medium for 24- and 48-hour periods. The technique used was described previously.[9]

Secondary cultures of a continuous line of mouse liver fibroblasts (Line L) were also grown as monolayers on glass coverslips and in 4-oz medicine bottles. The cells were grown in Eagles Minimum Essential

Medium supplemented with 10% foetal bovine serum. The medium also contained 200 units neopan/ml medium, 200 units dimycin/ml medium, 200 units penicillin G/ml medium, 200 units colistin/ml medium and 100 units fungizone/ml medium.

All cultures were exposed to 1·0 μg aflatoxin B_1/ml medium and 1·0 μg sterigmatocystin/ml medium, respectively for 24 hours, after which the medium containing the toxin was withdrawn. The cells were loosened from the glass surface by the addition of 0·25% trypsin. A cell suspension in fresh medium and serum diluted 1:2 was made and seeded into fresh bottles and into roller tubes containing glass coverslips. The cells were subcultured every 2-4 days. Aflatoxin B_1 and sterigmatocystin were dissolved in DMSO and a 0·1% DMSO solution was added to the medium.

In the first experiment the cells were studied for five consecutive passages.

In an additional experiment the same technique was followed as in experiment 1 but the cell cultures were exposed to 1·0 μg aflatoxin B_1/ml medium and 1·0 μg sterigmatocystin/ml medium for the second time, in the fifth subculture. After 24 hours the toxic medium was withdrawn and the cells subcultured once.

In a third experiment exposed cells were subcultured ten times and were then subjected to the toxins for a second 24-hour period. Two subcultures were made after the second exposure.

In every experiment one set of cultures was incubated in fresh medium (controls) and one in medium containing 0·1% DMSO.

The cultures were fixed in Bouin's fixative, stained with haematoxylin and eosin, dehydrated in alcohol and mounted with Canada balsam.

Electron microscopic preparations

The cultures were fixed in phosphate-buffered gluteraldehyde and washed in 0·1 M phosphate buffer pH 7·4. The cells were scraped from the glass surface of the 4-oz medicine flats with a silicone 'policeman' and made into a pellet by centrifugation at 30,000 r.p.m. for 30 minutes. The pellet was post-fixed in buffered 1% osmium tetroxide, dehydrated in a graded series of alcohol solutions and embedded in an Epon-araldite mixture. Sections were cut on a LKB ultramicrotome, stained with lead hydroxide and examined with a Philips EM300 electron microscope.

RESULTS

I. The effects on primary kidney epithelial cells

Light microscopy. The cells of the control cultures were uniform in size and shape with 1-4 prominent nucleoli (Fig. 1). A mitotic rate of more than 1·45% was observed after 24 hours incubation. The DMSO-treated controls were similar morphologically but there was a slight increase in mitosis.

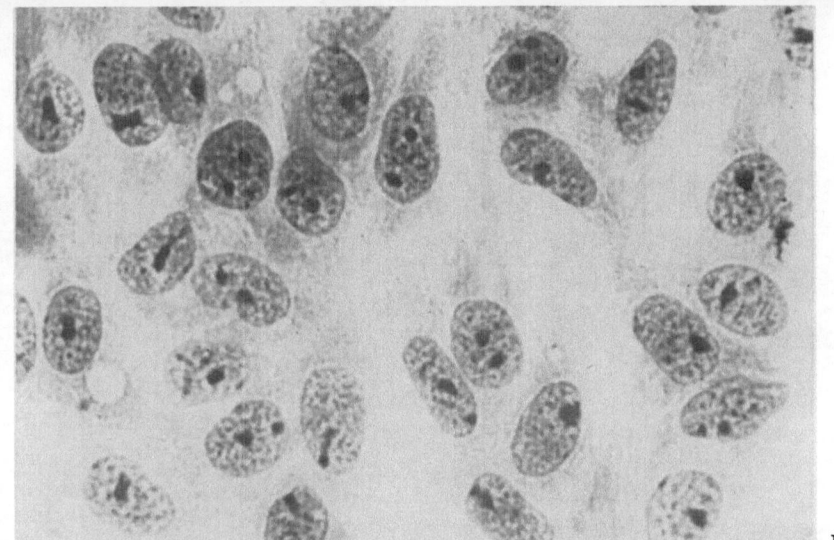

FIG. 1

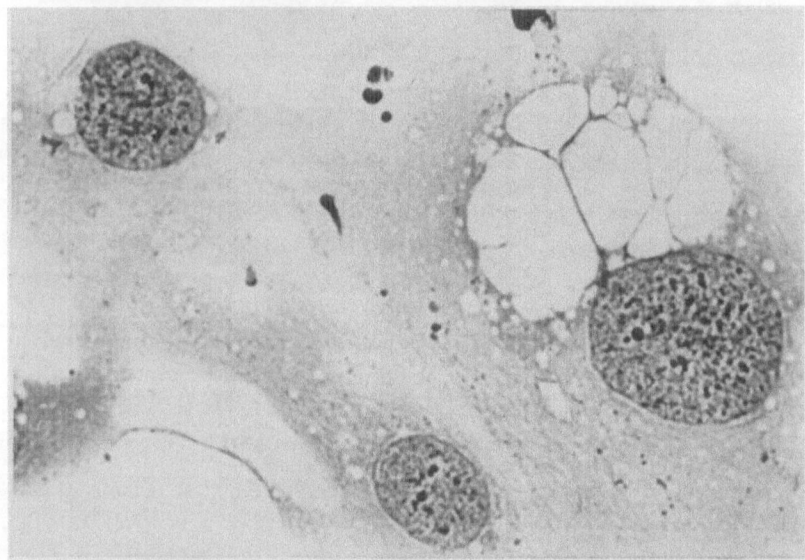

FIG. 2

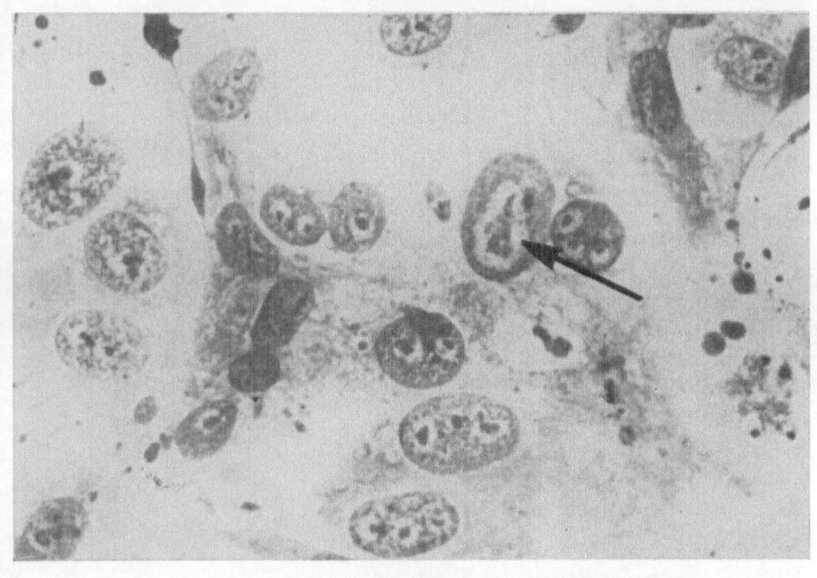

FIG. 3

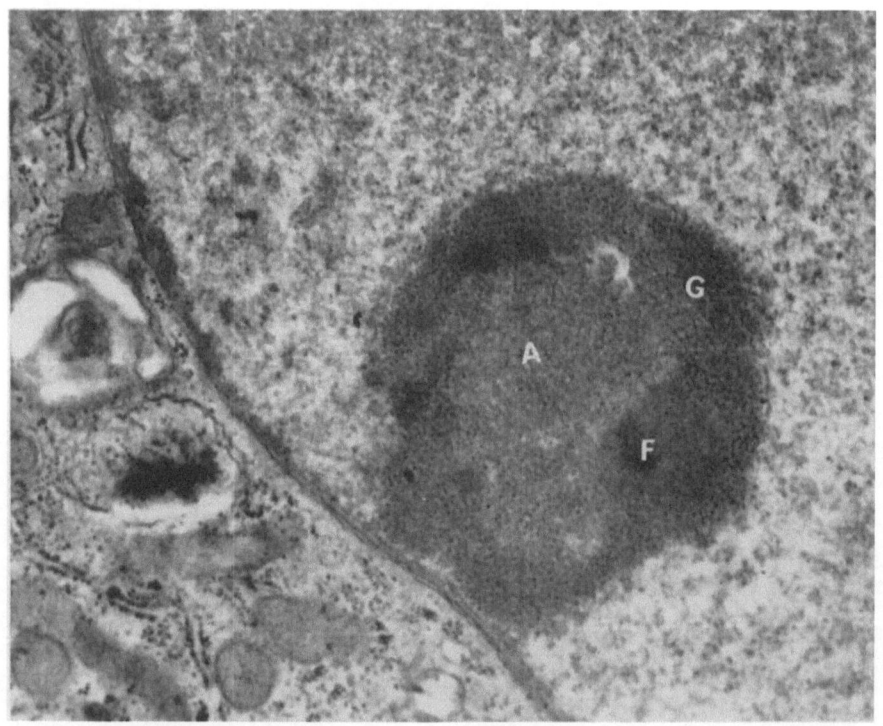

FIG. 4. A rounded nucleolus, after 24 hours' exposure to 1 μg aflatoxin B₁/ml; segregation into areas (G) granular, (F) fibrillar and (A) amorphous. (×35,000)

FIG. 1 (illustration overleaf). Control cell culture of green monkey epithelial cells. (H. & E. ×640)

FIG. 2 (illustration overleaf). Cell culture after 24 hours' exposure to aflatoxin, showing cytoplasmic vacuolation and fragmented nucleoli. (H. & E. ×640)

FIG. 3 (illustration overleaf). A cell culture treated with 1·0 μg sterigmatocystin/ml for 24 hours, showing nuclei with nucleoli (or nuclear bodies) surrounded by a halo. A nucleus with a large eosinophilic area and halo (arrow) is seen. (H. & E. ×640)

Aflatoxin B₁ 1·0 μg/ml medium. Treatment with aflatoxin B₁ caused many degenerative changes, including pycnosis, karyorrhexis and increased cytoplasmic vacuolation (Fig. 2). There was a marked decrease in the number of cells on the coverslips. (In actual cell counts of cultures (where a thousand cells per slide were counted) only 50% of the number of cells on the control slides were found.) Mitosis was completely inhibited, and many large cells were seen. The loss of chromatin was marked at 24 hours, giving the nuclei a 'ghost-like' appearance. Most noticeable, however, was the effect on the nucleolar morphology. Fragmented, small, numerous nucleoli were found in most nuclei. Halos were observed around the nucleoli in some of the experiments.

Sterigmatocystin 1·0 μg/ml medium. This toxin produced similar degenerative effects on the cell cultures. These included increased pycnosis, karyorrhexis, nuclear folds and a decrease in cell numbers (Fig. 3). Inhibition of mitosis, production of large cells and loss of chromatin from nuclei were also observed. Changes in nucleolar morphology were slightly different from those caused by aflatoxin B₁. Some of these nucleoli were very small, some were fragmented into basophilic and eosinophilic areas and some were large and eosinophilic and completely separated from the basophilic part. A halo usually surrounded these large eosinophilic nucleoli.

Electron microscopy. There was no difference in the ultrastructure of the two sets of control cells. The nuclei of these cells contained prominent but irregularly shaped nucleoli. The granular and fibrillar components were interspersed to form the nucleolonema.

Aflatoxin B₁ 1·0 μg/ml medium. All the nucleoli were round, segregated into fibrillar, granular and amorphous areas (Fig. 4). There were many areas of cytoplasmic degeneration.

Sterigmatocystin 1·0 μg/ml medium. The small and fragmented nucleoli observed with the light microscope were small and completely segregated. There was a variation in nucleolar size, most being relatively small (Fig. 5).

II. The effects on a continuous line of mouse liver fibroblasts

Cells of the control cultures were usually uniform in size and appearance, most being small and spindle-shaped. A few large cells were seen on scanning. Many mitotic figures were observed, of which the majority were normal (Figs. 6 and 8). There was no difference in morphology in the DMSO controls.

Experiment No. 1

Aflatoxin B₁ 1·0 μg/ml medium. There were no changes in morphology after 24 hours' treatment with aflatoxin B₁ or in the first or second passages. There was a tendency for the cells to grow in a disorientated fashion. In the third subculture many cells were larger and some showed a loss in chromatin material. In the fifth passage half of the cells consisted of large cells.

Sterigmatocystin 1·0 µg/ml medium. No morphological abnormalities were found after exposure to sterigmatocystin for 24 hours. The cells of the first and second subculture showed little change, except for a slight increase in cell size. In the third subculture many large and giant cells were seen. Half of the cell population of the fourth subculture were giant cells. Giant cells growing over each other predominated in the fifth passage. Some of these cells were multinucleated, some contained one giant nucleus and some showed a loss of chromatin material from the nucleus. Abnormal mitotic figures were frequently observed (Fig. 7).

Experiment No. 2

Aflatoxin B₁ 1·0 µg/ml medium. The changes in the cell cultures were similar to those observed in experiment No. 1, except that there were fewer large cells. When the cell cultures were exposed to aflatoxin B₁ for a second time, all the cells were detached from the glass coverslips and could not be studied.

Sterigmatocystin 1·0 µg/ml medium. No morphological changes were observed up to the second passage; there was, however, a tendency to dis-orientated growth. The cells of the second and third subcultures were larger, star-shaped and grew in a criss-cross pattern. The cells of the fourth passage showed a marked change. Giant cells predominated. Cultures of the fifth passage showed many giant cells and smaller spindle-shaped cells increased. After these cells were treated with sterigmatocystin for a second time cells of the first subculture were all in abnormal size and shape. Many cells showed extensive vacuolation of the cytoplasm. The cells were multi-nucleated or contained one huge abnormal nucleus. Only abnormal mitotic figures were seen.

Experiment No. 3

Aflatoxin B₁ 1·0 µg/ml medium. After 24 hours' treatment up to the third passage, the cultures were sparsely populated. The cells, which were star-shaped and fairly large, grew in a disordered way. From the third passage up to the tenth passage small spindle-shaped cells predominated. On scanning large cells were frequently observed. After a second exposure to 1·0 µg aflatoxin B₁/ml medium for 24 hours many giant cells and star-shaped cells appeared. In the first subculture after the second exposure, many giant cells, pycnotic cells and rounded cells were observed. Most cells were loosened from the glass coverslips in preparations of the second subculture. Of the cells which

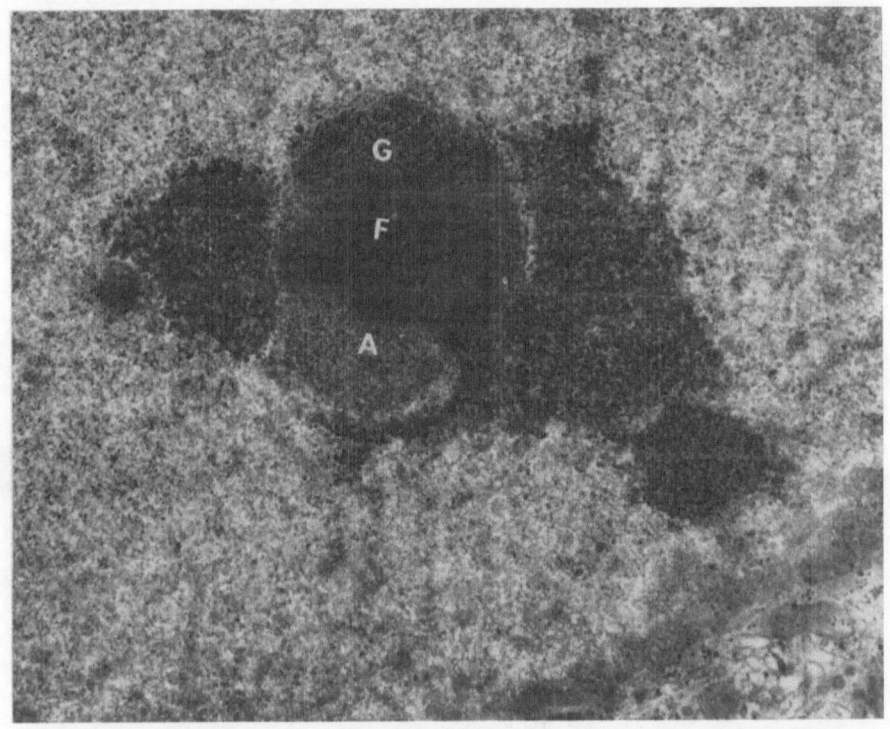

FIG. 5. This nucleolus is also segregated into (G) granular, (F) fibrillar and (A) amorphous areas after treatment with $1.0\,\mu$g sterigmatocystin/ml for 24 hours. (× 32,000)

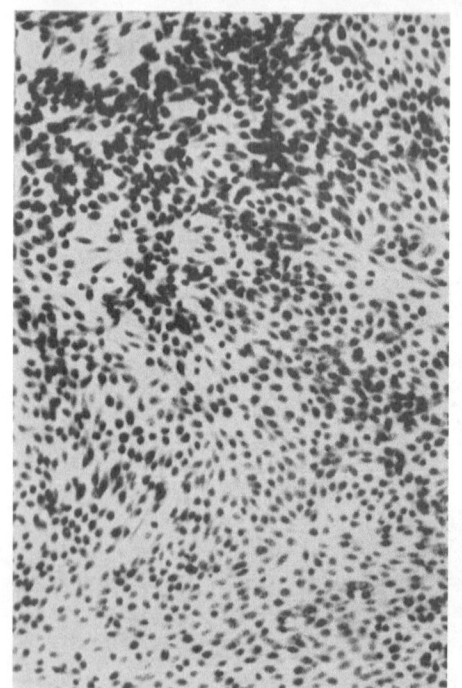

FIG. 6. A control cell culture of mouse liver fibroblasts line (L). (H. & E. ×160)

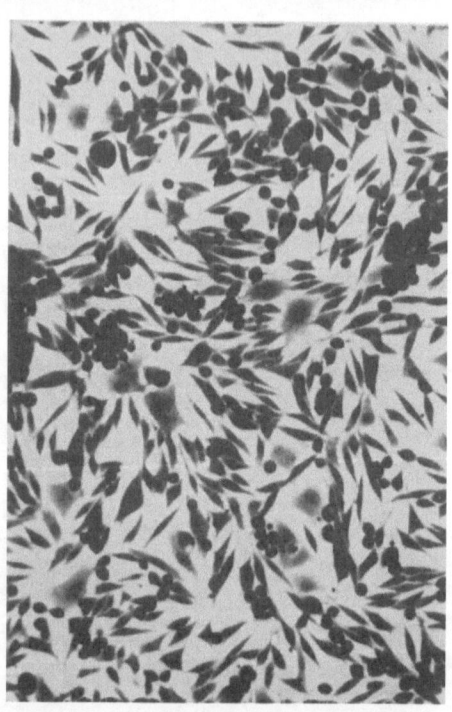

FIG. 8. A culture of MLF cells subcultured a second time after 24 hours' treatment with 1·0 μg sterigmatocystin/ml, showing multinucleated giant cells. (H. & E. ×160)

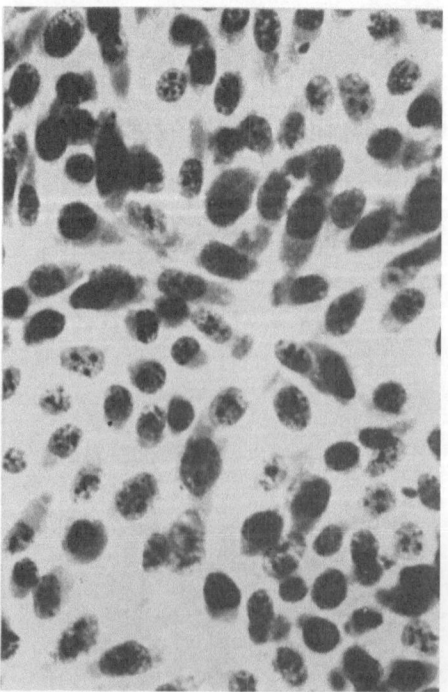

FIG. 7. A confluent layer of control MLF cells growing in an oriented pattern. (H. & E. ×640)

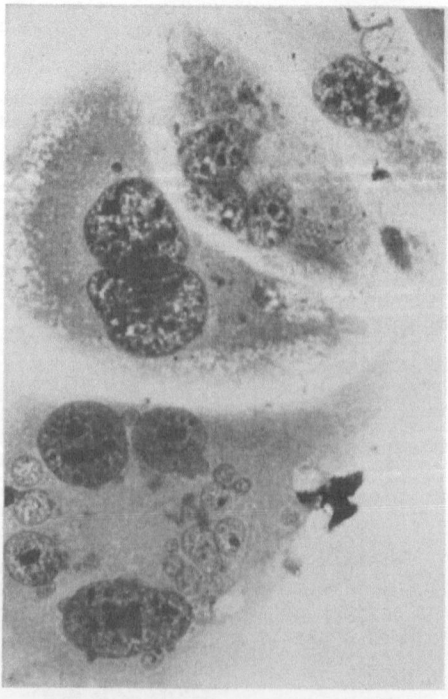

FIG. 9. Marked disoriented growth of cells were observed on the first subculture after a second exposure to 1·0 μg sterigmato-cystin/ml. Note the presence of many large cells. (H. & E. ×640)

remained, most were round and clumped into groups. These cells showed marked degenerative changes and were unable to grow when subcultured. *Sterigmatocystin 1·0 µg/ml medium.* Star-shaped large cells and giant cells were frequently observed up to the fourth passage. Abundant growth with mostly normal-sized spindle-shaped cells were seen in the fourth up to the tenth subculture. Cells of the first subculture after the second exposure to sterigmatocystin showed an increase in the number of large and star-shaped cells. In the second subculture many large binucleated cells or cells with 3-5 nuclei were observed. A large number of star- and spindle-shaped cells were growing in pronounced criss-cross pattern over the large cells (Fig. 9). On subcultures of these, cells were able to grow well.

Electron microscopy

The control cells were small and spindle-shaped. Most cells contained a large nucleus and relatively little cytoplasm.

Sterigmatocystin 1·0 µg/ml medium. Cell structures exposed for 24 hours and the cultures of the second and fifth subcultures after treatment were studied.

The cell membranes of all the cells exposed for 24 hours and those of the cells in the second subculture had numerous microvilli. Many of these cells were very large with multiple nuclei. Some of the cells showed a marked dilation of the granulated endoplasmic reticulum. Large dense membrane-bounded inclusion bodies were seen in the cytoplasm of many cells.

Cell cultures of the fifth subculture of experiment No. 3 showed smaller spindle-shaped cells with fewer microvilli, no inclusion bodies and a well-developed granular endoplasmic reticulum. No obvious changes in nucleolar morphology were noticed in any of the treated cells.

DISCUSSION

Aflatoxin B₁ and sterigmatocystin proved to be extremely toxic to the primary cell cultures. The cytotoxic effect was adequately illustrated by the degenerative changes observed in the treated cells.

Karyorrhexis and pycnosis were increased after 24 hours' treatment with aflatoxin B₁. Aflatoxin B₁ also caused a marked decrease in cell numbers. Cytoplasmic vacuolation increased in the remaining cells. There were also more nuclei with folds which would tend to implicate a loss in chromatin material. Many cells did indeed have a ghost-like appearance. Mitosis was completely inhibited. More large cells were observed. The most outstanding changes caused by aflatoxin B₁ were, however, the decrease in size of the nucleoli and fragmentation of the nucleolus into basophilic and eosinophilic areas. Zuckerman *et al.*[5] also reported a decrease in the size of the nucleoli in cultures of human embryo liver cells. Electron microscopic studies of these nucleoli revealed segregation of the fibrillar and granular parts of the nucleolus. Similar segregation was found in electron microscopic studies of rat and monkey liver cells from animals treated with aflatoxin B_1.[10]

The toxic effects of sterigmatocystin studied by light microscopy were similar, but not identical, to those of aflatoxin B_1. Sterigmatocystin also caused an increase in pycnosis and karyorrhexis, a loss of chromatin material and nuclear folds. More specific changes were inhibition of mitosis, fragmentation of the nucleolus and the formation of intranuclear eosinophilic nuclear masses. The latter may have been part of the nucleolar apparatus but they also may have been inclusion bodies or altered nucleoplasm. Many of the nucleoli were surrounded by a distinct halo. Cells treated with aflatoxin B_1 all showed nucleolar fragmentation. Electron microscopy revealed nuclear pleomorphism and segregation into two or three of the following components: amorphous, fibrillar and granular.

There are several chemically unrelated compounds which cause nucleolar segregation. These compounds are usually agents which interfere with DNA and RNA synthesis. According to Simard and Bernhard[11] inhibition of RNA synthesis is caused by agents which block RNA-polymerase. Actinomycin D may act as an example of a compound which inhibits RNA synthesis and also causes nucleolar segregation.[12] Other compounds which have a similar effect are 3'-methyl-4-dimethyl amino-azobenzene, 4-nitroquinoline-N-oxide,[13] mitomycin C[14] and amino nucleoside of puromycin.[15] Irradiation of cells also causes nucleolar segregation.

It has been reported that aflatoxin B_1 inhibits synthesis of several RNA's of which 45 S RNA is most pronounced.

According to preliminary work done in this laboratory, sterigmatocystin binds to some extent with DNA.[16] The incorporation of orotic acid into rat liver RNA is also inhibited.[17] These findings together with the nucleolar segregation indicate that the mode of action of sterigmatocystin on a primary cell culture may be similar to that of aflatoxin B_1.

The continuous line (L) of mouse liver fibroblasts were resistant to the cytotoxic effects of aflatoxin B_1 and sterigmatocystin after 24 hours' exposure. According to Diamond,[18] transformed rodent cells are usually resistant to treatment with carcinogenic polycyclic hydrocarbons.

On subcultivation two outstanding phenomena were, however, observed. In the sterigmatocystin-treated cell cultures a large number of giant cells appeared between the second passage and the fifth passage. Fewer giant cells were observed in aflatoxin B_1 treated cells. The second change was an increased tendency for a disorientated growth pattern in toxin treated cultures. After a second exposure to aflatoxin B_1 and sterigmatocystin in the tenth subculture, a marked criss-cross growth pattern was observed on subcultivation. The sterigmatocystin-treated cells were affected much more than those treated with aflatoxin B_1. This disordered growth pattern of the sterigmatocystin-treated cells was similar to that observed in cell cultures treated with other chemical carcinogens.[19, 20, 21, 22]

Neoplastic cells produced by carcinogens, or spontaneously transformed *in vitro*, were found to be unusually resistant to chemical carcinogens.[23, 24] Mouse L-line cells were resistant to the cytotoxic effects of 3,4-benzopyrene and 3-methyl cholantrene.[25]

ACKNOWLEDGEMENTS

I thank Mr N. Liebenberg and Mr M. J. van Wyk for the preparation of the photographs.

REFERENCES

1. BULLOCK, E., ROBERTS, J. C. and UNDERWOOD, J. G. (1962). *J. Chem. Soc.*, 4179.
2. DICKENS, F., JONES, H. E. H. and WAYNFORTH, H. B. (1966) *Br. J. Cancer*, **20**, 134.
3. PURCHASE, I. F. H. and VAN DER WATT, J. J. (1968). *Fd. Cosmet. Toxicol.*, **6**, 555.
4. HOLZAPFEL, C. W., PURCHASE, I. F. H., STEYN, P. S. and GOUWS, L. (1966). *S.A. med. J.*, **40**, 1100.
5. ZUCKERMAN, A. J., TSIQUAYE, K. N. and FULTON, F. (1967). *Br. J. exp. Path.*, **48**, 20.
6. LEGATOR, M. (1966). *Bacteriol. Rev.*, **30**, 471.
7. DANIEL, M. R. (1965). *Brit. J. exp. Path.*, **46**, 183.
8. HARLEY, E. H., REES, K. R. and COHEN, A. (1969). *Biochem. J.*, **114**, 289.
9. ENGELBRECHT, J. C. and PURCHASE, I. F. H. (1969). *S. Afr. med. J.*, **43**, 524.
10. SVOBODA, D., GRADY, H. J. and HIGGINSON, J. (1966). *Am. J. Path.*, **49**, 1023.
11. SIMARD, R. and BERNHARD, W. (1966). *Int. J. Cancer*, **1**, 463.
12. REYNOLDS, R. C., MONTGOMERY, P. O'B. and HUGHES, B. (1964). *Cancer Res.*, **24**, 1269.
13. FLOYD, L. R., UNUMA, T. and BUSCH, H. (1968). *Exp. Cell. Res.*, **51**, 423.
14. LAPIS, K. and BERNHARD, W. (1965). *Cancer Res.*, **25**, 628.
15. LEWIN, D. K. and MOSCARELLO, M. A. (1968). *Lab. Invest.*, **19**, 265.

16. SCHABORT, J. C. (1969). Personal communication.
17. NEL, W. and PRETORIUS, H. E. (1970). *Biochem. Pharmacol.*, **19**, 957.
18. DIAMOND, L. (1969). *Progr. exp. Tumor Res.*, **11**, 364.
19. BERWALD, Y. and SACHS, L. (1963). *Nature* (Lond.), **200**, 1182.
20. BERWALD, Y. and SACHS, L. (1965). *J. nat. Cancer Inst.*, **35**, 641.
21. HEIDELBERGER, C. and IYPE, P. T. (1967). *Science*, **155**, 214.
22. DIPAOLO, J. A., DONOVAN, P. and NELSON, R. (1969). *J. nat. Cancer Inst.*, **42**, 867.
23. ALFRED, L. J., GLOBERSON, A., BERWALD, Y. and PREHN, R. T. (1964). *Br. J. Cancer*, **18**, 159.
24. DIAMOND, L. (1967). *Int. J. Cancer*, **2**, 143.
25. ALFRED, L. J. (1964). *Br. J. Cancer*, **18**, 159.

RECENTLY DISCOVERED METABOLITES WITH UNUSUAL TOXIC MANIFESTATIONS

by

B. J. Wilson

Associate Professor of Biochemistry
Vanderbilt University School of Medicine, Nashville, Tennessee

This report will deal with but three of several interesting mycotoxicoses that have been studied in our laboratories at Vanderbilt University Medical School. These were selected, not because of the completeness of our knowledge concerning the causative agents, but because of the unusual nature of the toxic disease signs. I regret the paucity of information currently available on the respective toxic principles, but at least we are made aware of the need for further work and the direction that future research should take.

Toxin from Penicillium cyclopium

The first problem relates to the tremorgenic-diuretic toxin first reported 2 years ago from our laboratory.[1] This unusual substance is synthesised by *Penicillium cyclopium*, or *P. crustosum*, or *P. palitans*, or *P. viridicatum*, depending on which taxonomic authority you accept. Perhaps we should resolve the matter by referring to the organisms as the *P. cyclopium-viridicatum* group since apparently the differential criteria are not well defined.

This toxin is produced in and confined to the mycelium of the fungus as it grows as stationary cultures on various liquefied food substrates. The toxin occurs as a white, featherlike crystalline preparation. It appears to have the formula $C_{37}H_{44}O_6NC_1$ for a molecular weight of about 633 mass units. The bromo-toxin has been prepared by substituting KBr for KCl in the chemically defined medium, and traces of the iodo-toxin and the dehalogenated molecule have also been detected. Very little is known about the structure but we have reason to believe that the nucleus may be a steroid. It is definitely not the same as cyclopiazonic acid described by Dr Holtzapfel. It is not identical with viridicatin, cyclopenin or their derivatives which are well-known metabolites of this group of fungi.

The toxin is most effective when administered by stomach tube or by IP injection using propylene glycol or other suitable vehicle. Several different laboratory animals are susceptible to the neurotoxic effects, and sheep, cattle and horses died after eating feed naturally contaminated with the organisms. Most laboratory experiments have employed white mice and rats.

I

Some, but by no means all, of the behavioural effects of IP injected toxin are listed in Table 1 which also shows the dosages used. As you note, 250 µg/kg given in an acacia suspension caused perceptible tremors whereas ten times that dose produced convulsions and death in one of three animals.

Table 1

Pharmacological Effects of *Penicillium Cyclopium* Toxin Injected in Mice

I.P. Dose (mg./kg.)	Irritability / Respiration	Exophthalmos	Tremors	Limb weakness	Convulsions	Death
0·10	Neg. / Neg.	Neg.	Neg.	Neg.	Neg.	0/3
0·25	I / Neg.	+	+	Neg.	Neg.	0/3
0·50	I / D	+	+	+	Neg.	0/3
1·00	I / D and I	+	+	+	Neg.	0/3
2·50	I / I	+	+	+	+	1/3
5·00	I / I	+	+	+	+	1/3
10·00	I / I	+	+	+	+	1/3

I = increased rate.   D = decreased rate.

A considerable variation in resistance to the lethal effects is shown in the fact that two of three animals survived as much as 10 mg/kg. Other observed effects included increased irritability, rapid respirations, diarrhoea, diuresis, pinna loss, loss of corneal reflex, mydriases, and some lachrymation in which there is an exudation of formed elements of the blood. Figure 1 shows a mouse undergoing a convulsive seizure.

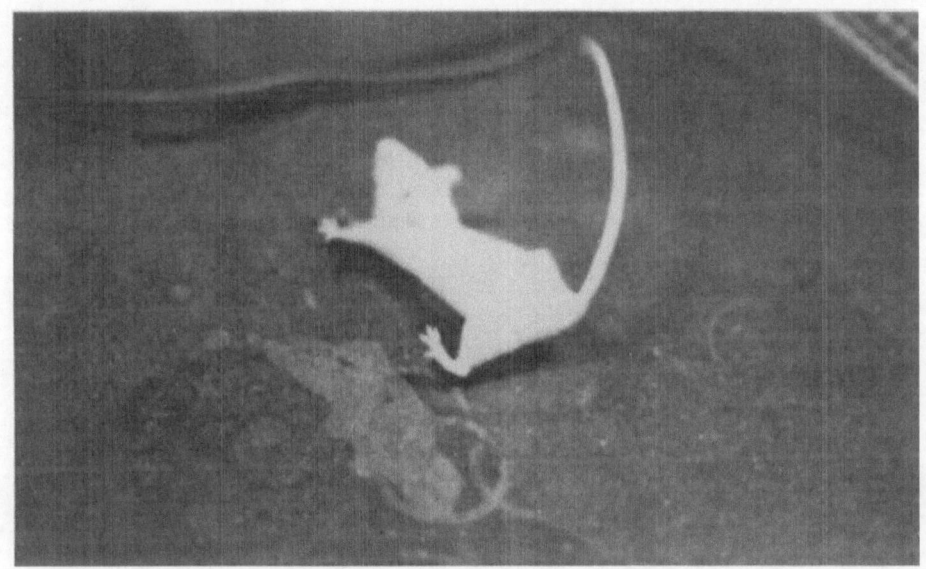

FIG. 1. Mouse exhibiting convulsive seizure after dosing with tremorgenic toxin.

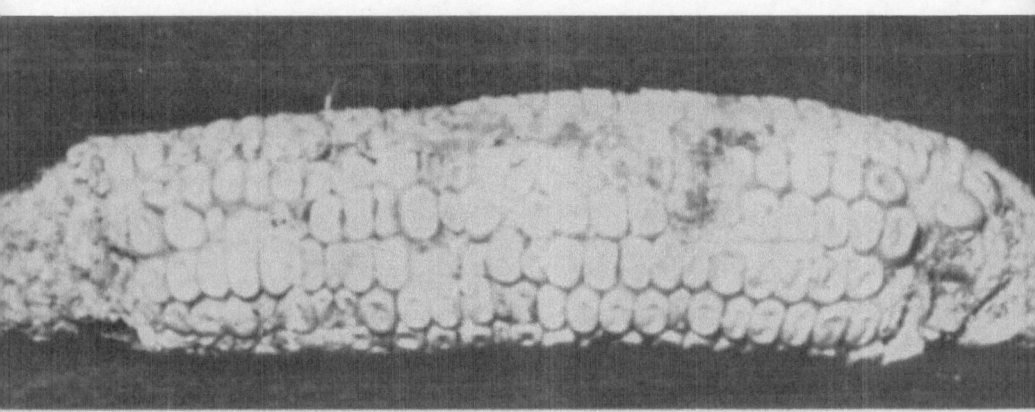

FIG. 2. Ear of Egyptian corn covered with mycelium of *Fusarium moniliforme*.

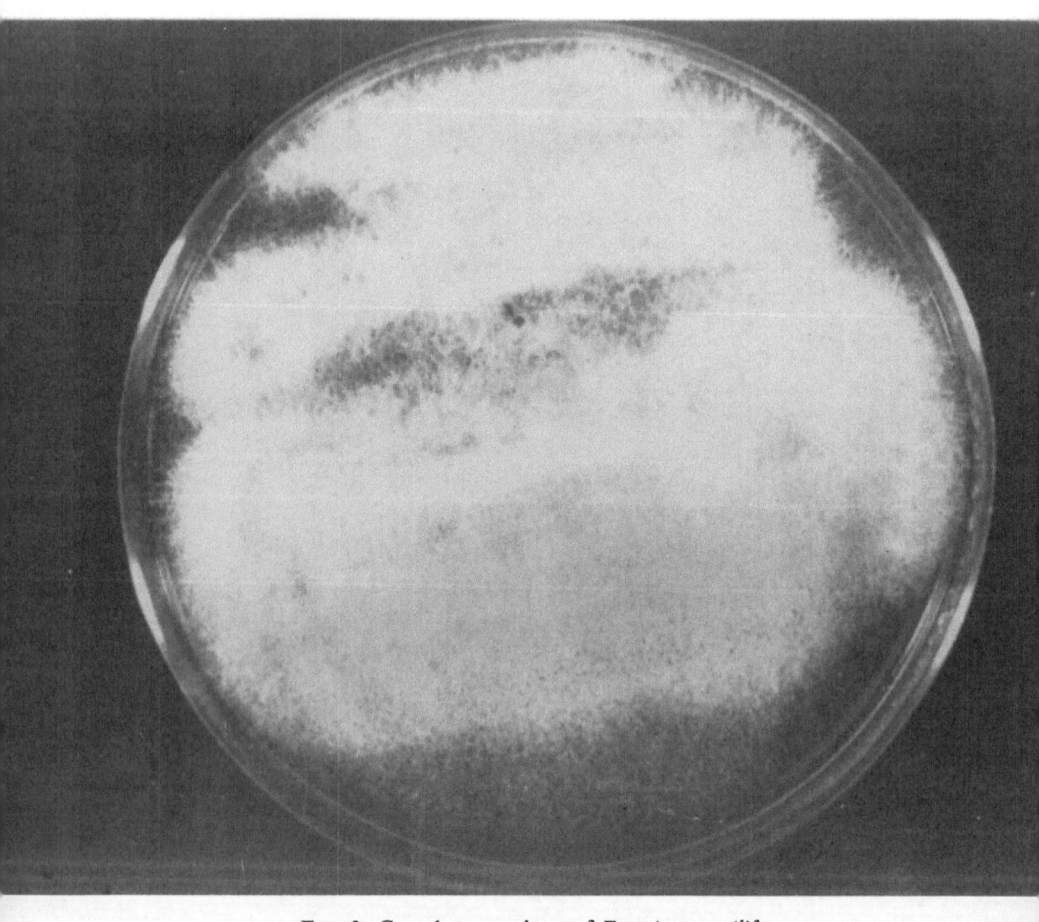

FIG. 3. Czapek agar culture of *Fusarium moniliforme*.

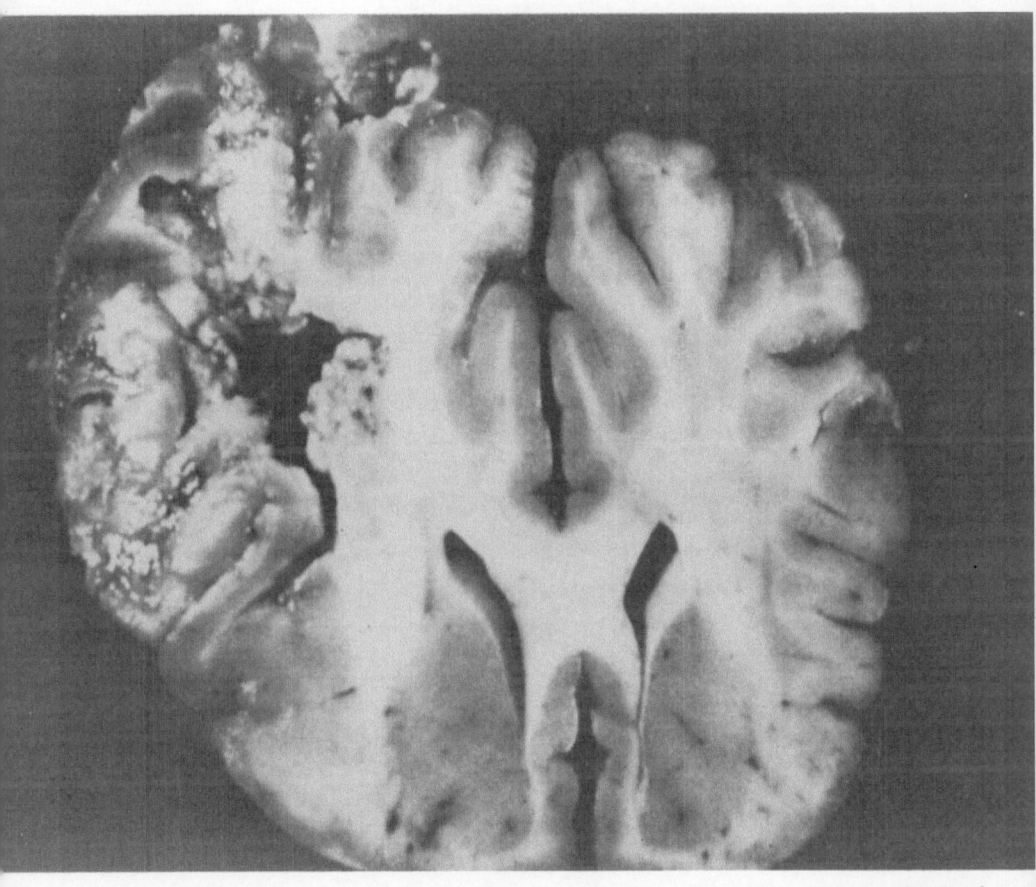

FIG. 4. Large necrotic lesion in right hemisphere of donkey brain. Animal was fed ten pounds of toxic corn.

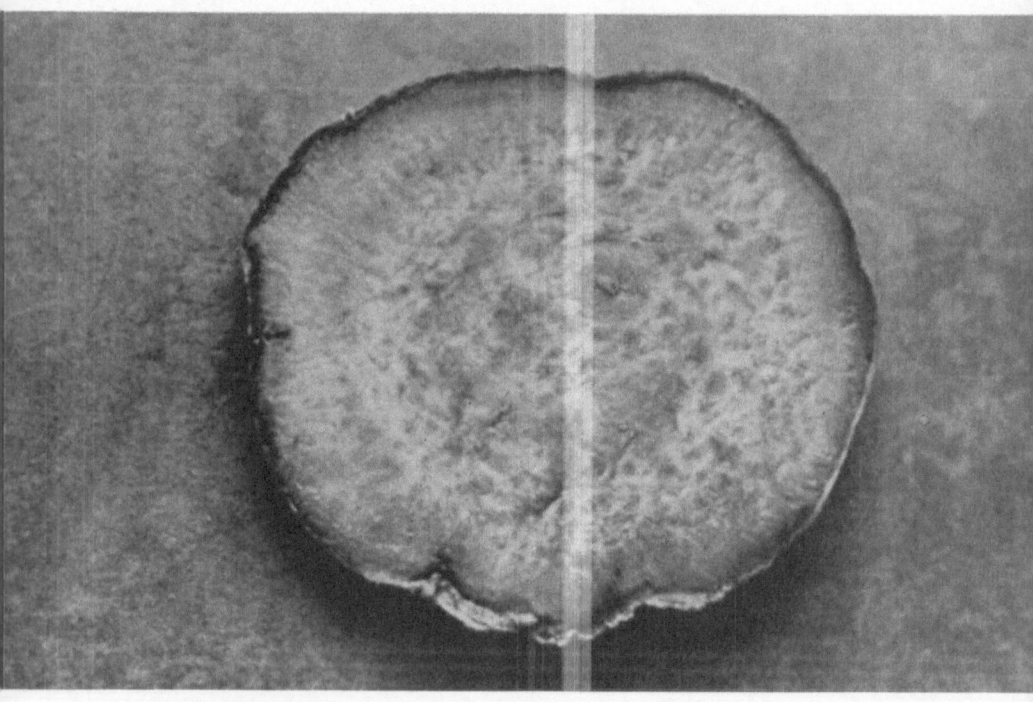

Fig. 6. Sectioned toxin-containing sweet potato showing slight subcortical discolouration.

The onset of fine body tremors in mice may begin within a few minutes depending on the dose and route. If the dose is large the tremors are soon replaced by convulsions. Should the animal survive the seizures, which may last several hours, he returns to the tremors which in some instances may persist for 3 days before apparent recovery. If he dies during a convulsive seizure the carcass shows an immediate rigidity.

The rat is also susceptible to the tremorgen but in this species the effect seems to be more severe and prolonged. For example, a dose of 2·5 mg/kg may cause difficulty in locomotion that can last for two or more weeks.

A few isolated experiments have shown the toxin to have no apparent anti-pseudocholinesterase activity but it does cause a substantial contraction of isolated longitudinal smooth muscle of the guinea-pig ileum.

Table 2

Effects of Orally Administered *Penicillium cyclopium* Toxin on Urinary Excretion in Rats

Test group	Quantity excreted in 4·5 hours						
	Na+*	K+	Ca++	Mg++	Cl	Gluc. (mg)	U. Vol. (ml)
Control	345	150	7	30	370	2	1·95
0·5 mg/kg	480	270	15	39	521	3	3·25
2·0 mg/kg	1830	505	81	151	1902	60	18·05

* Electrolytes estimated as microequivalents.

The tremorgenic potency of the toxin is approximately 10 to 20 times greater than that of arecoline and tremorine, two well-known tremorgenic drugs. Also, of several anticonvulsive drugs screened for their activity in countering toxic effects, only near-lethal doses of phenobarbital and curare abolished the neurological properties of toxin in mice.

A diuresis first noted in the mouse has been studied in some detail in the female rat. Table 2 illustrates an experiment in which two levels of toxin were given by stomach tube. The urinary volume increased and the absolute values for the various electrolytes and glucose excreted also increased as the dose of toxin was increased. The mechanisms behind these phenomena are not known with any certainty as yet. We do know that there is a hyperglycaemia induced by toxin that may be lowered to some extent by administration of insulin. Although there is some effect on the P:O ratio in rat kidney mitochondria, the effect on ATPase has been equivocal, and much additional work is needed. Current efforts are directed to the histopathology of the toxic state and to the effects of tremorgen on neurohormone levels in the brain.

The intoxication is especially interesting when we recall that there are at least two rare human afflictions that show separately something of the neurotoxicity and nephrotoxicity exemplified by this toxin. The first is a disease known as the 'Ilesha shakes', a temporary neurological condition occurring in the Western region of Nigeria and possibly related to consumption of yams or some other food.[2] I saw a case in a 9-year-old girl during a visit to a Methodist mission hospital at Ilesha in 1965. Dr Pearson, the hospital superintendent, recently informed me that these cases still occur.

The second condition was an unusual epidemic of polyuria affecting about 150 people in India in 1966.[3] This was attributed to mouldy millet and the condition was apparently reproduced in rats given the grain. A species of *Rhizopus* was implicated, but I have found no subsequent reports on the subject.

Equine leucoencephalomalacia

I want to make only brief mention of another mycotoxicosis—one that seems to be peculiar to certain equine species. I refer to the condition sometimes called equine leucoencephalomalacia, although several other names and epithets have been used throughout the world where this condition has been known for many decades.[4] Our attention was directed to outbreaks in the vicinity of Cairo, Egypt where flooding of corn (maize) fields of the Nile Delta has occurred in past years. The ears of corn believed responsible for the disease characteristically show a dull, pink film of mould mycelium overlying the ears of grain (Fig. 2). Black and green spots of mould damage are also seen, but the pink colouration is most commonly noted. Of several aspergilli and penicillia isolated, none was shown to be the cause of the toxicosis. Instead, as one would suspect, the pink-coloured organism, identified as *Fusarium moniliforme*, was found to be the culprit (Fig. 3).

Growth of the organism on both Egyptian corn and American whole grain corn for 2 weeks at 25°C causes the corn to become toxic to a lethal degree. In one such feeding study a male Egyptian donkey was fed only 10 lb of freeze dried corn, along with other staples, over a period of 11 days. On the 12th and 13th days the animal went off feed and began to show signs of neurotoxicity as evidenced by walking in circles. On the 14th day the lower lip drooped and the head was held facing downward into one corner of the pen. The right eyelid was insensitive to stimulation. After another 2 hours of walking in circles the animal fell down and struggled for about an hour before expiring.

Figure 4 is a photograph of the large necrotic lesion found in the white matter of the right hemisphere. Two remarkable things are readily apparent here. First, the rapidity with which this large lesion develops and the remarkable ability of the animal to live long enough for the lesion to form.

Gastrointestinal ulcers and other visceral lesions have been noted in animals dying from the disease, but they constitute inconstant findings and their relationship to the neural lesion is not clear. Incidentally, the older the donkey, the more susceptible he is to the disease.

We have fed toxic corn to goats, pigs, monkeys and several laboratory animals with negative results. We have also administered several types of extracts of the corn to donkeys without them getting the disease. We are continuing this work on an intercontinental basis—the toxic preparations are produced in the U.S.A. and shipped to Cairo where Dr Maronpot does the large-animal feeding trials at the U.S. Naval Medical Unit there.

We hope to have some more definite answers to this problem in the near future.

Sweet potato toxicity

This toxicosis is not really a mycotoxicosis, although moulds play a prominent role in the production of toxin. I am referring to a group of abnormal toxic metabolites of the sweet potato (*Ipomoea batatas*) which is formed by the tubers in response to various chemical and mechanical injuries. The classical black rot fungus, *Ceratocystis fimbriata*, is the best known, but it is by no means the only one which may be involved.

Our attention was brought to this problem by veterinary collaborators in the State of Georgia, U.S.A. where 50 head of cattle were lost last year as a result of consuming mouldy sweet potatoes. As with other such occasional outbreaks the animals became dyspnoeic after about 2 to 4 days and eventually died in an anoxic state. At autopsy the main findings were lung oedema, alveolar epithelialisation and other related phenomena.

On examining the samples of sweet potatoes provided we found that none of the dozen or so fungi or bacteria present on the potatoes were toxigenic. However, ether extracts from the sweet potato samples, fed or injected into mice, caused a gradually increasing dyspnoeic state occurring over a few hours that soon led to death—apparently from anoxia. Post-mortem examination showed a hitherto undescribed respiratory toxic condition consisting of hydrothorax and pulmonary emphysema that to some extent resembled the disease in cattle. An occasional animal showed liver damage and oedema of the kidneys and the myocardium.

To hasten on to a climax of the story, we found that there was more than one toxin present in the sweet potatoes. The first identified was the previously described ipomeamarone (Fig. 5) whose structure was described by Kubota and colleagues in Japan.[5] A most fascinating point here is the fact that ipomeamarone is the enantiomer of ngaione, a hepatotoxic oil (but a normal metabolite) of the Ngaio tree and certain shrubs in Australia and New Zealand.[6] We found, as one obscure Japanese report had indicated, that ipomeamarone was toxic to the liver but did not cause the lung oedema or pleural effusion in mice. A new compound isolated from toxic potatoes was found to be hydroxyipomeamarone which we call ipomeamaronol.[7] This also was hepatotoxic but was not the lung oedema factor.[8] This latter substance has been most elusive but has finally been isolated and is now being studied intensively.

Production of these toxins, along with several other related furan compounds, can be accomplished, we find, using a culture of *F. javanicum* to

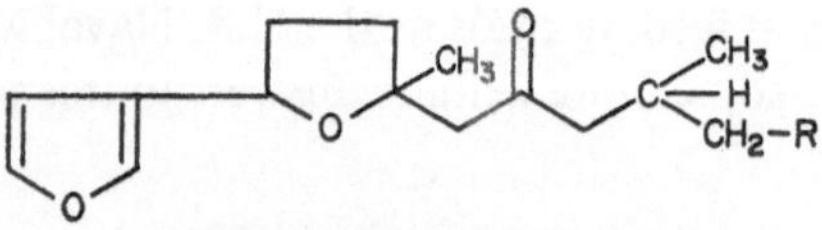

FIG. 5. Formula of ipomeamarone (R = H)
and ipomeamaronol (R = OH).

inoculate fresh slices of sweet potato which are then incubated at room temperature for about 6 days. Ether extraction followed by preparative column chromatography and then gas-liquid chromatography effects isolation of the various desired components.

A most disturbing finding is that sweet potatoes sold on the wholesale and retail markets in Nashville, Tennessee often contain these metabolites even when the tubers show only slight subcortical discolouration as the sole abnormality (Fig. 6).

Although African yams such as *Diascorea rotundata* have been implicated as a cause of liver disease,[9] neither this species nor two others tested were capable of forming these furanosesquiterpenes.

It seems that the further we look, the more naturally occurring toxicants we find, but it is not as yet clear whether any of these substances is currently playing a significant role in human health problems. We remain alert to this possibility, however, at all times.

REFERENCES

1. WILSON, B. J., WILSON, C. H. and HAYES, A. W. (1968). *Nature* (Lond.), **220**, 77.
2. WRIGHT, J. and MORLEY, D. C. (1958). *Lancet*, **1**, 871.
3. NARASIMHAN, M. J., GANLA, V. G., DEODHAR, N. S. and SULE, C. R. (1967). *Lancet*, **1**, 760.

4. BADIALI, L., ABOU-YOUSSEF, M. H., RADWAN, A. I., HAMDY, F. M. and HILDEBRANDT, P. K. (1968). *Am. J. vet. Res.*, **29**, 2029.
5. KUBOTA, T. and MATSUURA, T. (1958) *J. Chem. Soc.*, 3667.
6. HEGARTY, B. F., KELLY, J. R., PARK, R. J. and SUTHERLAND, M. D. (1970). *Aust. J. Chem.*, **23**, 107.
7. YANG, D. T. C., WILSON, B. J. and HARRIS, T. M. *Phytochemistry*. In press.
8. WILSON, B. J., YANG D. T. C. and BOYD, M. R. *Nature* (Lond.). In press.
9. GILBERT, C. and GILLMAN, J. (1963). *Nature* (Lond.), **198**, 196.

EPIDEMIOLOGICAL INTERACTIONS

by

M. A. Crawford

Nuffield Institute of Comparative Medicine
The Zoological Society of London
Regent's Park, London NW1, England

The study of epidemiology provides clues of a complex nature as to the aetiology of disease processes. In the experimental approach, we alter one factor and follow the consequences.

In epidemiology, we study populations which demonstrate a high incidence of a particular disease and attempt to establish which factors may be responsible by comparison with a low incidence population. Unfortunately, the diversity of human behaviour is such that seldom is only one factor, which can be studied by epidemiology, different, although the potential of different factors can be examined experimentally. The 'purists' criticise the epidemiological approach on the grounds that too many factors are involved for intelligible sense to be made of the disease patterns. Yet the pure experimental approach can similarly be criticised. The laboratory animals are distinctly different from the human animal in at least two important features, longevity and development of the central and peripheral nervous system. At the same time the design of many experiments are irrelevant to the human situation.

Again in experiment the addition of one factor, *ipso facto*, alters the

Table 1

Rabbit Liver Lecithin Linoleate with and without Cholesterol

	Standard diet	
	Without cholesterol	With 10% cholesterol
Linoleate in	Mean of 6±S.E.	Mean of 6±S.E.
lecithin	17±S.E.	8·3±S.E.
free fatty acids	11±S.E.	4·1±S.E.

Five month old white rabbits were fed a standard diet with or without 10% cholesterol added for 1 month after which the liver was extracted and analysed by thin-layer and GLC.

relative balance of every other biological factor—a simple consequence that is often overlooked. The presence of abnormal quantities may also produce a chain reaction effect on other cellular components with which it reacts, again altering the whole cellular balance. If, for example, cholesterol is fed to an animal not only does it increase in the tissue pools but also the pool size of linoleic acid decreases because it is trapped by the cholesterol (Table 1). This linoleate trapping assumedly reduces the amount available for lecithin synthesis.

Consequently both the experimental and epidemiological approach are difficult but the difficulties are frequently made worse by our training which fosters the narrow definition of the 'Eureka syndrome'. Much of our thinking and probably much progress is clouded by such attempts to narrow a problem to such a fine degree of definition that the interactions which go to make up the life and death of the cell may be almost entirely overlooked.

Dietary and climatic variations in Uganda

We became interested in the epidemiological approach through work in East Africa where the strong geographical and climatic contrasts make it possible to examine rural communities who by virtue of local custom, climatic and geographic considerations, are restricted to certain types of crops or food staples.[1]

The diets selected by certain groups of indigenous East Africans can largely be determined by the type of crops which the climate will support. Around the shore of Lake Victoria, where there is abundant rain and surface water, particularly in the humid enclave created by Lakes Victoria, Edward, George, Albert, Kyoga and the Nile Basin, fruits like the plantain, root crops like sweet potato and cassava together with groundnuts grow with ease and abundance (Table 2). However, in areas both north of the water enclaves created by Lake Victoria and the Rift Valley, where the climate becomes hot and dry, people cultivate grains such as sorghum, sim sim and maize.

Cancer incidence in Uganda

In 1962, Dodge[2, 3] reported the incidence of different cancers in Ugandan Africans (Table 3). As his survey was carried out at Kampala this really means the incidence in the population which the Kampala hospital served.

Bladder cancer

Two tumours were of direct interest to us; bladder and liver. Bladder cancer was investigated because those cases studied by Dodge were rarely infected with *Schistosoma haemotobium* which is thought to be responsible for the high incidence of bladder cancer in Egypt. Fripp[4] reported the urinary excretion of glucuronidase in *S. haemotobium* infection and

Table 2

Climatic, Ethnic and Dietary Variants in the Selected Geographic Locations
(From ref. 1)

Location	Mean annual			Ethnic group	Staples
	Temp. °C.		Rainfall in.		
	Max.	Min.			
North Shore Lake Victoria					
Mulago ⎫ Buganda ⎬ Busoga ⎭	27	16	50-70	Bantu	Plantain/root crops
Karamoja/Suk	32	14	20-30	Nilo-Hamitic	Sorghum/milk
Madi Opei	35	16	20	Nilotic	Millet
Gulu	32	16	40	Nilotic	Mixed, sim sim, millet, root crops
Kigezi	24	10	50-60	Bantu	Mixed, root crops, plantain

Buganda and Busoga can be considered to be regions in which the plantain and sweet potato play a dominant role as staples. Around the north shore of Lake Victoria the climate is suitable for the growth of plantain but, whilst this crop dominates, a wide variety of other crops such as cassava, maize and millet also contribute significantly to the diet. However, in the dry regions to the north and north-east the plantain cannot be grown and the people use cow's milk, blood and grains. Gulu represents a transitional region from the plantain-free area in the north with very little plantain in use, but some root crop. The mountains of the south-west cause the climate in Kigezi to be moist and groups using a wide variety of crops can be found.

Table 3

Types of Malignancy as a Percentage of all
Malignant Disease in Ugandan Africans—
1952-59 (3,172 Cases) (From ref. 3)

Malignant lymphoma	9·89
Carcinoma of cervix	9·42
Carcinoma of penis	7·15
Carcinoma of liver	6·65
Carcinoma of skin	5·04
Carcinoma of eye	4·76
Carcinoma of breast	3·87
Carcinoma of prostate	3·81
Kaposi sarcoma	3·65
Carcinoma of bladder	3·4
Carcinoma of bladder (Ghana)	2·5
Carcinoma of bladder (Port. E.A.)	7·9

suggested this enzyme could liberate from conjugates, free ortho-amino phenols which are known to be carcinogenic; we had found a high excretion rate of urinary indoles in Ugandan Africans from the plantain belt[5] and it

Table 4

Excretion Rates for Quinolinic and Intermediates in 24-Hour Morning Specimens (mg/24 hour) (From ref. 1)

	Group Composition			
	Plantain/root crop		No. plantain European	
Kynurenic acid	32	(30)	15	(18)
Xanthurenic acid	34	(30)	27	(18)
3-HOAA	32	(31)	6	(33)
Quinlinic	138	(12)	9	(20)
N-methyl nicotinamide	9·3	(7)	13	(5)
Kynurenine	19	(31)	8	(33)

was likely that other indolic metabolites would also be raised. As this group of compounds includes 3-hydroxyanthanilic acid (3-HOAA) for which there is good evidence of carcinogenic activity, we examined the actual urinary excretion rates and indeed found them to be high (Table 4).

Occurrence of mycotoxins in Uganda

Liver cancer was of interest because it was quite clear from our own purchases in the Kampala supermarkets that groundnuts were being sold

Table 5

Aflatoxin Content Throughout the Year 1965-1966 (From ref. 8)

Month	Total number of samples	Number of samples containing aflatoxin B_1 (mg/kg)			
		0-0·1	0·01-1·0	1-10	>10
January/February	12	10	2	0	0
March/April	15	11	3	1	0
May/June	15	8	4	3	1
July/August	15	11	2	2	1
September/October	12	10	2	0	0
November/December	15	11	4	0	0

which were heavily infected with mould and the incidence of primary hepatoma was high by comparison with European standards. Outbreaks of disease in domestic animals in Europe and East Africa has focused attention on the importance of food contamination by fungi and the induction of cancer in laboratory animals by fungal metabolites.[6, 7]

We established that aflatoxin was present in the samples which were being sold for human consumption and on examination of 250 samples in 1965-1966 we found 15% contained more than one part per million of aflatoxin B_1.[8]

We were able to culture *Aspergillus flavus* from all the samples which had little detectable aflatoxin and little mould. From these cultures we also isolated *Rhizopus* sp., *A. repens*, *A. niger*, *A. tamrii*, *A. ochraceus*, *A. terrens* and *Penicillium* sp., including *P. citrinium* and *P. patulum* both of which are also known to produce toxic metabolites. We also examined the effect of seasonal variations in climate on the accumulation of aflatoxin and found, as suspected, fluctuations with higher titres at the end of the rain seasons (Table 5).

In 1967, we repeated our analyses of Ugandan groundnuts and found that 12% of the 430 samples contained more than 1 mg/kg aflatoxin. Furthermore, it is also clear that *A. flavus* may invade the developing fruit of the peanut, in the soil, prior to harvesting.[1, 9, 10] This finding is consistent with our own observations that not one of the samples of peanuts was free from spores.

On incubation of groundnuts, with a low aflatoxin concentration, we found that little accumulation took place during 1 week's incubation at room temperature with a moisture content of 5-8%. However, at 15-30% a concentration of some 15-30 mg/kg was reached (Table 6). Diener and Davis[12] examined accumulation in relation to relative humidity and found that the growth of *A. flavus* was restricted at 85% but growth was rapid at 95-97%.

Aflatoxin and primary hepatoma

It is clear that aflatoxin is present in the food eaten by Ugandan Africans. In Uganda, groundnuts are frequently used as an accompaniment to plantain or other staple foods. The groundnut plays a valuable role in the diet of many African communities on account of the high protein content. Rutishauser[13] reported that the average consumption of groundnuts in five boys' schools in Buganda was 63 lb (29 kg) per 50 boys per week—i.e. 1·26 lb (570 g) per child per week. If the rate of contamination was 1 mg/kg a meal containing 100 g of groundnuts would result in a dose of 0·1 mg which would be 0·0025 mg per kg body-weight in an 88 lb (40 kg) child. The lethal dose (LD_{50}) of aflatoxin in ducklings is 0·4 mg per kg; to attain

Table 6

Aflatoxin Concentration in Relation to Moisture Content

Moisture content	Aflatoxin B_1 content (mg/kg) after storage for:		Fungi isolated	Growth
	1 week	1 month		
Dried	0·01	0·01	*Rhizopus* sp. *A. repens*	Scanty
As purchased (8% water)	0·01	0·03	*A. flavus* *A. niger* *Rhizopus* sp.	Scanty
Plus 2·5%	0·01	0·08	*Rhizopus* sp.	Scanty
Plus 5%	0·09	0·38	*Rhizopus* sp. *A. flavus* *A. niger*	Moderate
			A. tamrii *A. ochraceus* *A. terreus*	Scanty
			Penicillium sp.	Moderate
Plus 7·5%	0·62	0·95	*Penicillium* sp.	Moderate
Plus 10%	1·1	6·0	*Rhizopus* sp. *A. flavus*	Heavy
			A. niger	Moderate
			A. ochraceus *A. terreus* *A. tamrii*	Scanty
Plus 15%	15·0	destroyed	*A. tamrii*	Scanty
Plus 25%	31·0	destroyed	*Rhizopus* sp. *A. flavus* *A. niger*	Very profuse
			Penicillium sp.	Moderate
As purchased: incubated in 90% humidity	0·04	0·98	*Penicillium* sp.	Moderate

this a 40-kg child would need to eat 16 kg of nuts, which is unthinkable. However, if the nuts contained 10 mg/kg it would require little more than 2 weeks for a child to consume a duckling LD_{50} dose. It would seem difficult for a level of contamination of 10 mg/kg or more to escape unnoticed as at this level we found the nuts to be very heavily infected and many would discard groundnuts if there was an obvious growth of mould.

However, at a level of 1 mg/kg aflatoxin the fungal growth may not be sufficient to make it obvious to casual observation.

There is, however, a real danger that the mould may grow on the nuts during a damp period followed by an arrest in growth with a change in climate or storage conditions. The nuts may then appear relatively free from mould, although they may be dirty. With this last reservation it is probable that groundnuts could be regularly eaten with an aflatoxin content of up to 1 mg/kg. Whilst on the one hand it would take a considerable period of time for an LD_{50} dose to be consumed, it should also be pointed out that no sample examined by us was free of *A. flavus* spores. It is difficult to predict the cumulative effect at such levels, particularly as the effect of aflatoxin is so species-dependent. Insufficient is known about the cumulative effects of low doses to reach a conclusion regarding the implications to human hepatoma in Uganda except to say that if it does play a role, it is most likely to be intermittent and chronic. The probability of a toxic dose being consumed at one meal is almost negligible, and at 1 mg/kg it would require approximately 6 months to consume such a toxic dose. An analogy with current views on radiation hazards may provide some guidance to the situation. The maximum accepted safe cumulative dose throughout any given year is approximately 1/100th of a single lethal dose.[14] If the analogy is valid, it might provide a basis for considering the possible harmful effects of aflatoxin in foodstuffs.

The rate at which aflatoxin can accumulate in groundnuts, given the right conditions (the nature of cropping, length of storage, humidity and rainfall) requires a more detailed investigation than we have so far carried out. Furthermore, the report by Coady[15] on the isolation of toxin-producing fungi from other food sources in Ethiopia indicates that attention should not be confined to groundnuts. Moreau[16] lists 148 species of fungi which produce identifiable toxins. Jarvis[29] lists 15 species which produce severe proven effects in animals (Table 7).

Aflatoxin-producing strains have been isolated from oil seeds, grains pulses and even cassava,[17] and from rice stored at a moisture content of 24-26%,[18] and in maize containing 19·6-20% moisture.[19] In this respect it is of interest that people in North East Uganda also eat sorghum and actually use it when it is mouldy. What this really means is that with so many fungi capable of producing toxins occurring in different foods it will be difficult to incriminate a single causative factor.

Studies[20] have shown that aflatoxin B_1 rapidly inhibits RNA and DNA synthesis. Hence, in trying to unravel the epidemiology it would be useful to know why aflatoxin is an hepatotoxin as every cell in the body uses RNA and DNA. A possible answer may have come from our studies on the excretion of 3-HOAA and aflatoxin in Patas monkeys.

A possible factor in liver and bladder specificity

In the experiments on Patas monkeys, using a cannula in the gall bladder and urethra we found that aflatoxin could only be detected with difficulty

Table 7

Fungal Species known to produce Diseases in Man and Animals (ref. 29)

Species	Toxin	Disease syndrome	Animals affected
Aspergillus flavus	aflatoxins	Groundnut poisoning	Ducklings
A. clavatus	patulin	Hyperkeratosis	Calves
A. ochraceus	ochratoxins	Maize poisoning	Ducklings
A. oryzae var *microsporus*	Maltoryzine	Malt sprout toxicosis	Cattle
Fusarium graminearum	oestrogenic-Factor F_2	Barley scab poisoning	Pigs
F. poae	(various toxic glycosides and saponins)	Alimentary toxic Aleukia	Man, cattle, horses, pigs, dogs
F. sporotrichioides			
Cladosporium epiphyllum			
Penicillium citrinum	citrinin		Rats
P. citreoviride	citreoviridin	Yellow rice toxicity	Mice
P. islandicum	islanditoxin luteoskyrin		?Man
P. rubrum	rubratoxins	Hepatitis X	Dogs
		Haemorrhagic syndrome	Swine, poultry
Pithomyces chartarum	sporidesmin	Facial eczema	Sheep
Periconia minutissima	?	Photosensitivity disease	Cattle
Stachybotrys atra	stachybotryotoxin	'Massovie zabolivanie'	Man, cattle
		('Massive illness')	Horses

in the urine after administration by stomach tube, but was excreted in the bile. On the other hand 3-HOAA was excreted only to a limited extent by the bile and was largely cleared by the kidneys.

One reason for this different handling could be attributed to their different physical characteristics. Aflatoxin is lipid soluble and bound to plasma protein and is consequently not readily available to the body pools except when it is stripped from the protein by the liver. On the other hand the 3-HOAA is more hydrophylic and is excreted by the acid transport system of the proximal renal tubule. As a consequence, the blood level is kept low but the urine is concentrated. With aflatoxin the converse may be true, plasma-protein binding limits the size of body pools but release in the liver prior to biliary excretion may provide large pools to permit toxic action (Table 8).

Table 8

(a) Excretion Routes of 3-HOAA and Aflatoxin B_1

| | % Recovery in four hours | | % plasma content bound to protein |
	Urine	Bile	
Aflatoxin	0·1	32	87
3-HOAA	56	4	23

20 mg 3-HOAA/kg and 5 mg aflatoxin/kg administered by stomach tube 1 hour prior to a 4 hour collection.

(b) Renal Clearance of 3-HOAA in a Patas Monkey

Creatinine	20 ml/min
Para-aminohippuric acid	91 ml/min
3-HOAA	54 ml/min

Ten minute clearance samples with 3-HOAA infused at 1 mg/min/kg in a 6 kg male Patas monkey (*Erythrocebus patas*).

Frequency of liver and stomach cancer

If we now look at the incidence of liver cancer within Uganda we find from Burkitt's[21] figures that a similar high incidence of liver cancer occurs throughout the whole of Uganda but that there are district variations in the incidence of stomach cancer (Table 9). The same is also true for Tanzania. Burkitt[21] comments that the main difference in incidence between high and low humidity zones appears to be in stomach cancer, not liver cancer. Whilst groundnuts may be more frequently grown and consumed in the moist and intermediate zones it is also true that grains (sorghum in particular), can become mould infested despite the apparent dryness of the area. This infection may be accounted for by wide seasonal fluctuations in actual humidity although the average humidity is low, or by storage of wet grains, and in some instances the growth of fungus may be deliberately encouraged. As has already been mentioned, only a few days of exposure to high humidity is required for the accumulation of toxins in serious quantities.

All one can perhaps say is that a much wider variety of carcinogens is available than was originally thought and it is therefore possible that the picture is complex; although aflatoxin may be an hepato-carcinogen in experimental animals, this and other toxins may well act on other tissues

Table 9

Proportional Frequency of Stomach and Liver Cancer
by District

	Stomach	Liver
Uganda		
1. Plantain belt	17·7	40·3
2. East	4·3	45·3
3. West	13·6	30·2
4. North	6·5	50·3
Tanzania		
5. Kilimanjaro	44·2	41·9
6. West Lake	41·4	26·7
7. Tanga	37·3	38·8
8. Kigoma	7·5	47·5
9. Shinyanga	6·8	50·0
10. Tabora	5·9	28·4

N.B. Areas 1, 3, 5, 6 and 7 are high humidity zones.

in Man. A protection of internal organs might be expected to follow the manner in which aflatoxin is handled internally but we might also expect that, as the toxic food is eaten, tissues of the gastrointestinal tract may be exposed to the carcinogens.

In the case of bladder cancer, a high incidence of cancer in the aniline dye industry was corrected when it was discovered that orthoamino phenols, which are carcinogenic, were handled daily by the workers and human contact with these compounds was prevented. Theoretically the high incidence of liver cancer might also be preventable although technically extremely difficult at this stage.

Nutritional interactions

Finally, I would like to bring in the question of dietary background. Much has been written about diet and health in Africa because protein/calorie malnutrition is common in many parts of Africa. Various authors[22, 23, 24, 25, 26] have commented on the alterations in plasma amino acids in Kwashiorkor. We reported[27] that even young adult Africans showed differences that were

Table 10

Comparison of the Proportions of Plasma Amino Acids in
Europeans and Plantain Eaters

	Plasma content (molar %)				
	Plantain-root crop community (n = 12)		European community (n = 14)		Probability of difference
Amino acid	Mean	SE	Mean	SE	by chance
Leucine	3·7	1·9	5·9	2·6	<0·010 >0·005
Lysine	5·9	0·5	6·1	0·5	>0·1
Valine	6·9	1·0	9·3	2·1	<0·005 >0·001
Threonine	10·7	4·9	8·5	2·6	<0·050 >0·025
Isoleucine	1·8	0·1	2·5	0·3	<0·005 >0·001
Phenylalanine	2·8	0·5	2·9	0·5	>0·1
Methionine	1·2	0·1	1·1	0·1	>0·1
Histidine	4·9	4·6	4·7	0·7	>0·1
Glutamic	5·3	4·5	3·9	0·5	>0·1
Alanine	19·0	11·4	14·7	2·4	<0·005 >0·001
Glycine	13·4	1·9	9·7	2·4	<0·001
Serine	5·9	0·7	6·1	1·0	>0·1
Proline	8·4	8·9	10·9	4·6	>0·1
Arginine	2·9	0·3	3·0	0·3	>0·1
Tyrosine	1·8	0·2	2·6	0·3	<0·010 >0·005
Citrulline	2·0	0·5	3·1	0·3	<0·010 >0·005
Ornithine	2·0	0·5	2·9	0·1	<0·010 >0·005
Aspartic	1·1	0·2	0·6	0·1	<0·025 >0·010

similar though not so gross as those reported in Kwashiorkor (Tables 10 and 11).

During experiments on the relationship between diet and endomyocardial fibrosis, we found no evidence that aflatoxin at 1 mg/kg in the standard diet produced any severe damage to the heart. We did, however, discover that 12 weanling (1-month-old) guinea pigs fed a low protein

Table 11

Plasma Tryptophan Content (μg/ml) in East African Communities
of Different Dietary Habits

	European community	Grain-fish-milk A	Grain-fish-milk B	Plantain-root crop
Number	15	16	17	21
Mean	12	10	9·9	8·0
SE of the mean	0·7	1·0	1·1	0·7

Values for the European community and plantain-root crop groups
were significantly different (P < 0·001).

(6% casilan) diet died at an early age of 3 months whilst the low protein diet without aflatoxin supported the animals for 5-6 months.

Of course, any African who is exposed to a low protein diet will *ipso facto* be exposed to a low fat diet as both in animal and vegetable products structural fats and proteins are closely associated. Consequently the low-protein African consuming a low-protein diet may be exposed to a chronic complex nutritional imbalance. Recent work has demonstrated beyond doubt that all cells require both protein and fat for their construction but as in all biological situations it must be the 'correct kind' of protein or fat for optimum performance. Studies by Clausen[28] have demonstrated that fat malnutrition renders sensitive membranous tissues of the central nervous system very much more sensitive to attack by toxic agents and information is slowly accumulating on the relationship between nutrition and infection.[23] Consequently, it is not unlikely that the lowering of the nutritional plane in man will increase the possibility of successful attack by viral or toxic agents.

Where epidemiologists and laboratory workers combine we seem to be entering a new productive field of investigation, the apparent complexity of which should stimulate rather than deter. At one time the science of Natural Philosophy narrowly defined the atom and the electron. The 'Uncertainty Principle' destroyed that narrow definition and turned the electron from a definable pin-point to a wave form with statistical rather than finite properties. Medical science at one time enjoyed the narrow definition of the one vitamin or one hormone but like Natural Philosophy seems to be entering a new phase where interactions demand an integrated, statistical approach. This seems particularly true for epidemiology which seems to me to be the unravelling of a set of experimental results without knowing the conditions of the experiment.

REFERENCES

1. CRAWFORD, M. A., HANSEN, INGE L. and LOPEZ, A. (1969). *Br. J. Cancer.* **23**, 644.
2. DODGE, O. G. (1962). *Acta Un. int. Cancr.*, **18**, 548.
3. DODGE, O. G. (1964). *Cancer*, 17, 1433.
4. FRIPP, P. J. (1961). *Ann. trop. Med. Parasit.*, **55**, 328.
5. CRAWFORD, M. A. (1962). *Lancet*, 352.
6. SARGEANT, K., SHERIDAN, A., O'KELLY, J. and CARNAGHAN, R. B. J. (1961). *Nature* (Lond.), **192**, 1096.
7. ALLCROFT, R. and CARNAGHAN, R. B. A. (1963). *Chem. Ind.*, 50.
8. LOPEZ, A. and CRAWFORD, M. A. (1967). *Lancet*, 1351-1354.
9. ASHWORTH, L. J. (JR.) and LANGLEY, B. C. (1964). *Plant Dis. Reptr.*, **48**, 875.
10. DIENER, U. L., JACKSON, C. R., COOPER, W. E., STIPES, R. J. and DAVIS, N. D. (1966). (Abstr.) *J. Ala. Acad. Sci.*, **37**, 345.
11. NORTON, D. C., MENON, S. K. and FLANGAS, A. L. (1956). *Plant Dis. Reptr.*, **40**, 374.
12. DIENER, U. L. and DAVIS, D. N. (1966). *J. Am. Oil Chem. Soc.*, **44**, 259.
13. RUTISHAUSER, I. H. E., DEAN, R. F. A. and BURGESS, J. J. L. (1962). *E. Afr. med. J.*, **39**, 478.
14. ADRIAN COMMITTEE (1966). In: *Radiological Hazards to Patients*: *Final Report.* H.M. Stationery Office.
15. COADY, A. (1965). *Ethiop. med. J.*, **3**, 173.
16. MOREAU, C. (1968). In: *Moissures toxiques dans l'alimentation* (Eds. Lechevalier SARC). Paris.
17. WOGAN, A. (1969). In: *Alimentary mycotoxicoses* in *Food-borne Infections and Intoxicants* (Ed. Rieman, H.), p. 395. Academic Press, New York.
18. CALDERWOOD, D. L. and SCHROEDER, J. W. (1968). USDA., Agr. Serv. Rep., 52-26, 32p.
19. VAN WARMELO, K. T., VAN DER WESTHUIZEN, G. C. A. and MINNE, J. A. (1968). Tech. Comm., No. **71**, Dept. Agric. Tech. Serv., Pretoria, S.A., 5p.
20. RECONDO, DE A. M., FRAYSSINET, C. H., LAFARGE, C. and BRETON, LE E. (1966). *Biochem. Biophys. Acta.*, **119**, 322.
21. BURKITT, D. P. (1970). Personal communication.
22. HANSEN, J. D. L. and BROCK, J. F. (1964). *Lancet*, **1**, 1278.
23. BROCK, J. F., HANSEN, J. D. L., HOWE, E. E., DAVEL, J. G. A., PRETORIUS, P. J. and HENDRICKSE, R. G. (1955). *Lancet*, **2**, 355.
24. DEAN, R. F. A. and WHITEHEAD, R. G. (1964). *Lancet*, **2**, 98.
25. WHITEHEAD, R. G. (1964). *Lancet*, **1**, 250.

26. WHITEHEAD, R. G. (1965). *Lancet*, 2, 567.
27. CRAWFORD, M. A., GALE, M. M., SOMERS, K. and HANSEN, I. L. (1970). *Br. J. Nutr.*, 24, 393.
28. CLAUSEN, J. and MOLLER, J. (1969). Neurochemical Institute, National Danish Multiple Sclerosis Society and the Laboratory of Psychiatry (Neuropathology), University of Copenhagen, Denmark, 1-14.
29. JARVIS, B. (1971). *J. Appl. Bact.* In press.

DIETARY AFLATOXIN LOADS AND THE INCIDENCE OF HUMAN HEPATOCELLULAR CARCINOMA IN THAILAND

by

R. C. Shank

Department of Nutrition and Food Science
Massachusetts Institute of Technology, Cambridge, Massachusetts

In mid-1967, a research project was initiated to investigate the possible role mycotoxins may play in the aetiology of human liver disease in south-east Asia. This present report is concerned with the results of 3 years of study in Thailand. Thailand was chosen as the principal country of the study because climate and agricultural practices favour mycotoxin contamination of foods and foodstuffs and because several reports indicated that certain areas of south-east Asia, Thailand in particular, suffer from apparent high incidences of liver disease, especially hepatocellular carcinoma.[1-4]

The first phase of the project involved a survey of mould invasion and aflatoxin contamination of more than 170 different foods and foodstuffs obtained from Thai markets, mills, warehouses, distributors, processing sites, farms and homes. The results of this screening survey indicated that mould invasion of most food products was very frequent (50-80% of the 2180 samples analysed contained viable spores after surface decontamination), that *Aspergillus* was the most prevalent genus invading foods, that more than 50 toxigenic strains of moulds existed in common dietary sources, and that aflatoxins were frequent contaminants of many common food products.[5, 6] An exploratory survey of hospital records in Thailand suggested a geographical variation in liver cancer incidence which was similar to the geographical variation of aflatoxin contamination in market foods.

The second phase of the project was a 1-year epidemiological pilot study in which the daily aflatoxin consumptions of 144 families were measured during each of the three seasons, and the incidence of primary liver cancer in three comparable populations was estimated. This pilot study was designed to provide a basis upon which to execute a long-term definitive study to determine statistically whether an association existed between aflatoxin (and other mycotoxins) and human liver cancer and other liver diseases.

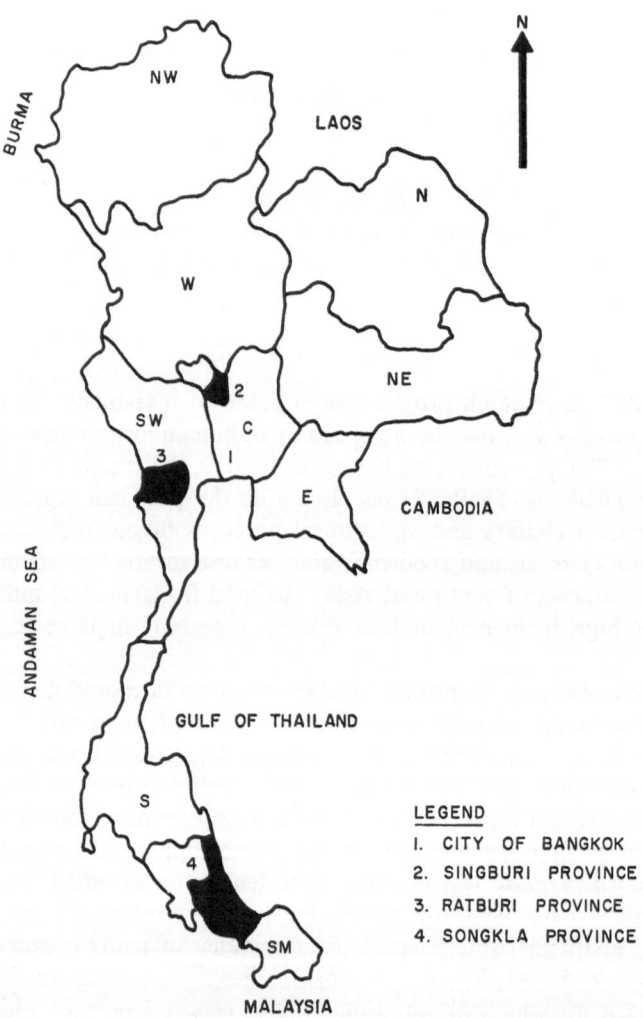

MAP OF THAILAND

FIG. 1

Consumption of aflatoxins

The market survey results indicated that Singburi Province (for a map of Thailand see Fig. 1), had a high degree of aflatoxin contamination in the food supply; the province of Ratburi was intermediate and Songkla was remarkably low. Therefore, these three areas were selected for the study.

After several discussions with the local health officials three villages in each province were selected for the survey. The villages were comparable on a socio-economic basis, contained 68 to 164 homes, and all had an average family size of six persons and average age of 22 to 31 years. Using a table of random numbers and maps indicating locations of individual houses, 16 families in each village were selected for the study. With the help of the village chiefs, the survey team was introduced to each family and the nature of the work was explained.

The survey team, made up of members of the technical staff in the Bangkok laboratories, observed each family for two consecutive days, three times a year (to study seasonal variation) for a total of 6 days, always on different days of the week. Each member of the family and their guests were weighed and asked their ages. The food prepared for each meal of the day was weighed before and after the family ate to determine the amount of each food consumed by the family. It was also recorded which foods were eaten by each family member and guest. Approximately 25 to 100 g were taken from as many cooked foods as feasible and placed in coded plastic bags and sealed. The samples were immediately frozen on dry ice or within 3 hours homogenised and stored under chloroform in glass bottles. As soon as the samples arrived in Bangkok, chemical assay for aflatoxins according to the method of Eppley[7] was initiated.

The market survey indicated that groundnuts could be a significant source of dietary aflatoxins. In Thailand most groundnuts are eaten between meals usually away from home, and their consumption could not be measured directly. Therefore, each family was questioned as to how many groundnuts its members consumed, and samples of all groundnuts and groundnut products were purchased from local vendors each day during the survey for subsequent aflatoxin assay. This, and all other pertinent information about each family, including the ingredients of each prepared food, were recorded on a dietary survey form printed in Thai.

In most cases 30-50% of the foods eaten by each family were analysed for aflatoxin content. Table 1 gives the average consumption of aflatoxins of the survey families in each of the nine villages and Table 2 gives the range of the daily aflatoxin consumption values. From these tables it can be seen that aflatoxin consumption from cooked foods (plate samples) was highest in the Singburi area, only slightly less in the Ratburi area, and much less in the Songkla area. For consumption of total aflatoxins, that is, forms B_1, B_2, G_1 and G_2, the year's average for Singburi is 10-14 times higher than for Songkla. Indeed, only 11 out of 922 plate samples collected in Songkla over the year had detectable amounts of aflatoxins, compared to 45 out of 1021 samples in Singburi and 159 out of 1005 samples in Ratburi. If the aflatoxin intake of one 75-year-old woman in Songkla, who for 2 days

Table 1

Average Daily Aflatoxin Consumptions of Survey Families Based on Chemical Analysis of Plate Samples (Nanograms Aflatoxin B_1 or Total Aflatoxins/kg Body Weight Family Basis)

Village	Aflatoxin	Hot Season	Rainy Season	Dry Season	Year's Average
C_1	B_1	0·2-1·5	353·0-376·0	67·0-74·8	140·1-150·8
	Total	0·3-3·0	513·6-554·6	67·7-81·5	193·9-213·1
C_2	B_1	2·6-4·8	nil-0·2	1·3-3·0	1·3-2·7
	Total	4·5-8·5	nil-0·4	1·3-3·0	1·9-4·0
C_3	B_1	31·0-31·2	0·1-0·3	5·2-5·4	12·1-12·3
	Total	61·8-62·7	0·3-2·6	8·3-8·5	23·5-24·6
Singburi Average	B_1	11·3-12·5	117·7-125·8	24·5-27·7	51·2-55·3
	Total	22·2-24·7	171·3-185·9	25·8-31·0	73·1-80·5
W_1	B_1	3·1-6·1	34·0-34·3	37·6-50·7	24·9-30·4
	Total	4·5-10·4	63·1-63·6	49·1-66·2	38·9-46·7
W_2	B_1	0·6-4·1	8·4-10·4	9·4-36·1	6·1-16·9
	Total	0·9-6·5	10·3-13·1	15·8-67·9	9·0-29·2
W_3	B_1	3·4-11·2	12·9-41·6	173·2-237·1	63·2-96·6
	Total	6·0-19·7	18·6-78·0	237·0-363·9	87·2-153·9
Ratburi Average	B_1	2·3-6·8	18·4-28·8	73·4-108·0	31·4-47·9
	Total	3·8-11·9	30·7-51·6	100·6-166·0	45·0-76·5
S_1	B_1	0·9-8·9	nil	nil	0·3-3·0
	Total	1·8-17·9	nil	nil	0·6-6·0
S_2	B_1	0·2-1·5	(45·4)*	nil	(15·2-15·6)*
	Total	0·3-2·9	(45·4)*	nil	(15·2-16·1)*
S_3	B_1	nil-0·4	nil	0·1-1·3	nil-0·6
	Total	0·1-0·8	nil	0·1-1·3	0·1-0·7
Songkla Average	B_1	0·4-3·6	(15·1)*	nil-0·4	(5·2-6·4)*
	Total	0·7-7·2	(15·1)*	nil-0·4	(5·3-7·6)*

* Of all the samples collected from this village during the rainy season, only one contained aflatoxin (B_1 = 71 ppb rice) and was eaten by only one person, a 75-year-old 31 kg woman. If her intake is excluded, the aflatoxin consumption for Village S_2 would be 'nil' for the rainy season and 0·1-0·5 ng B_1/day/kg body weight and 0·1-1·0 ng total aflatoxins/day/kg body weight for the year's average. Songkla's average then would be 'nil' for the rainy season and 0·1-1·3 ng B_1/day/kg body weight and 0·2-2·5 ng total aflatoxins/day/kg body weight for the year.

Table 2

Range of Daily Aflatoxin Consumptions for Survey Families*

Village	Aflatoxin B_1 ng/kg body weight (family basis)			Total Aflatoxins ng/kg body weight (family basis)		
	Hot Season	Rainy Season	Dry Season	Hot Season	Rainy Season	Dry Season
Singburi						
C_1	20·0	4251·0	638·1	40·0	6541·0	638·1
C_2	72·0	3·5	29·7	131·8	7·0	29·7
C_3	309·2	16·5	82·5	532·9	33·0	132·0
Ratburi						
W_1	77·7	460·0	123·0	127·7	866·5	123·0
W_2	19·0	65·3	114·0	30·0	65·3	227·0
W_3	88·0	135·5	1283·7	176·0	247·0	1701·0
Songkla						
S_1	57·0	nil	nil	114·0	nil	nil
S_2	23·5	nil†	nil	47·0	nil†	nil
S_3	6·5	nil	21·1	13·0	ni	21·1

* Minimum consumption in all villages during each season was 'nil'.

† Only one sample of prepared food collected from the 16 families in the survey during the rainy season in Songkla contained aflatoxin. It was a sample of rice eaten for 2 days by a 31 kg, 75-year-old woman eating alone; her daily aflatoxin consumption for that survey period was 1071·1 ng aflatoxin B_1/kg body weight for the first day and 380·2 ng aflatoxin B_1/kg body weight for the second day; the rice sample contained only aflatoxin B_1 (71 μg/kg).

during the rainy season survey ate a large amount of aflatoxin-contaminated rice (while no other contaminated foods were eaten by the survey families in the three villages), is excluded, then the average daily toxin consumption levels for the year for Singburi are 32 to 365 times higher than Songkla.

While the seasonal variation in total aflatoxin consumption in Songkla was minimal, there was considerable variation in Singburi and Ratburi (see Fig. 2). Maximum toxin consumption in Singburi was seen during the rainy season and in Ratburi during the dry season. During the survey period the three Ratburi villages experienced extensive flooding during the rainy season (especially severe in village W_3). The rainy season survey in village W_3 was done 1 week after the flood waters had receded and 22% of the food samples were contaminated with aflatoxins; the same families were surveyed again 4 months later during the dry season and 43% of the food samples were contaminated with aflatoxins. Flooding may have been responsible for the extensive contamination of the cooked food samples during the months following the rainy season.

Table 3 lists the consumption figures for some individual members of the survey families. These were obtainable when the exact amount of any one given food eaten by one person could be recorded. From this table it is important to note that six people consumed, during a single meal, at least 380-1072 nanograms of total aflatoxins per kg body weight on an individual,

Table 3

Aflatoxin Consumptions for some Individual Members of Survey Families

Season	Village	Sex	Age	Prepared food	Aflatoxin* B_1	Total aflatoxins*	Portion of single day's dose
Hot	Singburi						
	C_2	M	54	Ferm. fish c̄ chili	0·3-3·0	0·3-3·0	< 100%
	C_2	F	62	Boiled noodles	6·8-68	13·6-136	100%
	Ratburi						
	W_1	M	55	Sour curry	2·2-22	4·4-44	100%
	W_2	M	63	Fried mussels	0·2-2·0	0·2-2·0	< 100%
	Songkla						
	S_1	F	46	Shrimp c̄ garlic	0·1-1·5	0·3-2·9	< 100%
Rainy	Singburi						
	C_1	F	39	Fried bean sprouts	1·6-16	3·2-32	< 100%
	C_1	F†	47	Plaa tuu	452·7	536·7	100%
	C_1	F	16	Plaa tuu	528·1	626·1	100%
	C_2	M	58	Squash curry	0·6-6·0	1·2-12	100%
	Ratburi						
	W_3	F	45	Chili sauce	3·7	7·4	100%
	W_3	M‡	22	Fish curry	1·1-11	2·2-22	< 100%
	W_3	M‡	22	Chili sauce	0·1-1·0	0·2-2·0	< 100%
	Songkla						
	S_2	F§	75	Rice	1072·1	1072·1	100%
	S_2	F§	75	Rice	380·2	380·2	100%
Dry	Singburi						
	C_1	F	15	Chili sauce	0·3-3·0	0·3-3·0	< 100%
	C_1	F†	48	Boiled fish	12·2	12·2	100%
	C_1	M	11	Rice	14·2-142	28·4-284	< 100%
	C_2	F	58	Rice	5·9-59·3	5·9-59·3	100%
	Ratburi						
	W_1	M	84	Rice	557·1	728·6	< 100%
	W_1	F	80	Sadao	1·4-14	1·4-14	< 100%
	W_1	M	21	Rice	8·6-86	8·6-86	< 100%

Table 3—*contd.*

Season	Village	Sex	Age	Prepared food	Aflatoxin* B_1	Total aflatoxins*	Portion of single day's dose
Dry	Ratburi						
	W_2	F	54	Taro	24	36	100%
	W_2	M	12	Ridge gourd	2·4-24	4·8-48	<100%
	W_3	M‡	22	Beef curry	2·1-21	4·2-42	<100%
	W_3	F	54	Sour curry	1·6-16	3·2-32	<100%
	W_3	F¶	57	Rice	6·0-60	12-120	<100%
	W_3	F¶	57	Pork, vegs. and garlic	0·8-8	1·6-16	<100%
	W_3	F	49	Rice	8·6-86	17·2-172	<100%
	W_3	F	51	Rice	788·6	1028·6	<100%

* Nanograms per kilogram body weight.

† Two individual daily doses are available for this woman, one during the rainy season and the other during the dry season.

‡ Three individual doses are available for this young man, two during the rainy season representing individual intakes from two separate prepared foods eaten on the same day, and the third in the dry season; his total daily dose could not be calculated as he ate undetermined amounts of other contaminated foods at the same time.

§ This woman ate the same rice for two successive days and the individual daily dose for each was calculated.

¶ Two individual doses are available for this woman as calculated from known amounts of two contaminated prepared foods; her total daily dose could not be calculated as she ate undetermined amounts of other contaminated foods at the same time.

not family, basis. Eleven of these doses represent 100% of a single day's intake, that is, the total daily dose for the individual. In all other cases, the total daily dose could not be calculated as the individual ate undetermined amounts of other contaminated food at the same time. The amounts of these other toxin sources eaten by the individuals could not be determined because other family members also ate the same foods at the same time and only the total amount of food eaten by all consumers was determined.

The extent of aflatoxin contamination in the cooked foods prepared in the three survey areas is given in Table 4. It is clear that the Ratburi villages suffered a greater frequency of contamination and those in Singburi the highest levels of contamination. Only one sample collected in Songkla during the entire survey contained more than trace amounts of aflatoxin (71 μg B_1/kg).

In Singburi the most heavily contaminated samples were taken from a dish of cabbage fried with pork and garlic (748 μg aflatoxin B_1 and 1299 μg

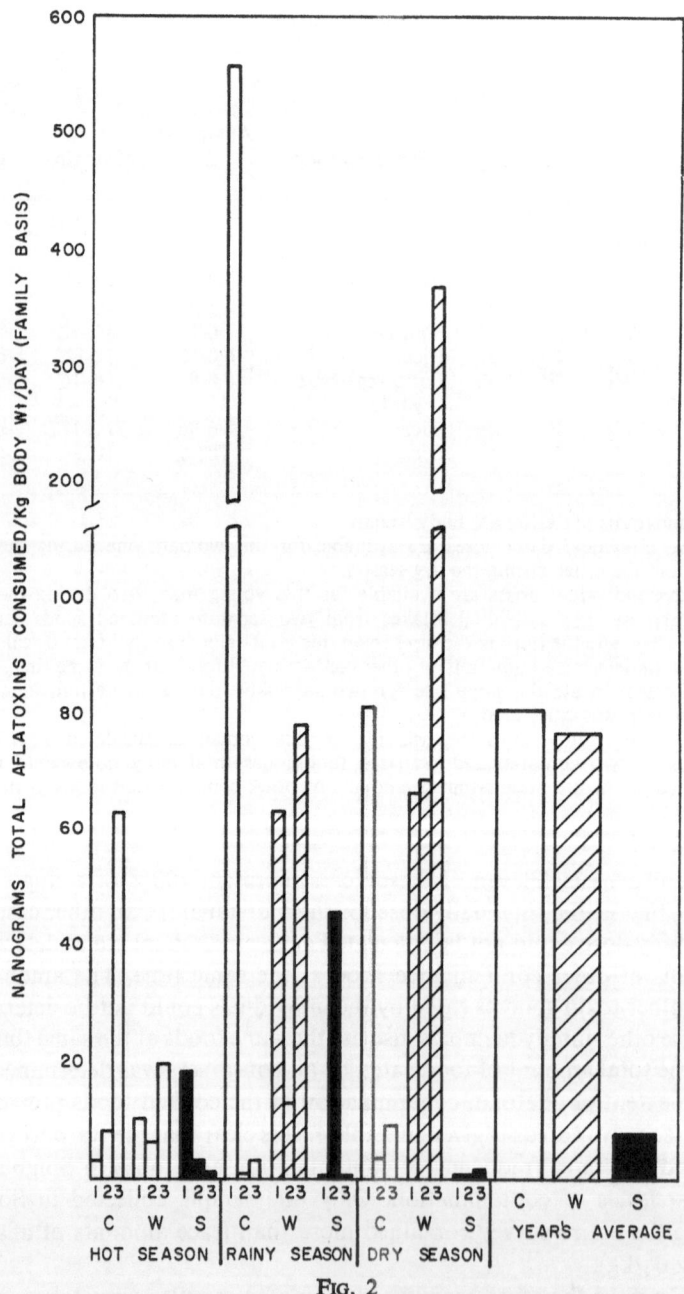

FIG. 2

Table 4

Extent of Aflatoxin Contamination of Cooked Food Samples

	Number of foods or samples		
	Singburi	Ratburi	Songkla
Foods eaten	2640	2943	2008
Samples assayed	1021	1005	922
Samples contaminated	45	159	11
Total aflatoxin conc., μg/kg			
Trace	22	129	10
< 50	4	19	0
50-100	10	7	1
100-200	3	3	0
200-300	1	0	0
300-400	0	1	0
400-500	2	0	0
500-1000	2	0	0
> 1000	1	0	0

total aflatoxins per kg food) and a dish of 'plaa tuu' (a fish similar to mackerel and preserved by sun-drying) which contained 679 μg aflatoxin B_1 and 795 μg total aflatoxins per kg food. In Ratburi the most heavily contaminated sample was taken from a dish of shrimp fried with pork, garlic and chili peppers; it contained 207 μg aflatoxin B_1 and 355 μg total aflatoxins per kg sample. In Songkla a sample of cooked rice was the most heavily contaminated; it contained 71 μg aflatoxin B_1 per kg sample.

Rice is the staple food in Thailand and Table 5 gives the frequency and extent of aflatoxin contamination of plate samples of cooked rice collected from the nine survey villages. While 1 % and 3 % of these samples were contaminated with low levels of aflatoxins in Songkla and Singburi

FIG. 2. Seasonal Variation in Daily Aflatoxin Consumption in Nine Villages in Three areas of Thailand.

Aflatoxin consumptions are expressed as the nanograms of total aflatoxins (B_1, B_2 G_1, G_2, consumed per kilogram body weight, per day on a family basis in Singburi central Thailand, C, villages 1, 2 and 3; open bars), Ratburi (southwestern Thailand, W villages 1, 2 and 3; hatched bars), and Songkla (southern Thailand, S, villages 1, 2 and 3; shaded bars). The mean total aflatoxin consumptions for the year for Singburi (central), Ratburi (west), and Songkla (south) are given on the far right. In Singburi and Ratburi the hot season occurs from March through June, the rainy season from July through October, and the dry season from November through February. In Songkla the hot season occurs from April through September, the heaviest rains fall from October through January, and the least rain falls in February and March.

Table 5

Frequency and Extent of Aflatoxin Contamination of Plate Samples
of Cooked Rice

	Singburi		Ratburi		Songkla	
Number samples assayed	201		214		210	
Number samples contaminated	6		22		2	
Average conc. in all samples*	$B_1 = 2$		$B_1 = 2$		$B_1 = t$	
	Total $= 3$		Total $= 2$		Total $= t$	
% Samples contaminated	3		10		1	
	B_1	B_2	B_1	B_2	B_1	B_2
Actual concentrations*	t(2)	—	t	—	t	t
	t(2)	t(2)	t(15)	t(15)	71	—
	50	—	12	12		
	390	210	19	16		
			23	12		
			65	20		
			93	28		
			138	42		

* Expressed as μg/kg sample; t = trace, less than 1 μg/kg sample; bracketed numbers indicate number of samples with that concentration when more than 1.

respectively, 10% of the rice samples collected in Ratburi contained aflatoxin. The average concentration of aflatoxin B_1 in all rice samples collected in each survey area ranged from less than 1 μg/kg to 2 μg/kg. It is suspected that the flooding in Ratburi may be responsible for the high frequency of contamination of rice; the rice in that area is almost always stored under the stilted homes.

These figures do not include the amount of aflatoxins consumed by eating groundnuts. Groundnuts are usually eaten between meals, especially by small children, and attempts to estimate family intakes of groundnuts were not successful.

Although the absolute exposures to aflatoxins appear to be very small, the potency of these compounds as carcinogens in animals must be kept in mind in order to put these data into perspective. The highest values, in Singburi, based on the yearly average total aflatoxin consumption, amount to 20-30% of the comparable intake values that induce nearly 100% tumour incidence in rats following continuous exposure.[8] Also, because these are family averages, exposures of individual family members are undoubtedly higher.

The incidence of primary hepatocarcinoma

A survey of hospital records and national health statistics indicated that Singburi had one of the highest reported liver cancer rates in Thailand and that Songkla had one of the lowest rates, ten times less than Singburi; Ratburi was also high, but not as high as Singburi. Unfortunately the incidence study could not have been done in Singburi without serious delay as a key figure in the study, the director of the provincial hospital, was called away for temporary assignment in another province. Therefore Ratburi and Songkla were selected for the incidence study and Singburi and Songkla were selected for a prevalence study which was executed later (see below).

Urban populations of approximately 70,000 to 75,000 were chosen in each province and three Thai physicians worked full time on the study in the nine hospitals located in the six cities selected. For the period of 1 year the doctors investigated all deaths occurring in the hospitals and at homes within the municipal boundaries. Hospitals in Bangkok also reported deaths of patients who were bona fide residents of the study areas. When a death occurred, the physician requested permission to take five liver viscerotomy specimens. Liver biopsies were done on all living patients (at the hospitals) provisionally diagnosed as having liver cancer. All specimens were examined histologically.

At the time this report was written the incidence study had not been completed. For the first 9 months of the study the leading causes of death in both areas were accidents, violence (mostly head injuries, gun and knife wounds, and motor vehicle accidents) and poisoning. These were followed by heart diseases, infections and infestations, respiratory diseases (mainly pulmonary tuberculosis) and non-infectious diseases of the brain (mostly reported as cerebral haemorrhages and undoubtedly includes some accidental head injuries). The sixth leading cause of death was liver diseases (principally cancer of the liver, cirrhosis, and infectious hepatitis, in that order).

Table 6 shows the age distribution of deaths occurring in both study areas for residents and non-residents alike for the first 9 months of the study, and the efficiency with which viscerotomy specimens were obtained from hospital and home deaths. While 67-70% of all hospital deaths were investigated by viscerotomy, only a few home deaths could be studied by this technique. This is because in most cases the deceased were sealed in coffins before the physicians could learn of the deaths and get to the homes to take the specimens. However, it is felt that few, if any, liver cancer cases were missed through home deaths as usually liver cancer cases in Thailand seek medical treatment from the nearest hospital where they are told of the nature of the disease. Thus when such cases die at home the family is often

K

Table 6

Age Distribution and Efficiency of obtaining Liver Viscerotomy Specimens for
all Deaths Occurring in Liver Cancer Incidence Survey Areas*

		Ratburi area		Songkla area	
Age (years)	Sex	No. of deaths	% histol. examined	No. of deaths	% histol. examined
15-20	T	65	66	20	40
	M	45	67	13	31
	F	20	65	7	57
21-30	T	65	62	62	61
	M	43	58	34	59
	F	22	68	28	64
31-40	T	101	60	65	72
	M	55	67	36	78
	F	46	52	29	66
41-50	T	79	62	48	73
	M	49	53	33	70
	F	30	77	15	80
51-60	T	112	54	92	52
	M	59	58	69	51
	F	53	49	23	57
61-70	T	95	39	79	44
	M	56	45	43	40
	F	39	31	36	50
over 70	T	148	19	79	32
	M	79	20	49	41
	F	69	17	30	17
All ages	T	665	48	445	53
	M	386	50	277	53
	F	279	45	168	53

* Includes deaths of bona fide residents in the survey populations and all other
deaths occurring in the survey hospitals, 15 years of age and older; report on only
bona fide residents awaits address confirmation.

able to inform the investigating physician that the deceased had liver
cancer. Liver viscerotomy specimens were obtained on only about 50% of
the bona fide residents dying in each area.

In the Ratburi area six bona fide residents died of primary liver cancer (proven histologically). In addition there were 13 histologically proven cases, four still living, who lived in the region but outside the municipal boundaries. There were also two cases outside the urban area that were diagnosed clinically but the pathology reports are still outstanding. In the town of Ratburi four residents died of liver cell carcinoma (proven histologically) in the first 10 months of the study. If no more cases are found then the incidence for the town (population of 32,634; 1970 census) will be 12·3 new cases per year per 100,000. The projected incidence of primary liver cancer in the Ratburi area (four municipalities) is ten new cases per 100,000 people per year.

In Songkla one case of a bona fide resident was confirmed by peritoneoscopy (no histology was done) and ten cases (six still living) from outside the urban area were diagnosed clinically but not confirmed histologically. The projected incidence of primary liver cancer in the Songkla area (two municipalities) is one new case per 100,000 people per year. The incidence study is scheduled for completion by the end of June, 1970.

The prevalence of primary liver cancer and hepatomegaly

While incidence is the desired form of expressing liver cancer rates, such a study was not feasible in rural Thai populations due to lack of medical facilities and problems related to a dispersed population. Therefore it was decided to measure the prevalence of the disease in large rural populations. Incidence figures can be calculated from prevalence data if the duration of the disease is known; duration was measured as will be explained below.

In view of the large expense and effort in performing a prevalence study for liver cancer, and because the overall objective of the long-term investigation is to determine whether mycotoxins are related to one or more liver diseases in Thailand, it was decided to expand the scope of the prevalence study to include all liver diseases discernible by hepatomegaly. Results of such a study would also be expected to make a significant contribution to the Thai medical community concerning liver diseases and their geographical variation.

In order to find statistically significant numbers of liver cancer and hepatomegaly cases by a point prevalence study, it was necessary to survey very large populations. It was anticipated that at most, 75% of any large village population could be palpated in a single examination study; therefore, two populations of 100,000 people each were selected in order to obtain data on 70,000 to 75,000 people per area, populations approximately the same size as studied in the incidence survey; this was as large as was feasible for the pilot study. A total of 337 villages took part in the study, 156 in Songkla and 181 in Singburi.

After several meetings with provincial and district health officials and a pretest of methods, it was possible to determine the size of the working staff, and obtain accurate population figures and maps of each area. The investigators attended the local monthly meetings of the village chiefs, explained the study, and asked for their help in preparing rosters of each village containing the house number, name, sex and age of each resident in each village; specially printed booklets were provided for this purpose.

Seventy medical students from the three medical schools in Bangkok were recruited to take part in the survey during their summer holiday. After a short orientation course, teams of two students each were given written sets of instructions, the appropriate village rosters, schedules and maps indicating the routes through the district to be taken.

Announcements of the survey were posted at several points in each village asking for the people's co-operation and explaining that the students would dispense free medicine where necessary. The students established

Table 7

Age Distribution of Prevalence Survey Populations in Singburi and Songkla and Extent to which the Populations were Examined

Age (years)	Singburi		Songkla	
	Number of residents	Per cent examined	Number of residents	Per cent examined
Under 1	1,048	62	1,858	65
1-5	9,355	70	12,948	63
6-10	12,889	73	14,442	64
11-15	11,738	60	12,298	54
16-20	8,716	37	10,268	34
21-25	5,654	41	7,775	37
26-30	4,691	45	6,450	44
31-35	5,307	51	6,065	48
36-40	4,769	53	5,926	51
41-45	4,103	56	5,024	55
46-50	3,492	58	4,144	55
51-55	3,189	60	3,401	58
56-60	2,820	61	3,305	57
61-65	2,256	63	2,595	56
66-70	1,713	65	2,396	56
Over 70	2,494	61	2,823	51
Total	84,234	58	101,718	52

temporary clinics in the villages and palpated all those who came in answer to the village chief's call. On the following day the students made house calls to examine those unable to attend the clinic. When hepatomegaly was found, it was so indicated in the roster and the liver size recorded in units of finger breadths.

Experienced Thai physicians checked with each team almost daily and obtained from them lists of hepatomegaly cases. The physicians then examined the cases to confirm and expand the diagnosis. Regardless of the nature of the disorder, a case report card was completed giving the details of the physical examination and physician's impression as to the nature of the ailment.

Table 7 lists the age distribution of both survey populations and the extent to which each age group was examined. At the time of this writing confirmation of hepatomegaly cases and histological examination of liver cancer suspects was incomplete. Conclusion of this study is expected by July, 1970.

The duration of primary liver cancer

The purpose of the duration study was to provide the information necessary to calculate incidence from the prevalence data; prevalence divided by duration expressed in years yields incidence.

The study was based on hospital records of primary liver cancer cases in major hospitals in the two largest cities in Thailand spanning the period 1963-1969. The study was explained to the doctors specialising in liver disease at each hospital, and they arranged to have the records collected and made available for examination. Pertinent information was transferred to individual case record cards, recording the patient's name, address, sex, age, ethnic group, admission number and date, hospital number and date, place and date of any previous diagnosis of liver cancer, discharge date, date and place of death, results from histological and clinical examination including liver size, consistency and surface, weight loss, location and severity of abdominal pain, whether cachexia, ascites, collateral circulation or metastases were seen, and the final diagnosis.

Cases were divided into four groups:

(1) Histologically proven cases of hepotocellular carcinoma.
(2) Histologically proven cases of primary liver cancer but not specified as to cell type.
(3) Cases of primary cancer of the liver clinically confirmed by peritoneoscopy, exploratory laparotomy, or autopsy.
(4) Cases of primary liver cancer clinically diagnosed without peritoneoscopy, laparotomy, or autopsy. Clinical diagnosis of cases in this last

group included hepatomegaly, hard or nodular liver, loss of weight, no cancer at other sites, pain over the liver area, ascites, collateral circulation and jaundice.

Duration in days was then calculated for all individual cases in each group; average duration for each group was expressed in months using 30·4 days per month.

Table 8

Average Duration of Primary Cancer of the Liver in 271 Cases

Basis of diagnosis*	Number of cases			Average age (years)			Duration (months)			Duration Range (days)	
	M	F	T	M	F	T	M	F	T	M	F
1. Hist. proven liver cell CA	64	13	77	48	48	48	1	1	1	1-357	10-87
2. Hist. proven 1° liver CA	22	10	32	45	53	48	3	1	2	4-1030	4-78
1 & 2 All hist. proven cases	86	23	109	47	51	48	2	1	2	—	—
3. Clin. confirmed	49	26	75	49	45	48	1	1	1	1-135	1-152
4. Clin. diagnosed	60	27	87	50	60	53	1	1	1	1-118	1-226
3 & 4 All clin. cases	109	53	162	50	52	50	1	1	1	—	—
All cases	195	76	271	49	52	50	1	1	1	—	—

* Classification is explained fully in the text; groups 1 and 2 are histologically proven cases but in group 2 the pathology report stated 'primary liver carcinoma' without specifying cell type. Group 3 is composed of cases stated to be primary liver cancer diagnosed by peritoneoscopy, exploratory laparotomy, or autopsy. Group 4 contains those cases where diagnosis of primary liver cancer was made without the aid of histological evidence or direct liver visualization.

Analysis of almost 2000 records provided complete information of 109 cases of histologically proven primary liver cancer and 75 cases of clinically confirmed primary liver cancer. In addition complete information was obtained on 87 cases clinically diagnosed but not confirmed by direct liver visualisation techniques. In all but nine of the 271 cases death occurred in hospital. Ascertaining death dates for those patients (much the minority) who died outside of hospital proved very difficult.

Table 8 lists the number of cases, the average age at death, and the average duration for males and females for each group. From this table it is clear that primary liver cancer in Thailand is more frequent in males, as has been reported previously.[4] The average age for all histologically proven cases was 48 years with 9% of the cases occurring before the age of 30. The average duration from the date of first recognition by a physician to the date of death for histologically proven cases, was 2 months. This reflects the fact that most patients exhausted home cures and herbal medicines and waited until the cancer was well advanced before they sought qualified medical help. Duration for clinically diagnosed and/or confirmed cases was only 1 month; in part this is due to the fact that many of the patients listed in this group died before a more thorough diagnosis could be made.

While the results from these studies are not yet complete, the data obtained so far do support the hypothesis that aflatoxins may play a role in the aetiology of human liver cancer in Thailand. Even though two areas of Thailand were studied in which the apparent minimum incidence of primary liver cancer differs by a factor of ten, the actual numbers are low and make statistical analysis of the data difficult. There exists in Thailand an area where the incidence of liver cancer is expected to be appreciably higher than in Ratburi. This area is the north-northeast of Thailand, the same area in which highest levels of aflatoxin contamination in market food samples were found.[6] This area was not studied in the pilot study as it has been reported that 70 % of the general population in north-eastern Thailand suffers from liver fluke infestation (opisthorciasis), and cholangio-cellular carcinoma is unusually prevalent; however the intentions are to study this area in the future in relation to aflatoxin consumption and liver cancer.

There is, of course, the problem of trying to relate aflatoxin consumptions measured today with the induction of liver cancer in the patients seen today. It is reasonable to assume that the induction period for human liver cancer is several years and the problem arises in assuring that the dietary aflatoxin levels now being measured represent those during the induction period. Almost no data are available to answer this question; however, it seems apparent from the market and diet surveys that groundnuts, garlic, dried chili peppers, dried fish, and leftover cooked foods are the main sources of dietary aflatoxins in Thailand, and there seems to have been little change in the eating habits associated with these particular foods. One possible exception to this may be usage of leftover cooked foods. Thai housewives today apparently are more aware of food poisoning problems associated with eating leftover foods, and since cold storage is rarely available to most Thai households, usually only enough food to supply the family for the immediate day is prepared. In most families, but certainly not all, any leftover foods, except curries, are given to farm animals or elderly people living alone.

ACKNOWLEDGEMENTS

The author wishes to thank Drs Pradith Siddichai, Natth Bhamarapravati, Boonchuay Subhamani, Stang Mongkolsuk, Amorn Poomee, Payup

Thajchayapong and Erb Pruangkarm, the provincial and district health officers in Singburi, Ratburi and Songkla, the staffs of the several survey hospitals, and the residents of the nine survey villages for their help and understanding in carrying out these studies, and especially Prof. Gerald N. Wogan, co-principal investigator of the project. This work was supported by U.S. Public Health Contract No. 43-67-93.

REFERENCES

1. BERMAN, C. (1951). In: *Primary Carcinoma of the Liver*. H. K. Lewis and Co., London.
2. TAKEDA, J. and AIZAWA, M. (1956). *Trans. Soc. Path. Japan*, **45**, 1,
3. BHAMARAPRAVATI, N. and NIMSOMBURNA, P. (1963). *Proc. 16th Assembly Japan Med. Cong.*, **3**, 376.
4. BHAMARAPRAVATI, N. and VIRANUVATTI, V. (1966). *Am. J. Gastroent.*, **45**, 267.
5. SHANK, R. C., GIBSON, J. B., CHONG, Y. H. and WOGAN, G. N. In preparation.
6. SHANK, R. C., GIBSON, J. B., CHONG, Y. H., NONDASUT, A. and WOGAN, G. N. In preparation.
7. EPPLEY, R. M. (1966). *J. Assoc. Offic. Anal. Chemists*, **49**, 1218.
8. WOGAN, G. N. and NEWBERNE, P. M. (1967). *Cancer Res.*, **27**, 2370.

PRELIMINARY RESULTS FROM FOOD ANALYSES IN THE INHAMBANE AREA

by

I. F. H. Purchase

Director: National Institute for Nutritional Diseases
South African Medical Research Council

and

T. Gonçalves

Director: Provincial Nutrition Commission Lourenço Marques Moçambique
Reporting on behalf of the Portuguese/South African
collaborative Research Group on Mycotoxins and Liver Cancer

One of the most interesting results of epidemiological studies conducted throughout the world is the wide variation in cancer incidence between different countries. This observation suggests that a large proportion of cancers are caused by environmental agents.

Liver cancer is no exception to this general observation and the incidence rate varies from less than 1 per 100,000 per annum in countries such as The Netherlands, Norway and Canada to 103·8 per 100,000 per annum in the male Bantu of Moçambique. Other countries with a high incidence in males are South Africa (Johannesburg Bantu) 19·2, Nigeria 9·8 and Hawaii 9·7 per 100,000 per annum. This variation in incidence has led many to seek for an environmental agent which might be responsible for the disease. Virus hepatitis, schistosomiasis, siderosis, cirrhosis, plant toxins (*Senecio* alkaloids and Cycad nuts), malnutrition, alcoholic beverages and bacterial toxins have all been implicated. More recently it has been suggested that mycotoxins may be responsible and the discovery of the carcinogenic properties of aflatoxin has given impetus to this hypothesis.

There are, however, some reasons for doubting this hypothesis.[1] Aflatoxin occurs in the South African groundnut crop more commonly in dry seasons than in wet seasons. The generalisation that hot humid conditions are necessary for mycotoxin production is shown to be incorrect by the temperature requirements ($<0°C$) leading to toxin production by moulds resulting in alimentary toxic aleucia. However, these objections merely make it imperative that studies should be conducted to try and confirm or disprove this hypothesis.

At our present state of knowledge, it is desirable that several factors should be considered before embarking on epidemiological studies. The first is that liver cancer is not an aetiologically specific disease entity, i.e. it may be caused by more than one environmental agent. This may apply particularly to liver cancer in different countries and it will render any comparative epidemiology liable to gross errors. If possible epidemiological studies of this sort should be concentrated in a small well-defined high incidence area, or, in other words, it should be 'micro-epidemiology'.[2] Another factor which must be taken into account is the paucity of information on mycocarcinogens.

Too much emphasis has been placed on aflatoxin in this regard[3] without consideration of other known carcinogenic mycotoxins—such as luteo-skyrin and sterigmatocystin—and unknown mycotoxins.

We have attempted to emphasize the importance of other mycotoxins by studying the mycotoxin sterigmatocystin. This compound is produced by a number of fungi and is hepatocarcinogenic in rats.[4] The type of tumour produced—hepatocellular carcinoma with varying degrees of fibrosis—morphologically more closely resembles Bantu hepatoma than does aflatoxin-induced tumours with their variable bile duct involvement. In addition, sub-acute sterigmatocystin poisoning in rats produced a morphological picture remarkably like that seen in hepatitis of unknown aetiology observed in the Bantu of Moçambique.[5] Thus, enough emphasis cannot be placed on mycotoxins other than aflatoxins.

METHOD

Technique for studying mycotoxin-liver cancer relationship

Because of the high cost involved in complete epidemiological, demographic, dietary and sociological surveys, we have decided to study the relationship in a high incidence area in the following way: All patients in hospitals and clinics in the Inhambane district were considered for inclusion in the study. Cases under the age of 30 years who have lived in one area for most of their lives and who have confirmed liver cancer were selected.

Food was sampled from the village in which the liver cancer patient had resided and resampling was planned to occur 3-4 times a year in order to cover possible seasonal variations. A field worker visited the village and purchased 2 kg samples of each foodstuff (unprepared) which was actually being used at the time of sampling. Cooked foods were not included in the survey. Samples were also obtained in the same way from several families living in the immediate vicinity of the patient's family.

Similar food sampling was undertaken from sex and age matched controls from the same hospital. These food samples were then sent to Pretoria for analysis in the following way:

i. The samples were chemically analysed for aflatoxin and sterigmatocystin.

ii. Toxicity tests were carried out using ducklings. The sample was included in the duckling diet as 50% by weight of the diet. The rest of the diet was made up of a standard chick growing mash.

iii. It was planned that toxic samples without sterigmatocystin or aflatoxin in them would be used for mycological studies. Unfortunately very few samples in this category have yet been received and thus a mycological survey of the non-toxic food samples is being planned.

Selection of the study area

In 1968, a group from the Moçambique-South African collaborative project visited hospitals in the south of Moçambique. From observations made during this trip, it was apparent that Inhambane was an ideal study area. Liver cancer is common, the population is relatively stable (more so than in an urban area) and it is served by hospitals and a regular scheduled air-service.

Subsequently, a follow-up of liver cancer in the area was made possible by the kindness of Dr R. L. Simpson (of the Methodist Mission Hospital at Chicuque near Maxixe), who made his excellent case records available to us. During the period January, 1968 to April, 1970, there are records of liver cancer at the Chicuque Hospital. These cases were diagnosed clinically in all cases, but a large number (all cases seen during the last six months) were confirmed by biopsy. The greatest number of cases were recorded in 1968 and fewer in 1969. Based on the 101 cases seen in 1968, and on the population statistics in the Anuario Estatistico de Provincia de Moçambique (1965) the crude liver cancer rate was 16·1/100,000/annum. The incidence according to administrative area (Circumscription) is given in Table 1.

The male/female ratio was 2·1:1 and the age distribution is given in Table 2. These figures confirm findings from other areas where liver cancer is common. They will have been influenced by a number of factors such as migration of males to Lourenço Marques and to the mines which will tend to reduce the male:female ratio. One of the most remarkable features is the high incidence figures which are obtained by one hospital. The incidence rates in Panda, for example, are second only to those reported for Lourenço Marques (103 for males and 30 for females) and considerable underreporting must occur in Panda. There are many other hospitals and clinics in the area and the Inhambane district is several hundred miles long, thus tending to reduce possible reporting of cases.

Table 1

Number of Cases of Liver Cancer (1968/70) and Crude Incidence Rate
(cases/100,000/year) for 1968 in the Inhambane District

Circumscription	Bantu Population	Cases (1968)	Incidence Rate	Total cases (1968-1970)
Govuro	38,884	0	0	0
Homoine	86,159	21	24	45
Inhambane	64,510	9	14	21
Inharrime	40,271	11	27	18
Massinga	108,676	8	7·4	19
Morrumbene	67,969	12	1·8	27
Panda	35,291	13	37	23
Vilanculos	67,069	5	7·5	7
Zavala	68,953	15	22	29
Others	—	7	—	9
Total	576,782	101	16·1	197

Table 2

Number of Cases of Liver Cancer According to Age

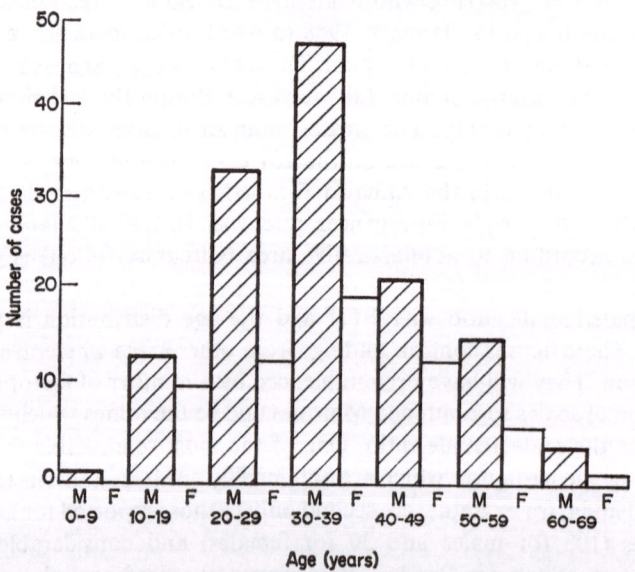

This study confirms that the Inhambane area is one of the most suitable
for studying liver cancer.

RESULTS

Results of the food sampling

Maize, peanuts, rice, beans, manioc and cashew nuts were the staple foods sampled during the first seven months of the project. Samples were

Table 3

Aflatoxin Positive Food Samples from 3 Cancer Families and their Matched Controls

Foodstuffs	Patients		Controls		Total	
	No. of samples	No. with aflatoxin	No. of samples	No. with aflatoxin	No. of samples	No. with aflatoxin
Peanuts	16	3	12	2	28	5
Maize	7	1	10	1	17	2
Beans	5	0	3	0	8	0
Rice	6	1	3	0	9	1
Manioc	2	1	5	0	7	1
Others	4	0	0	0	4	0
Total	40	6	33	3	73	9

Table 4

Aflatoxin Positive Food Samples in All Samples Received from Inhambane

Foodstuffs	No. of samples	No. with aflatoxin		% Contaminated
		< 1.0 p.p.m.	Total	
Peanuts	67	2	5	7·5
Maize	52	2	2	3·8
Beans	16	—	0	0
Rice	23	1	1	4·3
Manioc	8	1	1	12·5
Cashew nuts	4		0	0
Others	3		0	0
Total	171	6	9	5·25

drawn from nine families of liver cancer patients, but only the first three had matched controls. The results are given in Tables 3 and 4.

All samples positive for aflatoxin were collected in November and

December, 1969. All subsequent samples were free from aflatoxin. Sterigmatocystin was not detected in any of the samples.

Two of the peanut samples containing aflatoxin (more than 1 ppm) caused mortality in ducklings. Of the rest of the samples tested (156) five samples of beans, three of maize and one of peanuts caused limited mortality in the ducks (2/4). These samples are to be studied further. The mortality in the groups receiving beans could be due to the antitryptic factor present in raw beans.

DISCUSSION

One of the most difficult aspects of work executed in the field in Africa is obtaining completely reliable results. The diagnosis of liver cancer can only be considered confirmed on histological examination. Nevertheless, an experienced clinician in the area has no doubt in the majority of cases of the diagnosis of liver cancer and the clinical diagnosis cannot be disregarded, particularly when the clinician has biopsy facilities to confirm doubtful cases. Such is the case at Chicuque, and the figures quoted here are likely to be a good reflection of the actual situation in the area.

The significance of the crude incidence rates lies in the fact that they are so high in spite of the gross under-reporting of cases from the district. Patients would be seen at the hospitals and clinics in Inhambane, Govuro, Homoine, Inharrime, Massinga, Morrumbene, Vilanculos and Zavala as well as at mission hospitals and clinics. In fact there were ten other doctors in the district in 1965. This could account for the uneven distribution of cases, with none coming from some areas such as Govuro. In spite of this, the incidence in many of the Circumscriptions is higher than in any other country in the world.

The collection of samples of foods by field workers can introduce a number of errors. The absence of sorting of the foods, which would normally take place before cooking, could result in more mouldy grains in the food samples and selection of high quality foods by the local inhabitants to impress the field workers could reduce the potentially harmful foods. The latter criticism is not valid for all peanut samples, however, as some were stored and sampled in their husks. In spite of this a relatively low percentage contamination occurred at a relatively low concentration.

Unfortunately the comparison between patients and controls is not meaningful due to the small number of samples.

ACKNOWLEDGEMENTS

We wish to acknowledge the co-operation of the Moçambique government and the Research Group. Dr Peralta, Governor of the District of Inhambane, is thanked for his willing co-operation and for the provision of facilities in Inhambane. We would also like to thank Dr R. L. Simpson for access to records at the Chicuque hospital.

REFERENCES

1. PURCHASE, I. F. H. (1967). *S.Afr. med. J.*, **41**, 406.
2. PURCHASE, I. F. H. (1968). In: *Cancer in Africa* Symposium. Eds. Clifford, P., Linsell, C. A. and Timms, G. L., p. 327, East African Publishing House, Nairobi.
3. PURCHASE, I. F. H. and THERON, J. J. (1967). *International Pathology*, **8**, 3.
4. PURCHASE, I. F. H. and VAN DER WATT, J. J. (1968). *Fd. Cosm. Toxicol.*, **6**, 555.
5. TORRES, F. O., PURCHASE, I. F. H. and VAN DER WATT, J. J. (1970). *J. Path.*, **102**, 163.

AFLATOXIN INGESTION AND EXCRETION BY HUMANS*

by

T. C. Campbell and L. Salamat

Virginia Polytechnic Institute, College of Agriculture
Blacksburg, Virginia, U.S.A.

Although several workers have shown that the oral and parenteral administration of aflatoxin may cause liver cancer in a large number of experimental and domestic livestock animals (reviewed in Reference 2), there
remains only circumstantial evidence of the involvement of aflatoxin in the
aetiology of liver cancer in humans. Our original interest in this relationship arose about three years ago when we began to analyse certain food
products from the Philippines for the presence of aflatoxin. The first results
showed a very high level of aflatoxin in certain batches of peanuts and
peanut products and concurrent with these observations was an awareness
of a high incidence of liver malignancies.

The assays have been performed in the Philippines during 1967-1969 on
a variety of foods obtained from markets in or near Manila (Table I).
These data include only the samples that were analysed during the first
two years of our investigation and do not include a much larger number
run since the first of the year. However, these latter samples reflect the
same trends as the data reported in this paper. A very significant difference
is demonstrated between whole peanuts and peanut butter. Only 7% of
the 71 samples of whole shelled peanuts, which were most often being sold
as 'cocktail' peanuts, contained levels in excess of 30 μg/kg and the median
of the positive samples was a respectable 17 μg/kg. On the other hand, all
of the 29 peanut butter samples contained aflatoxin in excess of 30 μg/kg
with a median value of 155 μg/kg and (not shown in the table) a very high
mean of 500 μg/kg. Particularly noteworthy was one sample which was
being advertised as baby food which contained 8600 μg/kg.

After a few discussions with the processors and examination of their
facilities, it was our opinion that the choice or first grade peanuts were
being used in the cocktail or whole peanut preparations because of their
appearance. On the other hand, the lower grades, including the higher
levels of damaged, discoloured and presumably moulded nuts, were being
ground into peanut butter. Other peanut products such as candied preparations were intermediate in their level of contamination, perhaps
because of the fact that the nuts are partially hidden from the consumer's

* Portions of this paper have been presented in Reference 1.

eye and would allow the use of somewhat less than choice grades. Both Dr Shank and Dr Crawford have pointed out that most people probably do not consume obviously moulded nuts as they have observed that the average housewife will select and reject such contaminated material. Although such a practice is of obvious value, it may, however, be obviated in a situation where manufacturing practices do not make such careful selection.

A variety of other foods have been examined and none are found to be

Table 1

Aflatoxin Analyses of Philippine Foods (1967-1969)

Food	No. samples	No. greater than 30 μg/kg	Median and highest value of samples ($> 10 \mu$g/kg)
Peanuts (whole)	71	5	17 (100)
Peanut butter, Philippine, 1967-68	29	29	155 (8600)
Peanut butter, imported from USA	3	0	—
Other peanut products	32	11	37 (220)
Nuts and seeds	23	1	38 (64)
Tubers	59	6	68 (440)
Beans	29	2	45 (86)
Soybean products	24	0	16 (16)
Rice and rice products	72	1	16 (33)
Maize products (1967-1968)	14	1	12 (39)
Maize products (1969)	27	14	47 (400)
Cocoa	11	0	19 (29)
Livestock feeds	11	8	74 (103)
Fish products	27	0	—
Coconut products	7	0	21 (26)
Cooking oil	16	0	—
Mango	12	0	—

* All values expressed as μg/kg.

as contaminated as the peanut butter samples. Tubers (ubi, gabi, tugi and sweet potatoes) may be a problem under poor storage conditions. Ten per cent of these samples showed levels in excess of 30 μg/kg and levels were found to be as high as 440 μg/kg. Maize samples bought in 1968 during a prolonged drought showed only 1/14 to be positive with an aflatoxin content of 39 μg/kg. However, in 1969, during a heavier rainy season, over half of the samples were contaminated, with a median of 47 μg/kg and a high value of 400 μg/kg. Nearly all maize in the Philippines is grown in the south central island of Cebu. Noteworthy because of the relative absence of aflatoxin are the important rice samples. Only one sample of 72 was positive and contained a level of only 16 μg/kg. Livestock feeds used for swine and poultry and collected during 1969 showed alarmingly high levels, with 72% positives, and a median of 74 μg/kg. All appeared to contain maize most probably grown in 1969 and this ingredient may have been responsible.

Although it is a reasonably alarming public health problem with respect to the contamination of peanuts, maize and commercial livestock feeds, there is at present considerable progress being made on the aflatoxin problem. The Philippine Food and Drug Administration, the Department of Agriculture and the processors are co-operating to develop better harvesting, storage and selection procedures. Shown in Table 2 are results of peanut butter samples assayed on a continuing basis during 1969 shortly

Table 2

Aflatoxin Analysis of Peanut Butter Run After Institution
of Improved Selection Procedures* by Processors

Month	Number of samples	Number of processors	Mean level μg/kg
May	9	9	190
June	12	10	105
August	10	9	128†
September	13	11	91
November	6	6	77

    * These data made available through the courtesy of Commissioner Luzonica Pesigan.
    † Heavy rain.

after the processors and Food and Drug personnel were made aware of the nature and importance of the problem.

Of particular interest to us was the relationship of the aflatoxin contamination of the food samples and its ingestion by man. For example, recent cases were on record of children under four years of age undergoing surgery for primary liver cancer.[3, 4] Of the various types of cancer, liver malignancies register the highest incidence (Table 3), although, quite unfortunately, primary and secondary lesions are not distinguished in the available health records.[5] The relative incidences in the various health regions of the country are of interest in that the rates in health regions 3 and 6 are approximately 7-10 × those of the rest of the country. It is in health region 3, which includes the Manila metropolitan area, that most of the locally produced peanut butter is consumed. This product is essentially not distributed and consumed in the remaining health regions. On the

other hand, region 6 includes Cebu, where maize is consumed by approximately 90% of the people, almost to the exclusion of rice. These are, in
fact, the only people in the Philippines consuming maize as the basic
energy staple. Whereas other aetiological factors may certainly be operative,
the consumption of peanut butter in one health region and maize in the
other may be more than coincidental to the very high rates of liver cancer
in these two regions. There are, however, in these regions better medical
facilities and the case reports may therefore be more accurate. Undoubtedly,
a more thorough epidemiological survey will be required to substantiate
this suggestion.

Table 3

Liver Malignancy, Philippines

| | | Rate/100,000 Population | |
Region	Population	Primary	Secondary
1	3,860,000	0·39	1·58
2	1,310,000	0·15	0·30
3	9,770,000	1·17	4·24
4	3,020,000	0·20	1·45
5	3,850,000	0·54	1·87
6	5,810,000	1·12	4·35
7	2,320,000	0·34	1·51
8	3,450,000	1·01	2·32
Total	33,400,000	0·80	2·88

Because humans were obviously consuming relatively high levels of
aflatoxin, studies were initiated to determine whether aflatoxin B_1 or its
metabolic products is excreted, with first attention being paid to the
individuals consuming peanut butter. Some of the discussion of the last
two days has centred on a question of the appropriateness of measuring
specific foods or actual food consumption as an index of aflatoxin intake.
However, it was our aim in this project to determine whether it would be
feasible to measure excretion of aflatoxin or its metabolites, instead of
intake, in order to have a more accurate index of aflatoxin exposure. A
cursory investigation revealed that children were the principal consumers
of peanut butter. Subjects were asked whether peanut butter had been
consumed within the previous 72 hours. Some families who regularly
consumed local peanut butter volunteered urine specimens before and
during consumption of food samples randomly bought on the local market.

All urine speciments were extracted and chromatographed as published previously.[1] A number of fluorescent compounds may be seen upon chromatographic development.

Although three suspicious blue fluorescent spots were observed in urine extracts of subjects ingesting peanut butter, two were eliminated from further consideration for the following reasons. First, equivalent compounds were not detected in an extract of monkey urine prepared earlier[1] from animals administered B_1. Second, these two compounds were later detected in urine specimens of human subjects having consumed peanut butter known to be free of aflatoxin. Third, neither of these compounds was chromatographically equivalent to B_1, B_2 or B_{2_a}. (The latter compound, which is the water adduct of B_1, was kindly supplied by L. Stoloff and A. E. Pohland of the U.S. Food and Drug Administration.) Therefore, we concluded that these two compounds were not aflatoxin metabolites.

The third blue spot appeared to be aflatoxin M_1, the hydroxylated derivative of B_1. Its identity was confirmed as the M_1 reported in the literature according to the following procedures. First, sample extracts containing 'M_1' were chromatographically compared with an M_1 standard (supplied by L. Stoloff and A. E. Pohland) in four additional solvents: 100% ethyl acetate,[6] the benzene-rich phase of benzene:ethanol:water, 46:35:19,[7] 3% methanol in chloroform,[8] and diethyl ether:chloroform: acetic acid, 40:40:20.[9] In each of these solvents, as well as the original 10% acetone in chloroform, the R_f values of the suspected M_1 and the standard M_1 were identical as shown both by co-chromatography and by chromatography of adjacent spots. Second, the suspected M_1 was chromatographically identical to the M_1 observed in the monkey urine. Third, the thionyl chloride test of Andrellos and Reid[10] (which was originally intended as a B_1 confirmatory test) gave identical derivatives with both the M_1 standard and the suspected sample 'M_1'. Identical and single derivatives were formed with each of the acid catalysts: trifluoracetic acid, R_f 0·18, glacial acetic acid, R_f 0·30 and formic acid, R_f 0·30; the developing solvent was the benzene-rich phase of benzene:ethanol:water (46:35:19) and the R_f of the unreacted M_1 was 0·33. On the basis of the foregoing criteria, we concluded that the sample M_1 was the same compound as the aflatoxin M_1 reported in the literature.[11-13] This was the only aflatoxin compound found; B_1 was not found in any of the M_1-positive samples.

Because the concentration of our M_1 standard was not known at the time of the assays, no attempt could be made to quantitate accurately the M_1 in the extracts. But allowing for the threefold increase in fluorescent intensity of M_1 compared with B_1 earlier reported by Purchase and Steyn,[14] our best estimates indicated that not more than 1-4% of the ingested aflatoxin B_1 appeared as M_1 in the urine. Whether all of this M_1 resulted from the *in vivo* metabolism of B_1 or whether it was produced by the fungus[15] before ingestion could not be determined with certainty, although no M_1 was observed in the peanut butter samples. Furthermore, aflatoxin B_1 has been shown to be enzymatically metabolised to M_1 by oxidative NADPH-dependent rat and mouse liver microsomes.[16]

Table 4 gives data for seven families each of two to four children whose parents had told us that they regularly eat peanut butter and whose urine specimens were collected before and during consumption. Collections were made for 0 to 24 hours before and up to 72 hours after consumption began. Each subject, therefore, served as his own control. Only the amount consumed by the whole family was recorded and an average amount was assigned to each member. The minimum daily consumption of aflatoxin B_1 required to produce detectable levels of M_1 was 15 μg/day. Of thirty-five analytical 24-hour periods (after consumption began) for the fourteen subjects consuming at least the daily minimum, thirty were positive for M_1 and five were equivocal positives because of uncertain interpretations of streaked chromatographic developments.

To test the value of this methodology in general survey procedures, we made single urine collections. Information on peanut butter consumption was sought and, in many cases, assays for aflatoxin were possible. Aflatoxin M_1 was detected in only six out of forty-six such cases. However, none of the twenty-seven subjects who had not eaten peanut butter excreted M_1.

The consumption of aflatoxin by nursing mothers would be important because this compound is considerably more toxic for young than for older subjects.[17] Milk collected from eleven mothers known to be consuming peanut butter (three consumed 4·2-8·4 μg/day and eight consumed unknown amounts) were negative for either B_1 or M_1, although only small amounts of milk (5-20 ml) were obtained (Table 5). On the other hand, three urine specimens from these same mothers contained M_1 although the intake of aflatoxin was unknown.

Faeces collected from seven children who had consumed 11·2-15·0 μg aflatoxin per day contained no aflatoxin metabolites, but three out of seven urine specimens from the same children were positive, indicating the range of marginal B_1 ingestion required for detection.

With the methodology reported here, the minimum ingestion of B_1 required to produce M_1 in the urine depends on the amount of urine collected and, of course, the proximity of the collection period to the time of ingestion. Previous reports[11, 13] have indicated a fairly rapid passage of M_1 through the kidneys in experimental animals after administration of aflatoxin. If a collection is made over the total 24 hours, these data suggest that 10-15 μg of B_1 per day is the minimum required for detection of M_1.

Analysis of Human Urine for Aflatoxin M_1: Continuous Urine Collections

Family	Number Subjects	Period of consumption	P.B. consumed (gm/subject/24 hr.)	Aflatoxin consumed (μg/subject/24 hr.)	Collection Period	Presence of M_1 in Urine (No. of subjects)
I	3	Before	—	—	—	−(3)
		0–24	20	0*	0–24	−(3)
		24–48	20	0*	24–48	−(3)
		0–48†	—†	—†	48–72	−(3)
II	2	Before	—	—	—	−(2)
		0–24	30	4·2	0–24	−(2)
		24–48	30	4·2	2–48	−(2)
		0–48	—†	—†	48–72	−(2)
III	3	Before	—	—	—	−(3)
		0–24	60	15	0–24	+(2), SM
		24–48	60	15	24–48	+(3)
		0–48	—†	—†	48–72	+(1), SM
IV	4	Before	—	—	—	−(4)
		0–24	80	16	0–24	+(4)
		24–48	80	16	24–48	+(4)
V	4	Before	—	—	—	−(4)
		0–24	120	25	0–24	+(4)
		24–48	120	25	24–48	+(3), SM
		48–72	120	25	48–72	+(2), SM −(1)
VI	1	Before	—	—	—	−(1)
		0–24	200	85	0–24	+(1)‡
		24–48	200	85	24–48	+(1)
VII	2	Before	—	—	—	−(2)
		0–24	150	110	0–24	+(2)
		24–48	190	190	24–48	+(2)

Jars of peanut butter obtained and weighed; total peanut butter consumed and averaged for each family member; remaining peanut butter assayed for aflatoxin.

(+), presence of M_1 in urine; (−), absence of M_1 in urine; SM, smeared chromatoplate, equivocal presence of M_1.

* US product. † Consumption stopped at 48 hours.

‡ Two additional members of this family were initially assumed to have consumed some of the peanut butter and their urines were negative; however, additional questioning revealed that one had been sick and one was not yet old enough to eat an appreciable amount.

Table 5

Analysis of Other Human Excretions for Aflatoxin M_1

Sample	Number of subjects	Period of consumption*	P.B. consumed (gm/subject/24 hour)	Aflatoxin consumed (μg/subject/24 hour)	Collection period	Presence of M_1 (No. of subjects)
A. MILK—Aflatoxin intake unknown	8	0-24	40-60	?	24†	−(8)
B. MILK—Aflatoxin intake known	3	0-24	20-40	4·2-8·4	24†	−(3)
C. URINE—Aflatoxin intake unknown (Part A Subjects)	8	0-24	40-60	?	24†	−(5), +(3)
D. URINE—Aflatoxin intake known (Part B Subjects)	3	0-24	20-40	4·2-8·4	24†	−(3)
E. FAECES	7	0-48	45-60	11·2-15·0	24-48	−(7)
F. URINE—(Part E Subjects)	7	0-48	45-60	11·2-15·0	24-48	−(4), +(3)

* Consumption stopped at 48 hours.
† A single sample of urine taken one day following consumption.

(+) Presence of M_1 in urine.
(−) Absence of M_1 in urine.
SM Smeared chromatoplate, equivocal presence of M_1.

On the other hand, we could not determine with any degree of assurance how much B_1 must be ingested if single urine collections were made, although most certainly considerably more than 15 μg/day would be required.

To improve the utility of this procedure, the sensitivity of the assay procedure needs to be increased. In these studies, the final extract was reduced to 200 μl and might be concentrated even more, although from observations of several urine specimen extracts the need for an additional clean-up step is indicated if the M_1 were to be seen without considerable chromatographic interference.

The presence of M_1 and the absence of B_1 in the urine, together with the absence of either B_1 or M_1 in faeces in known cases of B_1 ingestion, indicated considerable metabolism of the ingested B_1. The presence of a yellowish fluorescent metabolite of B_1 which is produced by mouse microsomal preparations[18] also could not be detected in human urine. We have shown that this compound is a metabolite of B_1 using ^{14}C-ring-labelled B_1 and is produced by mouse microsomal preparations. We are presently determining its structure. This appears to be the same compound referred to on Tuesday by Dr Pitout and yesterday by Dr Butler in reference to Patterson and Allcroft's work.[19]

In these studies, the amount of B_1 ingested was fairly accurately determined; yet, the absence of B_1 or its fluorescent metabolites in the excreta suggests that the majority of the B_1 is being metabolised to non-fluorescent metabolites. Whether the 'metabolite x' of Patterson and Allcroft[19] could be present was not determined, although it is possible that this latter metabolite is the same as our yellowish fluorescent compound which we searched for but which is only faintly fluorescent. We have obtained additional urine extracts from subjects known to have ingested aflatoxin and are presently collaborating with Dr Jaqueline Verrett of the US Food and Drug Administration in the use of her egg embryo system and with Dr Russell Sinnhuber of Oregon State University in his trout bioassay system to determine whether there remains characteristic aflatoxin toxicity.

These findings indicate that epidemiological methods based on the detection of aflatoxin M_1 in human excreta would really be quite limited unless an assay technique with a greatly improved sensitivity could be developed. These data are, however, academically interesting in that they indicate extensive metabolism by the human and may indicate a lower order of toxicity of aflatoxin for man.

REFERENCES

1. CAMPBELL, T. C., CAEDO, J. P. (Jr.), BULATAO-JAYME, J., SALAMAT, L. and ENGEL, R. W. (1970). *Nature* (Lond.), **227**, 403.
2. WOGAN, G. N. (1968). *Fed. Proc.*, **27**, 932.
3. PASCUAL, C. Personal communication.
4. CAEDO, J. P. (Jr.). Personal communication.
5. *Vital Statistics of the Philippines*, Disease Intelligence Center, Department of Health of the Philippines (1967).
6. STOLOFF, L. and POHLAND, A. E. Personal communication.
7. Anonymous (1966). *J. Assoc. Offic. Anal. Chem.*, **49**, 229.
8. PONS, W. A. (Jr.), and GOLDBLATT, L. A. (1965). *J. Am. Oil. Chem. Soc.*, **42**, 471.
9. LIJINSKY, W. and BUTLER, W. H. (1966). *Proc. Soc. Exptl. Biol. Med.*, **123**, 151.
10. Anonymous (1967). *J. Assoc. Offic. Anal. Chem.*, **50**, 214.
11. DE IONGH, H., VLES, R. O. and VAN PELT, J. G. (1964). *Nature* (Lond.), **202**, 466.
12. ALLCROFT, R. and CARNAGHAN, R. B. A. (1963). *Vet. Rec.*, **75**, 259.
13. ALLCROFT, R., ROGERS, H., LEWIS, G., NABNEY, J. and BEST, P. E. (1966). *Nature* (Lond.), **209**, 154.
14. PURCHASE, I. F. H. and STEYN, M. (1967). *J. Assoc. Offic. Anal. Chem.*, **50**, 363.
15. PURCHASE, I. F. H., STEYN, M. and PRETORIUS, H. E. (1968). *Mycopath. Mycol. Appl.*, **35**, 239.
16. PORTMAN, R. S., PLOWMAN, K. M. and CAMPBELL, T. C. (1968). *Biochem. Biophys. Res. Communs.*, **33**, 711.
17. WOGAN, G. N. (1966). *Bact. Revs.*, **30**, 460.
18. PORTMAN, R. S., MERRILL, A. S. and CAMPBELL, T. C. Unpublished observations.
19. PATTERSON, D. S. P. and ALLCROFT, R. (1970). *Fd. Cosmet. Toxicol.*, **8**, 43.

THE INCIDENCE OF FUNGI IN FOODSTUFFS AND THEIR SIGNIFICANCE, BASED ON A SURVEY IN THE EASTERN TRANSVAAL AND SWAZILAND

by

P. M. D. Martin,* G. A. Gilman† and P. Keen‡

There has been little detailed fungal analysis of foodstuffs collected in Southern Africa, especially as regards the diet of the rural Bantu. This is a

Table 1

Foodstuffs Collected

Name	Number of samples
Maize	256
Groundnuts	180
Sorghum	39
Assorted legumes including various kidneys beans, jugo beans (*Voandzeia subterranea*), mung beans (*Phaseolus aureus*) and cowpeas (*Vigna sinensis*)	45
Maize meal	67
Groundnut meal	48
Total	635

preliminary report of a survey conducted in eastern Transvaal and Swaziland between 1966 and 1969. Table 1 summarises the foodstuffs collected.

I. DETERMINATION OF THE INCIDENCE OF FUNGI

Method

Fifty seeds of each sample were planted, four to an agar plate, after surface sterilisation in 5% sodium hypochlorite for five minutes. The external husk was broken open by exposing the interior tissue in the case of hard seeds, or the grain was simply cut in pieces when the tissue was soft. In the case of large seeds such as maize and groundnuts, each one

* University of Botswana, Lesotho and Swaziland, Roma, Lesotho.
† South African Institute for Medical Research, Johannesburg. (On secondment from the Tropical Stored Products Centre (TPI), Slough, England).
‡ South African Institute for Medical Research, Johannesburg.

could be divided between three plates of different media; blood agar, malt salt agar and Sabouraud's dextrose agar with chloramphenicol. In the case of small fruits, however, such as sorghum, the material was too small to be divided easily, although the grains could still be crushed to give maximum exposure. In the case of meal prepared from cereal grains or groundnuts, a small quantity was distributed over 13 plates of each medium, which equates with the number used for whole seeds.

Results

Altogether 80 species were found associated with the foodstuffs. However, there was a considerable problem in determining which were true inhabitants of the substrate apart from transients and incidentals. Consequently one was led to reject such ubiquitous species as *Rhizopus nigricans* and *Rhizopus arrhizus* which occurred with almost 100% frequency, probable soil contaminants such as *Trichoderma lignorum*, as well as various species with exceedingly low frequency. Forty-one species were eventually considered to have some special ecological relationship to foodstuffs, and could be classified into four groups:

(i) *Species regularly present in all foodstuffs, though varying in frequency*

Species	Maximum affinity	Least affinity
Alternaria chartarum	Beans	Groundnuts, Maize meal
Aspergillus flavus	Sorghum malt	Beans
Aspergillus glaucus group	Groundnut meal	Jugo beans
Aspergillus ochraceus	Groundnut meal	Maize meal
Fusarium moniliforme	Maize	Beans
Penicillium citrinum	Jugo beans	Groundnuts
Penicillium cyclopium	Maize meal, beans	Groundnuts
Penicillium meleagrinum	Maize	Maize meal
Penicillium purpurogenum	Sorghum malt	Sorghum grain
Penicillium crustosum	Jugo beans	Sorghum malt

(ii) *Species distributed widely, but with marked substrate dislike or preference*

Species	Maximum affinity	Least affinity
Streptomyces griseus	Modifications or preparations from raw foodstuffs	
Aspergillus clavatus	Sorghum malt	
Aspergillus niger		Maize meal
Aspergillus versicolor		Beans
Aspergillus wentii		Beans
Cladosporium cladosporioides	Groundnut meal	Sorghum malt
Cladosporium sphaerospermum	Sorghum grain	Sorghum malt

Species	Maximum affinity	Least affinity
Fusarium equiseti	Groundnuts, sorghum grain	Maize meal, sorghum malt, jugo beans
Mucor circinelloides	Modifications or preparations from raw foodstuffs	
Penicillium frequentans		Groundnut meal
Penicillium rubrum		Groundnut meal
Penicillium rugulosum		Groundnut meal
Penicillium variable		Groundnut meal, sorghum malt, beans
Penicillium viridicatum		Maize meal Groundnut meal
Phoma herbarum	Millet, sorghum, sorghum malt	Groundnut meal
Yeast	Modifications or preparations from raw foodstuffs	

(iii) *Rare species with no apparent preferences*

Botryodiplodia theobromae
Epicoccum purpurascens

(iv) *Rare species with narrow specific preferences*

Species	Preference
Aspergillus candidus	Sorghum
Chaetomium sp.	Maize, sorghum, beans
Cladosporium oxysporum	Beans
Coniothyrium fuckelii	Maize, beans, jugo beans
Diplodia maydis	Beans
Fusarium semitectum	Sorghum
Fusarium sporotrichioides	Beans
Gliocladium catenulatum	Groundnuts
Gliocladium roseum	Maize, groundnuts
Nigrospora oryzae	Maize, jugo beans
Penicillium islandicum	Maize meal
Trichothecium roseum	Groundnuts, sorghum
Verticillium sp.	Maize, maize meal, groundnuts

From the foregoing it is apparent that many of the various species characteristic of foodstuffs have sharp preferences in their choice of substrate. This conclusion is abundantly confirmed when the substrates themselves are compared as a whole with respect to fungal flora. Although the various substrates have a large number of species in common, the frequency of the species often varies enormously; in fact, comparisons between any two substrates show that the number of species in common with a less than 10% difference in incidence never exceeds half the total number of species, and is usually much less. Furthermore, there is no species, whatever its general frequency, that does not demonstrate an inclination for or against one of the substrates investigated.

Thus, simple estimates of similarity between the substrate microfloras are not easily made, since such comparisons are multidimensional. There are no clear differences between floras of all the substrates, and an interesting feature is that there is as much difference between the floras of a raw substrate and its product (e.g. maize and maize meal) as there is between the raw substrates themselves. One consistent trend noted, however, is the increase in incidence of three species, *Streptomyces griseus*, *Mucor circinelloides* and an *unidentified yeast* when the raw substrate is converted into a more refined product, i.e. maize meal, groundnut meal, sorghum malt and millet malt. It must be remembered, however, that surface contaminants are also being estimated here.

The following are a number of specific comments on the fungal flora of the various substrates:

A. Whole foodstuffs
    (i) Maize
        This has the highest general level of infection by all species as well as complete representation. Dominant species are *F. moniliforme*, *A. niger*, *P. crustosum*, *P. rubrum* and *A. flavus*.

    (ii) Groundnuts
        In contrast to maize, groundnuts support a slightly lower number of constant species and the general level of fungal invasion is also less. Three species present on maize have not been found on groundnuts: *A. candidus*, *Chaetomium* and *Coniothyrium fuckelii*. Twelve other species have lower incidences. However, four other species *A. ochraceus*, *F. equiseti*, *G. catenulatum* and *T. roseum* prefer groundnuts to maize, and *G. catenulatum* obviously has its greatest affinity for this substrate.

    (iii) Sorghum
        This substrate is also slightly less rich in fungi than maize. The flora is characteristic in that there is a relatively low incidence of *A. flavus*, and a relatively high incidence of *A. candidus*, *G. sphaerospermum* and *Phoma herbarum*.

    (iv) Beans
        On the basis of a relatively few samples it would appear that there are fewer species inhabiting this substrate than others. The dominant species are *Alternaria chartarum* and *P. crustosum*.

(v) Jugo beans

The number of samples of jugo beans is also much less than that of other foodstuffs. The flora is hard to characterise; there are not as many species as on maize but the missing species are of minor importance. The dominant species appear to be *A. glaucus*, *A. niger*, *F. moniliforme* and *P. crustosum*. *F. sporotrichioides* characteristically occurs on this substrate.

B. Prepared foodstuffs (relatively few samples have been examined so far)

(vi) Maize meal and maize bran

In addition to the increase in species noted above, three other species are enhanced by conversion of maize into meal. These are *C. cladosporioides*, *P. cyclopium* and *P. islandicum*. On the other hand 16 species including *A. flavus* show a decrease and five further species are eliminated.

(vii) Groundnut meal

Preparation of meal from groundnuts also results in increase of a small number of species, including *C. cladosporioides*, and the decrease or disappearance of a much larger number. Possibly the latter is due to liberation of free fatty acids. Surprising is the appearance of *A. candidus* which is absent from raw groundnuts, and the complete disappearance of *G. catenulatum*.

(viii) Sorghum malt

Conversion of sorghum to sorghum malt results in the reduction or elimination of several species such as *C. sphaerospermum* balanced by the increase of a smaller number, including *A. clavatus*.

(ix) Other substrates

These have not been investigated fully, so a complete spectrum cannot be presented. There are no striking features to record at present.

Observations on the distribution of Aspergillus flavus

Previous work by Keen and Martin[1] showed that groundnuts from Swaziland were frequently invaded by *A. flavus* and that the proportion of infected samples rose with a higher degree of total invasion by other fungi. Furthermore, it appeared that a relatively high proportion of samples containing aflatoxin came from an area with a hot and humid climate of low altitude, in contrast to lower proportions from cooler, higher areas.

Aspergillus flavus occurred fairly frequently in the foodstuffs studied here, having a general incidence of about 50%. It was higher in sorghum malt and lower in sorghum grain and beans. As is well known elsewhere,

Table 2

Incidence of *Aspergillus flavus* and of Aflatoxin above 0·05 ppm
in Foodstuffs

Foodstuffs	Number of samples	% frequency of A. flavus	% frequency of samples with aflatoxin
Maize	256	53·5	1·6
Groundnuts	180	49·4	11·1
Groundnut meal	48	50·0	8·3
Sorghum	39	33·3	7·7

Table 3

Geographic Incidence of *Aspergillus flavus* in 395 Samples
collected in Autumn and Spring 1968-1969
(all foodstuffs equally represented)

Area	Number of samples	Number with A. flavus
Low veld, E. Transvaal	178	88
Middle veld, E. Transvaal	15	3
Low veld, Swaziland	29	23
Middle veld, Swaziland	93	39
Lebombo, Swaziland	80	53

Table 4

Incidence of *Aspergillus flavus* according to storage method

Type of storage	Foodstuffs	Number of samples	Number with A. flavus
Underground pits	Maize, rarely sorghum	46	38
Tins, drums or tanks	All crops	60	29
'Silulus' (grass baskets)	All crops—usually maize or groundnuts	36	20
Jute sacks	All crops	81	34
Separate cribs (thatched)	Maize cobs	25	9
Cribs inside huts	Maize cobs	49	20
Other	All crops	11	5

the formation of aflatoxin is not inevitable, even in heavily invaded samples. In the 1968-69 season, for example, although *A. flavus* was frequently isolated from visibly undamaged foodstuffs, only two samples (less than 1 % of those examined) contained aflatoxin B_1 at levels greater than 0·05 ppm, although smaller amounts may have been present. Differences between years may therefore be considerable. Table 2 shows the overall incidence of aflatoxin in the various foodstuffs tested. It should be noted that, although *A. flavus* occurred with equal frequency in maize and groundnuts, the proportion of samples containing aflatoxin was considerably lower in maize.

Tables 3 and 4 summarise the distribution of *A. flavus* in the most recent part of the survey, both geographically and from the storage point of view. *A. flavus* appeared most frequently to invade grain stored on the Lebombo (middle veld) and in the low veld areas of Swaziland. This is probably because of the high incidence recorded in maize pits (most of which were present in these geographic areas) as opposed to other methods of storage. It is not certain, however, whether *A. flavus* always originated in the pit or whether it invaded the grain immediately after its removal while it was still moist. In a full pit, visible (surface) damage by moulds appears to be confined to the neck where air is more readily available.

II. DETERMINATION OF THE TOXICITY OF FOOD STORAGE FUNGI

Method

A total of 531 strains of fungi isolated from the foodstuffs analysed above were tested according to the standard duckling method.[2, 3] The proportion of markedly toxic strains was determined for each species. As many fungi as could be isolated in pure culture directly upon culture of the substrate were tested, but owing to difficulty of recovery of many of the species and difficulties experienced in keeping them viable, the number of strains tested fluctuated from one species to another.

RESULTS

The proportion of markedly toxic strains was found to vary widely from one species to another, but the most notable single fact that has so far emerged is that 45 of the 52 species tested so far are toxic to some degree, implying that toxicity among the fungi as measured by this test, is general rather than unusual.

The species can be grouped in five classes according to discontinuities in the order of ascending degree of toxicity.

L

Group I   *Species non-toxic or weakly toxic (0-11% of strains)*

	Number of strains tested	Number markedly toxic
Mucor circinelloides	5	0

Group II   *Species with low degree of toxicity (12-31% of strains)*

Penicillium purpurogenum	8	1
Aspergillus tamarii	5	1
Penicillium meleagrinum	19	5
Penicillium cyclopium	21	6
Rhizopus stolonifer (nigricans)	38	11
Penicillium viridicatum	13	4

Group III   *Species with moderate degree of toxicity (37-56% of strains)*

Penicillium variabile	8	3
Cladosporium sphaerospermum	16	6
Phoma herbarum	5	2
Trichoderma lignorum	10	4
Trichothecium roseum	5	2
Penicillium crustosum	17	7
Penicillium frequentans	16	7
Aspergillus niger	19	9
Aspergillus repens	19	9
Rhizopus arrhizus	15	7
Aspergillus candidus	6	3
Aspergillus ochraceus	10	5
Aspergillus ruber	26	13
Cladosporium cladosporioides	6	3
Fusarium oxysporum	63	32
Penicillium charlesii	11	6
Aspergillus wentii	16	9

Group IV   *Species with high degree of toxicity (63-67% of strains)*

Fusarium equiseti	39	25
Penicillium rugulosum	14	9
Penicillium citrinum	6	4
Penicillium rubrum	9	6

Group V   *Species with very high degree of toxicity (80-100% of strains)*

Aspergillus flavus	15	12
Nigrospora oryzae	8	7

Group VI   *Species requiring further strains for study*

Alternaria chartarum	4	2
Aspergillus auricomus	2	2
Aspergillus biplanus	1	1
Aspergillus clavatus	2	1
Aspergillus echinosporus	1	1
Aspergillus granulosus	1	1

	Number of strains tested	Number markedly toxic
Aspergillus melleus	1	0
Aspergillus terreus	1	1
Aspergillus ustus	1	1
Botryodiplodia theobromae	2	0
Curvularia sp.	3	1
Diplodia maydis	2	0
Fusarium sporotrichioides	3	0
Gliocladium catenulatum	3	3
Gliocladium roseum	2	0
Penicillium implicatum	3	1
Penicillium islandicum	2	1
Penicillium jenseni	1	1
Penicillium roseo-purpureum	1	0
Scopulariopsis brevicaulis	3	1
Yeast sp.	1	1

The results are in general agreement with those obtained by Scott.[3] The response of these strains to the duckling test does not appear to be conditioned by the type of substrate from which they were isolated nor by the geographical location of the substrate. We can assume that toxic and non-toxic strains are universally distributed in nature, only requiring an optimum set of conditions to produce toxin. Yet there is probably some subtle environmental factor governing the ability to produce mycotoxins. Laboratory tests showed that on the whole fungi tend to lose their original toxicity when retested one month later than the first trial. Of 25 assorted strains of *Aspergillus*, *Cladosporium*, *Fusarium*, *Penicillium* and *Rhizopus*, 11 retained their original level of toxicity or non-toxicity. Five strains, mainly Aspergilli and including *A. flavus*, increased slightly in toxicity and one strain of *A. ruber* increased markedly. Six strains of all these genera lost markedly in toxicity and two slightly.

The role that these mycotoxins may play with respect to the human body is, as yet, obscure. Aflatoxin has been shown to alter human liver cells cultured *in vitro*[4] but it is not yet known whether other mycotoxins have similar effects, or whether this is even of practical significance. However, two conclusions may be drawn. Firstly, that this work has shown a high proportion of strains of *A. flavus* to be toxigenic in comparison with strains of other fungi, and secondly that improved storage practice should certainly reduce the level of fungal contamination in the diet.

REFERENCES

1. KEEN, P. and MARTIN, P. (1970). *Trop. Geog. & Med.* (In press.)
2. PURCHASE, I. F. H. and THERON, J. J. (1967). *Bull. Int. Acad. Path.*, **8,** 3-6.

L*

3. Scott, de B. (1965). *Mycopath. et Mycol. Appl.*, **25**, 213-222.
4. Zuckerman, A. J., Rees, K. R., Inman, S. R. and Robb, J. A. (1968). *Br. J. exp. Path.*, **49**, 33-39.

ACKNOWLEDGEMENTS

We wish to thank Dr I. F. H. Purchase and Mr D. M. T. Tagg for the toxicity tests on ducklings and the Commonwealth Mycological Institute, Kew, England, for some of the fungal identifications. We are also indebted to Mrs C. Miller and others at the Cancer Research Unit, SAIMR, for undertaking the aflatoxin analyses. Financial support is gratefully acknowledged from the National Cancer Association of South Africa (G. A. Gilman), the National Institute of Health (grant C.A.07003) and D.P.I.F. grant (P. Keen).

BIOLOGICAL SCREENING AS A LABORATORY AID IN DETERMINING CANCER AETIOLOGY

by

I. F. H. Purchase

Director, National Institute for Nutritional Diseases
South African Medical Research Council

and

H. J. B. Joubert

Division of Toxicology, National Institute for Nutritional Diseases
South African Medical Research Council

Epidemiological studies aimed at elucidating the cause of cancer have been undertaken in the past and are currently being undertaken in many areas in the world. These studies attempt to define a relationship between the distribution pattern of the cancer and that of a given agent suspected of being aetiologically associated with the cancer. There are, however, many drawbacks to this approach. In the first place epidemiological studies can only provide evidence on the existence or non-existence of a relationship between the cancer and the aetiological agent; conclusive proof can never be obtained. Secondly, cancer of a particular organ, although because of a consistent histological picture it is often considered as a disease entity in itself, may merely be the common end result of the individual or combined action of a number of different aetiological agents.

Some of the drawbacks inherent in epidemiological studies of the aetiology of cancer can be overcome by confining the epidemiological studies to limited geographical areas—'micro-epidemiology'.[1]

This approach should reduce the variables introduced by dietary habits, customs, food taboos and usage, climate and genetic variations in the population which are inherent in 'intercontinental' epidemiology. Even when the micro-epidemiological approach is used, however, the problem of selecting the likely environmental agent from the myriads available is only reduced from a random selection to an inspired guess.

The logical approach would be to attempt to localise the agent in one of the major environmental groups such as: food-borne, water-borne, climatic or infectious. Once the agent has been so localised, some form of screening technique may be devised which will identify the aetiological agent. This technique will have to be capable of identifying an unspecified agent (i.e. unspecified in terms of chemical or physical properties) unless some very good evidence is available that a specific agent is involved; in other words it is desirable to use a biological screening test, which may be relatively non-specific, rather than a chemical test which must be highly specific in order to be accurate.

The presence of an area in South Africa with a high incidence of oesophageal cancer provided an ideal situation in which to test these ideas. Oesophageal cancer is extremely prevalent in the Bantu of the Transkei,[2] which has a population of 1·5 million and an area of 16,440 square miles. The incidence of the disease is uneven over the Transkei, with the largest number of cases occurring in the south-east. The population is largely rural, living for the most part on foods produced in their own gardens. A survey of the gardens supplying foodstuffs to families which have had members dying of oesophageal cancer and to families without reported cancer cases was undertaken.[3]

It was found that the former gardens ('cancer gardens') all showed signs of mineral deficiency whereas the non-cancer families' gardens were relatively free of deficiency signs. The deficiency was found to be mainly a lack of molybdenum and to a smaller extent of copper and iron. These findings suggested that, if an environmental agent was responsible, it was likely to be food-borne or water-borne. It has been suggested that the molybdenum deficiency might result in disturbances in nitrogen metabolism in the plant with a resulting production of nitrosamines. Accordingly various plants have been assayed for nitrosamine content and the first plant analysed, *Solanum incanum*, was found to contain dimethylnitrosamine.[4]

In 1967, it was decided to institute biological screening of the foodstuffs from cancer gardens to determine whether carcinogens were present. This decision was based on the description of 'cancer gardens' and the conclusion that the carcinogenic agent was likely to be located in the food rather than in other parts of the environment. BD IX rats were selected as the biological screen because of their known susceptibility to oesophageal cancer and the fact that oesophageal cancer was not found in untreated controls over many years of observation.[5]

METHOD

Ten adult male and female rats were imported from Germany and placed on the experimental diets for one week before conception. The offspring from these rats were allocated to two groups of 40 rats. Group one received a diet consisting of 64% maize + 32% beans + 4% salt mixture. Group two received the same diet with the addition of imifino (vegetables—mainly *Solanum nigrum* and thistles) when available. All staple foods were obtained from cancer gardens; the maize was a mixture of white and yellow varieties and the beans were Haricot beans.

The food was cooked using a technique shown to us by a Bantu from the Butterworth area. The beans and milled maize, and imifino in the diet for group two, were cooked together for 20 minutes in an iron pot. This mash was too wet to feed to rats and so it was dried at ± 50°C in a forced draught oven. The dried material was re-milled and fed to the rats *ad libitum*.

It was planned to produce a second generation of rats from parents on this diet, but all attempts to breed the rats have been unsuccessful.

No control group was introduced because of the shortage of space and because oesophageal cancer is unknown in this strain.

The rats were kept in an air-conditioned room maintained at 27°C and with a minimum relative humidity of 50%.

RESULTS

Survival

The mortality in the two groups is presented in the graph (Figure 1). At 125 weeks from the commencement of the experiment only 3 rats on diet 2 were alive while 23 on diet 1 were alive.

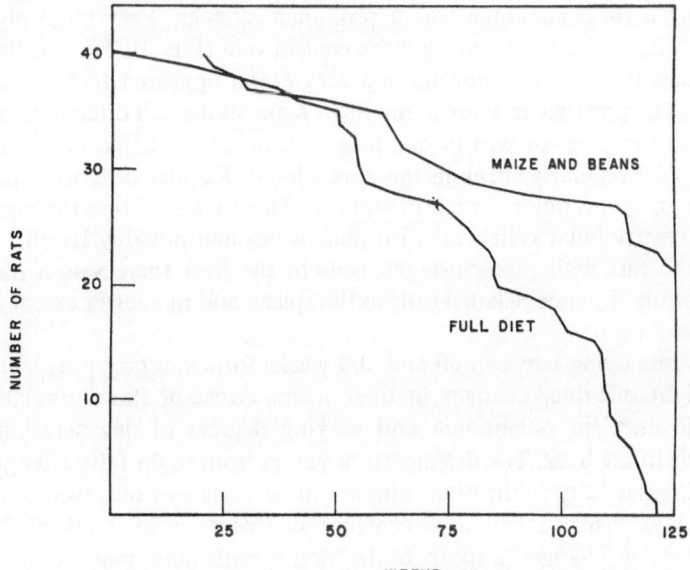

FIG. 1. Survivors in the two groups of rats up to 125 weeks.

Clinical symptoms

During the spring of 1968 and 1969 the rats appeared unthrifty and had a staring coat, irregular skin, xeropthalmia and haemorrhage into the anterior chamber of the eye. These periods (50-60 weeks and 105-120 weeks) were also the periods when mortality occurred in group 2.

Post-mortem examination

In most rats mortality was associated with chronic purulent pneumonia. In addition to this the rats dying from week 105-120 often developed ascites and many of them had hard nodular livers with circumscribed translucent nodules up to 5 mm in diameter.

Histo-pathology

The histo-pathological changes occurring in the kidney, lungs and other organs were due either to infections or to dietary imbalance. Most kidneys showed chronic glomerulo-nephritis and extensive nephro-calcinosis. Most lungs showed purulent broncho-pneumonia.

The most significant changes occurred in the liver. Three distinct types of pathological changes could be distinguished in the rats on diet 2.

Those rats dying between 50 and 60 weeks had minimal liver changes. Reduplication of the bile-ducts in the immediate vicinity of the portal tract forming a focal adenoma was a prominent change. Very large pigment laden cells were situated around the central vein (Fig. 2). These cells were 3-4 times the size of a normal hepatocyte and appeared to have several nuclei. The presence of large amounts of pigment made it difficult to decide whether the pigment was in one large cell or several adjacent small cells. Scattered irregularly through the parenchyma Kupffer cells were present with pigment granules in their cytoplasm. This suggested that the pigment-laden centrilobular cells were also phagocytes and possibly Kupffer cells.

In the rats with pigment-laden cells in the liver there was a massive infiltration of pigment-laden cells in the spleen and to a lesser extent in the lung.

The rats dying between 60 and 100 weeks formed a group by virtue of the slight bile-duct changes in their livers. Most of these animals had chronic purulent pneumonia and varying degrees of degeneration and necrosis in the liver. The degeneration varied from slight fatty change to a centrilobular fatty infiltration. Single cell necrosis was observed in 2 rats and an extensive coagulative centrilobular necrosis in 2 others. These degenerative changes appear to be non-specific and may result from toxaemia following on extensive purulent pneumonia.

The third group of rats consisted of those animals dying after 100 weeks (16 rats). Between 100 and 110 weeks there was a massive bile-duct cell proliferation and bile-duct reduplication which was so extensive that in some cases an estimated 60-70% of the liver consisted of bile-duct cells (Fig. 3). Fibrous reaction in these livers was limited to a moderate increase

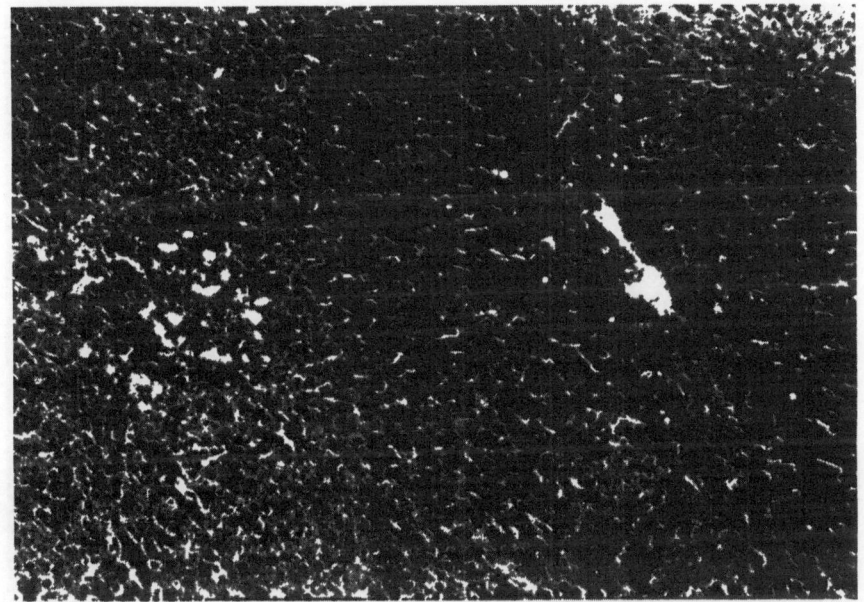

FIG. 2. Focal bile duct adenoma and centrilobular pigment deposition. (H. & E. × 160)

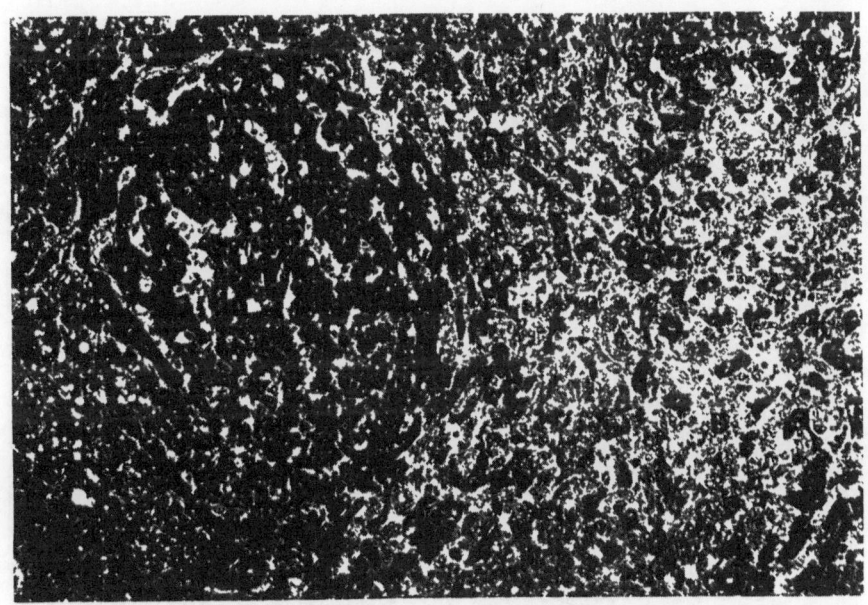

FIG. 3. Bile duct proliferation and hepatocellular nodule in the liver of a rat receiving diet 2. (Masson × 160)

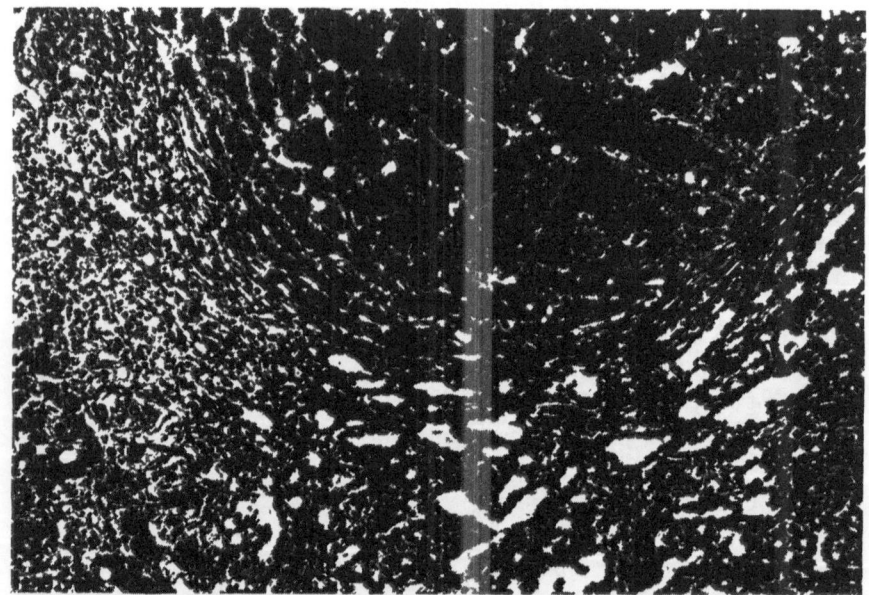

FIG. 4. The liver of a rat showing hepatocellular and cholangiocellular components of the carcinoma. (Reticulin × 160)

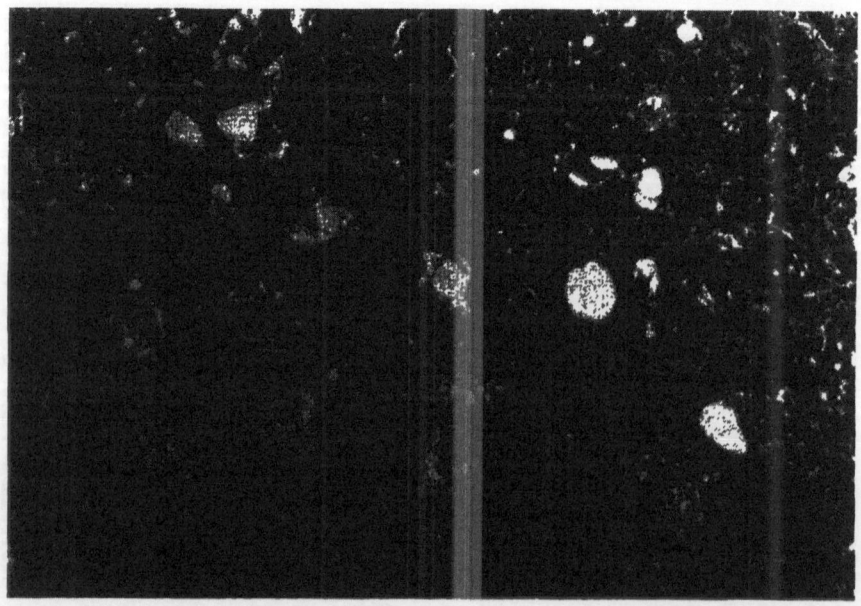

FIG. 5. Section of rat lung showing a bronchial carcinoma. (H. & E. × 160)

in reticulin fibres in and around the proliferating bile-duct cells and a less prominent increase in collagen.

The rats dying in the latter part of this period had more advanced changes. The bile-duct changes were so prominent that they presented as cholangio-carcinomas. Nodules of proliferating hepatocytes were frequently present and these varied from nodules containing a few cells to those up to 5 mm in diameter. The hepatocytes were atypical and appeared similar to those seen in hepatocellular carcinomas in rats (Fig. 4). Occasionally fatty changes were present in the cytoplasm but no fibrosis was seen in the nodules.

Four out of the 16 rats developed tumours in other organs. The rat dying at 108 weeks had a fibrosarcoma of the wall of the bladder. One rat dying at 113 weeks developed a bronchial carcinoma (Fig. 5). Two rats dying at 127 weeks developed a subcutaneous adenofibroma and a rectal fibrosarcoma respectively.

The rats in the group receiving diet 1 had less marked changes in the liver. A group of 4 rats died between 50 and 60 weeks. These rats had pigment-laden cells in the liver and other organs but nö bile-duct changes.

A second group of 4 rats died between 100 and 120 weeks. The changes in the livers of these rats were similar to these occurring in the rats on diet, 2 dying between 50 and 60 weeks, namely bile-duct adenoma and centrilobular pigment-laden cells. No tumours were seen in these rats up to 130 weeks.

DISCUSSION

This experiment indicates that a hepatoxin exists in the diet normally used by the Bantu in the Transkei. It appears from the type of changes produced that this toxin is also a hepato-carcinogen.

The major difference in the pathology between the group receiving maize and beans only and the group receiving a 'full' Transkei diet appears to be one of degree. It would thus appear that the additional item in the 'full' diet, namely imifino, contributed substantially to the lesions in the rats eating that diet.

It is noteworthy that the mortality in both groups was greatest simultaneously and that these periods were one year apart. It seems from this that there was a seasonal variation in the foodstuffs with the toxic component occurring in November-December. This seasonal effect was much more marked in rats receiving the full diet with the possibility that the mortality in each case in the maize and beans diet was coincidental.

No control group was present in this experiment as the end-point was expected to be oesophageal cancer. In fact the end-point was liver damage which makes it desirable to compare the livers of rats on a normal diet with the changes seen in this experiment. The cholangio-carcinomas and hepatomas are certainly the result of treatment as they did not occur in the group on maize and beans. Comparison of the liver lesions with that of breeding stock of the same strain but kept in Pretoria suggests that the bile-duct adenoma and pigment deposition were also a result of the diet used in the experiment.

It is difficult to pin-point the actual cause of the liver lesions from these results apart from concluding that imifino contributed substantially. Nevertheless the rats on maize and beans did develop lesions suggesting that they too contributed to the toxicity. Several possibilities for the toxicity are apparent. Mineral deficiencies have been postulated as contributing to the aetiology of the cancer in man. A direct mineral deficiency is unlikely to have been the cause as the salt supplement contained adequate amounts of Cu, Co, Mn, Mo and Fe. This does not, however, exclude an indirect effect such as the formation of nitrosamines.

Much of the maize used in these studies had been damaged by mould growth. It appears that mineral deficiencies can render maize more susceptible to mould growth. Several samples of foods have been analysed chemically and no aflatoxin or sterigmatocystin was detected. This does not exclude the possibility of other unidentified toxins being involved, although it seems unlikely that the imifino is mould contaminated as it is picked green and used within hours of harvest.

Another possibility is that the toxin is a nitrosamine. Analysis of water distilled from the cooked food by polarography and gas chromatography did not reveal any nitrosamines, which would be expected to distil over with the water. The only way in which nftrosamines could be formed is by the reaction of secondary amines and nitrite in the acid pH of the stomach. The seasonal effect of the diet could thus be explained by variations in nitrite content of the imifino, with the secondary amines being formed by the cooking of proteins.

The final possibility is that the imifino was toxic *per se*. This possibility is currently being investigated.

The production of liver cancer came as a surprise in this experiment. However, this does not invalidate the results or detract from their importance. If we postulate that nitrosamines are the final cause of the liver lesions, this organ specificity could be explained in several ways. Firstly, nitrosamines may change their organ specificity with change in dose; secondly, nitrosamines may change organ specificity with change in species. Either of these two possibilities may explain the presence of liver lesions. In addition, the Bantu of the Transkei are known to suffer from a very high incidence of liver cancer—the rate is approximately half that of oesophageal cancer in young adult males. Possibly this biological test system has indicated a carcinogen which could theoretically be responsible for both cancers.

In terms of the original problem—that of determining the presence of carcinogens—this experiment has demonstrated that biological testing of foods can, in certain instances, be a useful adjunct to epidemiology in determining cancer aetiology. The problems of the diet are but a few which will influence the result. In general, however, the technique has great promise when used carefully and with discernment.

ACKNOWLEDGEMENTS

I wish to thank Dr E. Rose for her continued help and co-operation during the whole of this experiment. This work would not have been undertaken without the support and encouragement of Dr J. J. Theron.

REFERENCES

1. PURCHASE, I. F. H. (1968). In: *Symposium 'Cancer in Africa'*. Eds. Clifford P., Linsell, C. H. and Timms, G. L., p. 327. East African Publishing House, Nairobi.
2. ROSE, E. F. (1965). *S.A. Med. J.*, **39**, 1098.
3. BURRELL, R. J. W., ROACH, W. A. and SHADWELL, A. (1966). *J. Nat. Cancer Inst.*, **36**, 201.
4. DU PLESSIS, L. S. and NUNN, J. R. (1969). *Nature* (Lond.), **222**, 1198.
5. DRUCKERY, H. (1967). *Z. für Krebsforschung*, **69**, 103.

AUTHOR INDEX

SUBJECT INDEX

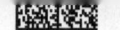